Watching EMERGENCY!
A Viewer's Off-the-Wall Guide

Seasons 4-6

May Fair

Copyright © 2015 May Fair

All rights reserved.

ISBN: 1981468714
ISBN-13: 978-1981468713

This books deals with *Emergency!*, the 1970s TV show about paramedics and firefighters at the fictional Station 51, and the doctors at Rampart General's emergency department.

What this book IS NOT: This book is *not* an "official" episode guide, or an "official" anything. It doesn't discuss the background of the show or recount the history of the paramedic program. There are no "behind the scene" interviews with cast or crew, no program notes, no filming locations or listing of guest stars, writers, or directors. Such details can be found elsewhere, on fansites, media sites, Wikipedia, books, interviews, etc.

What this book IS: Instead, this book is simply the random and unprofound thoughts and comments about episodes of this fun, enjoyable show. ***The comments were originally posted on a public message board, hence the informal nature of the writing.*** For legal reasons, the entire discussions, including other users' comments, are not part of this book; with the exception of brief excerpts (quotes) provided for context, this book represents one person's views. Again, these comments were written as a "just for fun" activity and meant to be enjoyed in that context.

Some of these commentaries are more in-depth than others, and have been geared toward those who are already fans of the series. Quite a few comments mention continuity errors in the episodes; however, far from denigrating the series, these goofs actually tend to endear fans to the show all the more, so please take these comments in the (loving) spirit in which they're intended.

With the exception of the first part of the fourth season, most episodes are reviewed twice, on successive viewings over the run of the series. Follow-up comments, and replies to comments of others, are separated by a row of three asterisks, and may include a brief quote. ***Please note* that many of the thoughts captured the first time around are touched upon again in the second review, along with 'new' insights as well. The two commentaries (old and new) are separated by a "three-peat" appearance of the tilde (~ ~ ~).

The thoughts/ideas/comments/opinions/theories expressed here belong to the writer, and are not concrete proof of anything. If those thoughts/opinions are off-the-wall, so be it, get the virtual tomatoes ready for hurling; if instead they're perceived to be brilliant, then the writer is either an extremely insightful thinker… or simply has too much time on her hands. You decide.

Watching EMERGENCY! Seasons 4-6

Main characters on the show:

Roy DeSoto – played by Kevin Tighe
John Gage – played by Randy Mantooth
Captain Stanley (Cap) – played by Mike Norell
Mike Stoker – played by Mike Stoker
Chet Kelly – played by Tim Donnelly
Marco Lopez – played by Marco Lopez
Dixie McCall – played by Julie London
Dr. Kelly Brackett – played by Robert Fuller
Dr. Joe Early – played by Bobby Troup
Dr. Mike Morton – played by Ron Pinkard

CONTENTS

Season Four . . . . p. 1

Season Five . . . . p. 98

Season Six . . . . p. 238

Author's Note . . . . p. 406

Season Four

Changes on the show in Season 4:

~ Guest stars are listed immediately after opening credits, rather than at the end of the episode.

~ Dixie wearing her hair down, pulled back in a ponytail, rather than pinned up. I don't think she's done that before.

~ Paramedics now have the patches on their left sleeves.

~ The numbers on the paramedics' helmets are now teal/green, instead of white.

4.1 The Screenwriter

So this episode gets a little meta... I wonder if Cinader had any input as Art Frommich is (more or less) basically a stand-in for Cinader himself; Mr. C originally went to Harbor General to research emergency medicine procedures and that's where he learned about the paramedic program, and we know what the result of *that* was. And he probably said "hey, we can mount a camera on the hood of the squad, just like they do in my 'other' show, Adam-12."

Anyway, Art has grand plans for his movie, and they may or may not begin with a "routine" motor vehicle accident between an apparently-drunk man and a motorcycle rider. Roy mentions popliteal pulse, which I always have to look up after I hear it. And the injured man falls into the same category of other victims who have jugular wounds, or nicked arteries: five drops of blood seems to represent 500 drops. At Rampart, there's all sorts of drama about Mr. Porter and his supposedly falling off the wagon, but, this being Emergency, there's actually a medical explanation for his seemingly bad/illegal behavior. And I have to say, I thought Mrs. Porter was all sorts of cute, and I just love the blouse and skirt she's wearing. I know this was 40 years ago but I think it's pretty timeless. Meanwhile the motorcyclist's wife looks like she belongs on a beach playing Annette Funicello's younger sister.

Getting back to the action, the Station 51 guys are at a construction site (I guess?) and have to deal with Al, a huge mountain of a man exhibiting the effects of some sort of inhalant. Al goes nuts on the guys until Roy can inject him with diazepam. (Fun fact: as he's yanking Chet around like a salt-shaker, we see Larry Csonka's Super Bowl ring.) Once the three FFs get him on the ground (Johnny holding one arm, Marco holding the other, and Chet trying to cover Al's legs) it looks like Chet is either in pain or getting a whiff of something he'd rather not smell.

I love it when Cap's telling Art about the fire department logs: they're confidential and can't be reviewed by anyone without a court order or something. Based on this I'm assuming that the show's writers never actually see the log-books, but probably just worked from some Cliff's Notes version. Maybe...?

Now, about Renee.... I honestly don't think she was that attractive. Yeah, she was pretty well built, but from the neck up—not so much. But the guys, of course, are all eyes, and when Johnny walks in and sees her, well, I was sort of impressed that he manages to keep *his* eyes above *her* neck. For the most part, anyway. He does give her the up-and-down once-over, but to his credit his gaze does *not* linger on the Grand Tetons. Unfortunately, she is the perfect stereotype of the dumb blond, and also of the dumb female actress. You'd think these writers would know better.

Then comes the baby delivery—on a public sidewalk, no less. I really like this scene. I do think the couple, who are both deaf—would probably have cards already printed explaining that they're deaf and can read lips, but that's a minor point. I just like the delivery scene and the fact that the biophone line is left open and Dixie, Early, and Brackett are all listening as it happens. I couldn't tell about Roy, but I don't think Johnny's wearing the OB gloves they usually wear during deliveries. And once again I have to wonder exactly what Kevin and Randy are doing for real between the actress's legs in these delivery scenes. And imagine what kind of funny ad-libs and pranks they could do in that situation that might end up in a blooper reel (but, sadly, didn't).

Last comes the fire at the Kiddytime Toy Company. I had to laugh when Cap tells the foreman guy to "get these cars out of here," and the guy says OK. How's he gonna move those cars himself?? And we already know there have to be people stuck inside... apparently every fire or explosion in LA County is required to leave at least one person stuck inside a building or otherwise unaccounted for. Otherwise, the paramedics wouldn't have anything to do at these scenes except to back the FFs with the hoses, and heaven knows they don't want to do *that*.

Every time I see this particular fire, and I see Art watching the firemen and the paramedics at work, I can't help hoping that he's finally seeing the light about what FFs and PMs do and how they risk their lives every day and do all sorts of dangerous stuff without a second thought. But nooooo, he's thinking about dolls that eat the world. *sigh*

Oh, a final note: I seem to remember seeing a picture that was obviously filmed during the Larry Csonka scene, of Kevin and Randy at the top of the pit. It's very much like a scene that's in the episode, except that Kevin is wearing sunglasses. I'd love to find that pic again.

* * *

May Fair

> Why did they keep talking to the husband if she could lip-read too?

The wife was a little too distracted and she'd have to 'happen' to be looking in their direction in order for them to talk to her. With John and Roy being at the other end of the table and not in her immediate field of vision, I imagine it was easier to get the attention of the husband. That way she could keep her focus on him and not be looking back and forth all the time.

Yeah, Cap's reaction to Miss October was funny. He didn't seem to be eye-goggling in the same way as Chet and Marco, but he seemed to be more... bemused. Almost as if he was trying to figure out if she was real (or could really be that empty-headed).

While seeing Larry Csonka in this episode, and Dick Butkus, Mark Spitz, Kareem, and other athletes who've been on this show, I'm trying to think if there are any current TV shows that have sports stars on as regularly as this show did. Interestingly, Butkus appeared late in season 3, and Csonka, Spitz, and Abdul-Jabbar all appeared in early Season 4 (Spitz and Kareem are in back-to-back episodes). Can the proximity of their appearances possibly be a coincidence??

Going back to the scene in the day-room.... Have we seen that awful-looking chili before? Maybe that concoction that Johnny was making in that one episode?? Eh, I don't remember.

* * *

> I thought the rescue of Al, the monster man was OK, however, I couldn't figure out why Roy was so slow to act? He just stood there like he didn't know what do to? Give him the damn diazepam Roy!!!!! It's like he froze.

Yeah, I noticed that, too. Sort of made it look like Roy doesn't care that his friends are getting hurt, or like he's afraid to get near the crazy-man, which is silly because we've never seen him hesitate during a rescue before.

Every now and then they write a scene in which Roy looks like a good-natured bumbler, and that's just not him. Good-natured, yes, always. But Roy's never been a bumbler, especially not on a rescue.

4.2 I'll Fix It

Cliff's Notes version: A broken motorbike.... Johnny says he'll 'fix' it.... Chet volunteers to help.... Enough said.

First call is to a home that's overrun by an old oil well. Yeah, lady, your house is ruined, but on the plus side, you got a heckuva settlement coming to you from the oil company. I mean, Jed Clampett found oil on *his* property, and look how well *he* did, right? In any case, regarding this rescue, I have to wonder how three otherwise smart, capable firefighters (Roy, John, and Chet) are trying to do something under that filthy house with all those broken wooden beams, nails, wires, and cracked china, *without gloves*. Makes no sense to me. But this is a truly dirty, awkward, and uncomfortable rescue. And I know I've said it before (in the thread that disappeared) but this one obviously couldn't have been rehearsed, so that makes it that much more realistic. Which I love; those are the best rescues, in my opinion. Also, in the very first scene, in which we see the wife walking out of her oily house, she slips and she appears to mouth a four-letter word. We don't hear it, of course, but it sure does look like that's what she says.

At Rampart, the same brainy kid who made a rocket ship a few episodes ago is back, and this time he's a medical nerd and thorn in Brackett's side. (He's also dismissive of Dr. Morton.)

May Fair

After some annoyance and a bunch of heavy sighs, Brackett ends up having one of his patented private chats with the child's father (who had been an insensitive bully) and all's well that ends well.

The PMs' next call is to help a little boy stuck in a large pipe. This is a cute rescue, although probably kind of scary for the boy in the pipe. But I do have doubts about Johnny rigging one of those dog-catcher type sticks. The real ones use some sort of vinyl or plastic-y 'noose' which is sort of easy to position as needed. On the other hand, Johnny's contraption used ordinary rope, which is limp and inactive and unless you happen to throw it exactly correctly, isn't going to do any good. But it's a TV show, so I'll give that a pass. Anyone notice that the older boy's name is Kevin? And Kevin—er, Roy—is awfully good with him and gets to be his special friend.

Next the boys are called out to a deli to retrieve a woman's wedding ring from some idiot doofus's hand. The woman is tall and dressed to *ahem* maximize her physical attributes, but her husband is an ogre who'll hit the roof if he finds out what happened. While Roy's getting the ice, the fearsome husband returns and just as he confronts the idjit guy, Johnny pulls the ring off. WHY he doesn't just slip it to the woman right then, I'll never know. She was standing right next to Johnny, for heaven's sake! Also, in theory I think I know why Johnny wanted the string, but not sure how that would work with the kid holding his hand over his head. In any case, Johnny leaves it to Roy to distract Gigantor so that he (Johnny) can slip the woman back her ring. Although their plan seems unnecessarily complicated, and I'm pretty sure any 17-year-old would be able to do it more easily. As it is, Roy serves as the distraction for Johnny, and thus is put in the position of fearing for the safety of his sausage. So to speak.

Last is a fire at a chemical plant. Quite dangerous but—hallelujah!—nobody is trapped inside!! Amazing. This time the drama comes from another source. For one thing, all six members of the engine company are hands-on... including Stoker. (Yay!) The other four guys have to cover Roy and Cap while they work to turn off some valve or other. (Meantime, we get to see 165s use the applicators, which look like heavy-duty garden waterers, or hose wands or whatever.) But after the unsuccessful first attempt, Cap and Roy try again. Note to self: if I ever need to open a stuck valve, all I have to do is hit it with a pipe, one of which is sure to be handy nearby. Incredibly, that's what Cap does—he hits the stuck valve it with a pipe, and *ta-da!*, that does the trick and the valve is loosened. Must work on the same principle as tapping the lid of a stuck jar with a knife, maybe?? In any case, it works, but not before Roy's turnout coat catches fire and Johnny looks concerned and rallies the troops to "Get Roy!" But the flames on his back are put out easily enough and Roy soldiers on so that he and Cap get the valve turned and call it a day. Seriously, they call it a day: the very next scene has Cap telling LA the fire under control. No idea how much time elapsed between the two events, though. And also, where was the Battalion Chief on this one? Shouldn't he be on site??

By the way, one thing that the baby-delivery scene in The Screenwriter got me wondering: how do they leave the biophone open so that Rampart can hear everything? When the paramedics talk, they have to press down a button on the handset, specifically so that Rampart *doesn't* have to hear everything. So I wonder if there's some way they can lock the handset into place and don't have to manually hold it open. Or maybe they just tape the button down....??

4.3 Gossip

(Another episode directed by Kevin.)

May Fair

There's a reason we're cautioned against "telling tales out of school." Or out of Rampart, as the case may be, as Nurse Ann Ridgely starts spurious rumors about Dr. Morton. Of course, we've never seen her before, and after this, it's obvious why we never see her again: I'm sure Dixie "disappeared" her right out of the Emergency Department. And yes, she really is nasty. I can't imagine how she lasted six years in *any* hospital if that's how she acts on the job.

At the station, Roy's trying to talk Johnny into competing in the Fireman's Olympics. (This conversation begins after Johnny hears the odd calls over the intercom. Ya just never know when a Samoan Fire Dancer's torch is going to result in a call to the fire department.) But the Olympics conversation is interrupted by a real call, to an MVA resulting in smashed vehicles a block apart. Cap and the guys handle the passenger car (non-serious injuries) while Roy and John travel a quarter-mile away to the wrecked armored car. (Their brief ride is complete with lights and siren... to a scene on the same block.)

At the armored car, the startled and shaken-up driver pulls his gun when John and Roy appear. To what end, I wonder? Not sure why he would shoot anyone who approached him, it's not like anyone can just open up the door and take any money. But the paramedics are only there to help and he's extricated from the vehicle and fixed up and sent away. Vince mentions calling more units to help secure the money, but we don't see the reinforcements, or anyone from the armored car company, either.

Like Kevin's last directorial effort, in this one we see more overhead shots at Rampart, as well as shots from unique angles. Apparently he liked to think outside the box, and it was somewhat refreshing. Although to be honest, I don't always care for the overhead shots in the treatment rooms.

Watching EMERGENCY! Seasons 4-6

The little boy who was unconscious... I may have led a sheltered childhood, but am I the only one who never heard of these peach-pit baskets?? And the making of them involves carving... as in with a pen knife. Doesn't sound like the best/safest pastime for an eight-year-old boy. Note: this case gives us a chance to see Joe Early doing his little penguin-y quick-walk; always adorable!

I know the highlight of the episode for a lot of viewers (*cough*women*cough*) is the sink-side conversation between Johnny and Roy. I wonder if the location of this chat was specifically written into the script, or if the director (Kevin) had any say about where it took place. It's just a simple conversation... could've taken place in the squad on the way back from Rampart, or during one of their regular tweaking-under-the-hood scenes, or while sitting in the day-room with a cup of coffee. But instead it's at the bathroom sink... while they're both half-dressed. Director or writer or whoever made that decision, all I can say is....*thank you!!*

Drama of a different sort unfolds at Rampart with the two Mrs. Johnsons. One of them, the brunette, is apparently the actress who played Batgirl on the show Batman. So E! can boast it had both Batman and Batgirl as guest stars. In any case, I wouldn't want to be *Mister* Johnson when he recovers from his accident. D'oh!

I'm a little confused by the timeline in one scene. It's nighttime and Roy and Johnny are in the dayroom, with Johnny lounging on the couch. It's where he tells Roy that he went to a local running track and ran early in the morning, and now he's sore. But he's just telling Roy this *now*, after they'd worked together for 12 hours? That doesn't make any sense to me. You'd think he'd mention his soreness earlier in the shift. In any case, Johnny is just about to tell Roy about his soreness when the alarm goes off. He'd just mentioned that he was hurting "from my toenails up to my—" Looked like his next word was going to start with a "b." Or I guess it could have been an "m." Imaginations do run wild!!

The alarm that interrupts his very interesting statement sends them to a hotel where a guy decided to climb up an electrically-lit sign... at night... to do some work for which he wasn't trained. Sounds reasonable, right? When he's hanging from the sign and goes into cardiac arrest, it occurred to me that they could just touch his arm to one of the electrical wires, and defib him the 'cheap and easy' way. (Just kidding!)

Last rescue is an explosion and fire at a place with a pineapple logo. But even though we don't know exactly what the company does, of course they carry all sorts of things that could blow up and be dangerous. Because doesn't every building store various chemicals inside?? Anyway there's the ubiquitous MM (Missing Man) that they have to find, and this time Cap goes in with them. You have to admire Cap for going in with the guys when he doesn't have to. (And where is the Battalion chief? Second ep in a row in which he should have been on scene. Can't remember if he was called out in I'll Fix It, but he was definitely called on this one, but we don't even see him.) Anyway, after Cap and Roy find the missing man, they assume Johnny's following them out, but for whatever reason, Johnny gets lost like a day-dreaming six-year-old. As soon as Roy realizes Johnny's not with them, he runs back, not really even waiting for Cap's permission. He finds Johnny without too much of a problem and just as they're running out of the building, things begin to blow up. Talk about hitting the deck!

Afterwards, we see the squad back into the station, and see the engine start to back in as well, with Marco on the tailboard. Sooty-faced, Roy and Johnny get out and joke about the Fireman's Olympics. Not surprisingly, they look very appealing. *sigh*

Note: I meant to mention in I'll Fix It that the numbers on their helmets were white instead of teal. Not sure why. But in this episode they're back to the teal numbers. Also, in this episode, Gossip, I thought Dixie looked especially attractive. Lastly, even though we didn't hear where Johnny said he was sore, we heard two—count 'em, *two!*—instances of a four-letter word. The first was the car accident, when the man said the armored car came at him "like a bat outta hell." The second was in the building fire, when Cap says "let's get the hell outta here." So two instances of the word hell, and Johnny didn't say either one.

4.4 Nagging Suspicion

Not sure why this one is called "Nagging Suspicion." No real nags, and nobody has any real suspicions. Anyway, Roy's checking out the sports pages because he follows the ponies— not at the track, for money, but just for fun. And apparently he's pretty good at picking winners. Obviously there's someone (who shall remain nameless... at least in this paragraph) who won't let the matter go at that, and the background plot is set. (Hmm, I guess the episode title could refer to the horses... although race horses aren't exactly the kind you'd refer to as 'nags.') We also see a kind of cute scene of Cap admiring the engine, and he'll always "be nuts about these engines," and Roy agrees that the firefighting bug "kind of gets in your blood." Just kind of cute to see grown guys get the same kind of excitement about fire engines that little boys do.

First call is for an "animal bite victim." Sounds pretty innocuous, right? Well, when the location of the call is at a zoo, not so much. Turns out some overzealous gawker leaned over too far to see the lion and fell over the fence. And the lion bit her or clawed her or something. Looks to me like the way she was, um, posed, doesn't quite match how it *should* look if she fell over, but hey, it's a TV show, so I'm gonna let it go. But the zookeeper guy is quick to utter (repeatedly) those four famous words we sometimes hear on this show: "It wasn't our fault." I can understand not wanting to be blamed for something bad that happens to someone, but if you're going to repeatedly profess your innocence about something, you should at least be sure you're professing it to the right person, someone who actually *cares* whose fault said incident actually is.

I have to say, it's kinda dumb for Roy to toss some things down to Johnny in the pit, as we all know how much cats (big ones as well as little ones) like things that are moving quickly, and the lion does almost come after Johnny because of it. Must admit, they did a pretty credible job of making it look like Johnny is in the lion's pit with the big cat not far away. But he gets the woman loaded into the stokes and the guys pull her up. Just about then the lion apparently "smells the blood of a fireman" and lunges forward; Johnny does some lunging of his own and climbs that rope up the wall of the pit in record time. As Roy checks the woman's vitals and John's on the phone to Rampart, it's kind of cute to see Chet shade the woman's eyes with his helmet. Such a thoughtful guy, that Chet! (Fun fact: call this fourth season the "yellow brick road," as in this season the guys will come up against "lions and tigers and bears." Oh my! Seriously—lions and tigers and bears. This episode we see the lion.)

As soon as the guys leave the victim in the treatment room at Rampart, Johnny starts in on Roy. How good are you at picking horses? How many times do you 'win'? How do you do it, you gotta have a system, etc. The least interesting storyline of the episode, imho.

Next call is right up Chet's alley: "Person sick in a bar." And not just any bar—an exotic dance club. Or... something.

Personally, I don't think it was very exotic, and it wasn't a strip club... not sure exactly what it was. Someplace where women serve drinks in their bikinis, apparently. But there is a scantily-clad girl dancing on stage. If you can call what she's doing up there dancing. I danced better when I was fourteen years old than she does. Seriously, all she does is put one foot behind the other one. And she's wearing some sort of clear vinyl mini-raincoat over a bathing suit. Not terribly titillating, if you ask me. (But then, this is a family show, and aired at 8pm on Saturdays, so I guess that's as risqué as it got.) Anyway, this call ends up being Chet's worst nightmare, as Cap tells him to wait with the engine... which I imagine is the equivalent of being banished to the kids' table at Thanksgiving. Usually Cap doesn't mind Chet tagging along at his side and yet this time, not so much. A bit of a (funny) cruel streak in the beloved Captain?? Anyway, maybe Chet and Marco and Stoker get a craps game going while the Cap and the paramedics are inside.

When Johnny calls Rampart from inside the bar/club, we see Brackett do a double-take and stare at the radio as if he thinks it's haunted. So they hear loud music in the background—it's happened before. And yet Doc looks so startled and confused. Back at the club/bar/discotheque/whatever-it-is, the guys load the stricken dancer onto the stretcher: Roy carries her feet while Johnny gets the interesting part (wink, wink), with his hands right under her breasts. (Hey, he's on duty and still manages to get to first base!) Outside, Chet asks "How was it in there?" Johnny plays it off: "Good thing you were out here, it would have been too much for you." Johnny, you devil!!

At Rampart, the dancer (Susie, I think?) is all tucked in wearing a hospital gown in the treatment room. I don't think I've ever seen them do that before. Heck, I remember in Brushfire, they were doing surgery on Conway (again in the treatment room), and they didn't even bother removing his turnout coat. But get a pretty dancer in there and she gets a gown and sheet pulled up over her and everything. By the way, I totally thought she and

Brackett had a bit of a thing between them. Quite a spark, I thought. I can see it now: The doctor and the dancer. Hey, another few days and she won't be his patient anymore; maybe she could show him how she earned her money at that club.

Next call is for Cactus Dad, the guy who thought he was cool enough to ride a skateboard. Downhill. Into cactus. Needless to say (see what I did there? *"Needles"*??), it didn't work out quite the way he wanted, and after the guys chat with him and convince him to go to his own doctor for a tetanus shot, what does Johnny do but the exact. Same. Thing. Yeah, and he wonders why people sometimes don't take him seriously. So next scene is Johnny getting needles removed at Rampart and Dixie administering the tetanus shot. Two things: 1) I thought Dixie looked especially beautiful in this scene, and 2) wouldn't Johnny have been required to keep up with all types of vaccinations and boosters as part of his job?

After more of the filler "picking the ponies" story, Station 51 is called out to assist the police department. Turns out there's a sniper in what is obviously an abandoned building, and the cops want the FD on hand when they shoot in some tear gas in there, in case it ignites a fire. I have a couple of problems (questions) about how this plays out. First of all, the cops open fire to provide cover for an officer to get into position to shoot the tear gas into the building. That seems a bit odd to me; if the cops fire on the sniper, even if they purposely try *not* to hit him, to me it seems like they're just inciting him to fire even more. (Am I right or is there something wrong with my logic??) We know how this strategy turns out—pretty much exactly as I thought—as the sniper snipes and Tear-Gun Cop is shot. The head cop in charge (who doesn't seem to be very much in charge) asks if Cap can help and the paramedics get ready to go in and help the fallen officer. Also, Cap tells the cop "I have an idea that might help." This is my second objection. Cap's idea is a good one—I think it should have been used in the first place. Instead of the cops providing "cover fire" so Tear-Gun

Cop can get into position, Engine 51 could have run a hose at the sniper; I don't think he'd have been able to see, much less shoot, with that force coming at him.

In any case, Cap's idea works and Roy and John are able to move the injured officer and treat him behind a nearby vehicle. While under active fire. Meanwhile, Vince picks up the tear-gas gun and successfully gets two cartridges into the building. As expected, the tear-gas does indeed start a fire and soon the sniper tosses his weapon out the window and surrenders. This brings up an instance of, "Do you hear what I hear?" Right after the sniper tosses out his rifle, Cap, Marco, and Chet stand up from where they've been crouching. We *see* Cap say something, but a voice that doesn't match the action says, "Put on your air masks." Thing is, it sounds like Johnny's voice. The line is obviously dubbed in, but why would they dub in *Johnny's* voice rather than Cap's? Or am I crazy for thinking it's Randy's voice?? Anyway, I like the whole rescue after that. Cap ushers in the rest of the first-alarm assignment and assigns them in the efficient Cap-like fashion we love so well. Johnny and Roy can work on the victim without fear of getting shot, and all the firefighters are doing great firefighter-y things in a very professional manner. So they finally get the injured cop to Rampart where he's being treated in a treatment room. Oddly, one of the nurses is wearing scrubs while the other two… aren't. Similarly, Dr. Morton is wearing scrubs, while the other two doctors… aren't. Wonder what's up with that?? In any case, they do end up doing surgery on the guy, right there in the treatment room. A thoracotomy. Must be a simple surgery, because Johnny and Roy have just finished telling Dixie about the rescue when Brackett comes out, all finished and cleaned up and everything. Quickest. Surgery. Ever.

So, I guess I better close the loop on Roy's pony-picking career. Johnny hounds and 'nags' Roy (hmmm….) about his "system" (or lack of) until poor Roy is second-guessing himself, so that when he does go to the track with all the guys' money (really?

they sent him by himself?? I thought "TV friends" did everything together), he went against his first instinct and chose another horse. Which didn't win, of course, so they lost their money. Fortunately—and the best part of this whole sorry storyline—the guys totally relate to the situation and admit it "sounds like something *I'd* do." So it all ends happily enough.

Quickly:

~ At the dance club, that was a cute little double-take Johnny does after he packs up the biophone, turning as if he expected Roy and the ambulance guys to still be there.

~ Those "flak vests" they wear at the sniper scene… they just look like quilted vests.

~ Why does the firefighter *carry* the sniper down the ladder? Not only could it have been dangerous (if he decided to hurt or threaten the FF), but the man isn't even injured. Would have been quicker if he'd been ordered to come down on his own.

~ The cop who'd been shot. When he's in the treatment room at Rampart, his belt buckle is undone. Poor Conway has to wear his turnout coat during surgery, and the go-go dancer gets a complete change of clothes. Guess they couldn't decide what to do with the cop, so he's halfway in between the two.

4.5 Communication Gaffe

So first we get an extreme close-up of Chet's face as he grooms his mustache, and then we find out Roy's going to be on a game show. Why does nobody at the station ask him *which* game show, much less mention whether they've seen it. If someone I knew said he/she was going to be on a show, I'd darn well ask which one—The Price is Right? Wheel of Fortune? Family Feud?

So the first call is to a crime scene, in which a LEO was shot while responding to a robbery or something. Hmm, that's two episodes in a row with cops being shot. In this case, though, one of the bad guys was also shot, and Detective Crockett (the first time we've met him) is a hard-nose who wants his cop treated first instead of the more-critically injured perp. I'm glad Roy stood up to him, but I wish he'd been more forceful, perhaps reminding the detective that they (the paramedics) don't answer to him. Later on Dixie is the one who lays it on the line: they deal with life-threatening injuries first. Anyway, I find it curious that at the scene, Roy is the one to go in the ambulance with the criminal/victim, since Johnny's the one who had been the one treating him up 'til then. Also, wouldn't we have seen more of the 'blue wall' at Rampart if a detective had been shot? Instead of a single other police officer who leaves after just a few minutes??

Cut back to Rampart to Mrs. Caine who brings in her son Robbie. (Robbie, Tommy, Billy... where are all the kids named Daniel or Jason or Eric?) Unless I misheard, the mother says of him "He's my only and my favorite"??? Seems kind of like a backhanded compliment to me. (That actress who plays the mother has been in a couple of episodes of E!) And we learn that just because you smack your kids around doesn't mean you're a bad person. It means you probably have a blood clot on the brain; in other words, an excuse. Because yeah, I'm sure that's what causes most abusive parents to hit their kids. (insert eye-roll icon here) And I notice that Brackett simply mentions having tests performed on the mother; he never really explains *what tests* or *why* he's suggesting them.

Meanwhile Roy and Johnny get a call for a "man down," and we hear some good tire-squealing as the squad drives past—*ta da!*—the house with white columns, one of our stock footage favorites. I don't recall if we've seen it yet in the series. This call isn't serious and doesn't even require a trip to Rampart; in fact this call is today's version of yesterday's skateboard call. In any case, we get to see Johnny as he deals with the ultimate Gage distraction: attractive women in bikinis, diving into a pool.

Roy's mother's name is Harriet? Harriet DeSoto? Poor woman!

I like the call on which Crockett joins Johnny and Roy. Although I do have to wonder who called this one in, as the two kids involved are miles from anywhere. And did you see all the signs on the empty lot? I guess they *really* didn't want anyone trespassing. But it's nice to see Crockett take charge of the situation. Have to wonder, though.... I guess they transported the kid on the back of the squad? I didn't see an ambulance on the scene. Getting back to the call, I hear Early prescribe 50 milligrams Benadryl, and Johnny confirms, "1 milligram epinephrine." I guess those are comparable, or was that just poor editing??

We get a brief scene of Roy and Johnny talking while working under the squad: each working separately and talking the same way—separately; each assumes the other is listening to him. Also, what could they have been doing under there? Nothing too involved, I'm sure. What if the tones sounded just then? And what would Charlie say about their doing whatever it is they're doing??

The final call is for a large accident, again in the middle of nowhere, for a truck and station wagon crash. (Once again, I wonder who put in the call.) But the resulting collision (because of course the truck is carrying kerosene drums) causes a couple of explosions—which are still occurring—which in turn causes a brushfire. I have to laugh when Cap tells the other engine to cover the "east side" of the fire. Should they all check their compasses to determine which is the east side? (I've noticed this same thing in other situations as well; these LACoFD captains must have an innate ability to tell north from south from east from west at any given moment.)

And while I appreciate that Marco was in charge of one of the victims, what if the driver had had a neck injury? I don't think Roy or Johnny even look at the guy before he is (clumsily) moved out. Lastly, I see Battalion Chief 5 is here on the scene. I thought Station 51 was under Battalion 14??

4.6 Surprise

For fans of classic (old) sitcoms, this episode has both Millie Helper (The Dick Van Dyke Show) and Helen Crump (The Andy Griffith Show).

And there's another instance of an Unfortunate Encounter with Cactus. Don't these Angelenos have enough sense to stay away from the prickly stuff??

Then there's the rescue with the runaway sign... that's a good one.

Dixie's birthday... meh. They made a huge deal over something that happens every year. Unless she signs their paychecks or is leaving Rampart for good, making such a big deal over one person's birthday is silly and unrealistic. (IMO, at least. But then, I can be a party-pooper at times. Plus, this *is* a TV show, after all, where the unrealistic happens every day.)

* * *

I do think that the birthday thing for Dixie was *way* over the top. Anyone who's ever had a work situation in which birthdays were recognized in some way knows that what was discussed in this episode is totally unrealistic for one individual's birthday. (If they have this huge party for Dixie, will they do the same for Brackett and Early? Morton? Cap? Just playing devil's advocate....)

* * *

Yeah, it was kind of disappointing not to see all the Johnny-explosion drama in that last rescue, but my thought is that maybe the show didn't want to focus on that this time, since we've seen other drama surrounding him (although not from a fire/explosion). Sometimes this show doesn't always show every step of a rescue (rescues in general, not just those relating to our FF friends), which I can understand on one hand, even though on the other hand I like watching some of the drama.

Which makes me wonder sometimes how often scenes were filmed and then not put into the final episode. I'd love to see all the "cutting-room floor" stuff. Wonder if that exists somewhere??

Isn't there an episode in which Roy is in a building when it blows and they all go in to find him?? Or am I imagining things again??? I could swear there is, but I don't recall when or how I saw it. Which really makes me wonder if I'm confusing it with something else, or some other show.

~ ~ ~

So this episode doesn't open with any light-hearted scene, setting up the "theme" of the day. Instead, a 'cold open' with the bay doors opening as the call goes out: "woman injured in motorcycle accident." Yeah, it's Millie Helper (from The Dick Van Dyke show), butt-side down in a cactus patch. She's in pain, but she's also sort of annoying and a little unpleasant; however, the idea to use the ladders to get her out is pretty ingenious. Funny, but when the scene ends and we go to opening credits, they had mentioned a few ways they *couldn't* get her out (i.e., ideas that wouldn't work), but after the credits, when the show resumes, they're already implementing the ladder plan. So we don't know how they came up with it. (Fun fact #1: did anyone know that the actress, Ann Morgan Guilbert, also played Grandma Yetta on The Nanny? I had no idea!!)

At Rampart, we finally get the set-up of the episode: Dixie's birthday, and a "surprise" party... that she totally knows about, of course, including Roy's "stealthy" attempt to come up with a gift for her (a hair dryer).

Next call is a construction accident, with a large sign gone wild in high winds. (Really? LA is known for its wind? Since when??) In any case, the wind is important for the purpose of this storyline, so ¡voila! we have a lot of wind. Convenient, right?? Speaking of convenient... at these rescue sites there's usually a malfunctioning winch or stuck pulley or something that makes the rescue difficult, and necessitates the call to the Fire Department. In this case it's a "busted hydraulic line." In any case, Cap orders them to take all their rope and a hose roller to the roof of the building. When 95s comes along, Cap asks for their rope and crew on the roof. He doesn't mention a hose roller, yet 95s brings theirs to the roof as well. Good thing, too, as the guys end up needing it. Roy and Johnny aren't wearing their usual safety belts, either; they're wearing a harness sort of thing, that also goes between their legs. I wonder how it's determined when they wear one thing and when they wear the other? Anyway, once the guy he's helping is pulled up, I like how Johnny sort of hops onto the runaway sign; that's a really cute hop. And didn't someone mention how Johnny often calls for "more slack!" and he sounds almost angry when he does it? He does that here, too. As previously noted, it almost sounds as if he's yelling angrily, as if the others didn't hear him the first two or three times he made the request. And it's a good thing Stoker can read minds, otherwise he wouldn't have known what to do when that line was thrown down. I don't think that part had been decided when all the rest of the guys went up to the roof.

Next disaster is Dixie… she's broken her ankle by dealing with an errant shopping cart. Horrors! The party is now in jeopardy! This part of the story is supposed to create an amusing chaos because Nurse Betty can't get the nurse's schedule right, which is always dangerous, because, as we all know, "It's not *nice* to fool Mother Nature!" *thunderclap* (Fun Fact #2: for several years, this actress lived in Newtown, CT. Yes, *that* Newtown.) In any case, I don't personally find the nurse-scheduling chaos part of the episode all that amusing.

So Squad 51 is next sent to a house for a man stuck in a sauna. Guess who we see: another actress from a groundbreaking '60s sitcom: Aneta Corsault. Better known as Helen Crump from The Andy Griffith Show, of course. Anyway, her husband is locked in his brand new sauna and in distress. Even more amazing is the fact that Johnny IDs him as being "about 30 years old." Wha—??? Is Miss Crump going after younger men now?? In any case, as things ironically turn out, his heat prostration saved his life, so all's well that ends well with him.

Meanwhile, Johnny's psyched about the party for Dixie (to take place in her hospital room, of course) and he's got a tape recorder, and some cassettes to provide music for—get this—dancing. (Insert eye-roll icon here; in fact, be sure those eyes don't just roll out completely.) Hey, Johnny boy, hang onto that tape recorder… you can use it when you get your "bright idea" for how to keep up with your written reports. (*Much* better and easier than rewiring the squad's radio.)

Final call is the gas leak in the apartment building. The paramedics are sent inside to search the rooms and also to ventilate the building. (Notice how when they open windows, they both stick their heads out and look around? What's up with that??) Anyway, Roy kicks down the door of one of the apartments, and then does a double-take when he notices an old woman in the bedroom. He's real sweet with her, trying to convince her she has to leave, even though she's refusing and fearfully protesting. But Roy calls in Chet (and a stretcher) and he firmly but politely and kindly goes ahead and gets her out of there. Johnny isn't quite as lucky, as he's at the top of the stairs when the place explodes, and he ends up taking a big tumble.

So the next scene is at Rampart, with Johnny's leg in traction and him forlornly reading a magazine. (I guess he hasn't discovered the soap opera on cable TV yet.) Roy comes to visit, which cheers Johnny up (yay!) until Roy turns right around and leaves again (boo). But it's a fake-out and next thing you know, the only people who work full-time at Rampart come into Johnny's room, thus leaving the Emergency Department totally unattended. Dixie shares her birthday cake and Doc Early hands Johnny his own tape player, and they all have a good, heartfelt laugh.

4.7 Daisy's Pick

I can't believe we lost the Season 4, Part One thread to the abyss a while back. I was busy today and I thought I could at least reread the comments for this episode and refresh my memory of it, but nooooo, can't do that; the thread is gone for good. So I zipped through the episode this evening.

First off, everyone talks about Daisy as if she's the most stunning thing in a nurse's uniform—Marilyn Monroe plus Halle Berry with a little Angelina thrown in. But really, she's no prettier than some of the other nurses we've seen on this show, and a big deal hasn't been made out of *them*. (Except for the one nurse who had some orderlies following her around.

But even she didn't have a dozen hunky paramedics drooling over her, much less putting money into a kitty.)

Anyway, I like the ice house rescue, although I wonder why Roy and John didn't wear their turnouts in there. And the victim was lying in a suspiciously plain pose. Then as they were wheeling him into Rampart we hear a page for "Stat Ident doctor in Treatment 3." Which of course is exactly where they took the ice-man. And then Brackett says something about "let's get him on the Byrd." Yay, the Byrd got name-dropped.

I also like the Captain Larson ship rescue. It was funny when Dixie held the door open and told Morton "Your ship has come in." Too funny!

As far as Daisy's concerned.... which paramedics actually worked on Friday, since Roy was busy and a whole bunch of other paramedics were out on their "date" with Daisy??

The last rescue (fire at the theatre) was good, too. Although I thought it odd that, just as Roy and Johnny went into the icehouse without their bunker coats, they went into the theatre without their air masks. I repeat: they went into *the burning building...* without breathable air. To me that makes no sense.

Well, that's all I got on this one. Hopefully tomorrow I'll be able to give the show the attention it deserves.

~ ~ ~

So this ep begins with Tom Dwyer backing the squad into the bay and "handing it over" to Roy. (We never see his partner, or even an unidentified person who could possibly *be* his partner.) Anyway, this is how the topic of Daisy is raised: while Johnny was on vacation, a new nurse started at Rampart and she has all the men abuzz. As I said before, she must be blindingly beautiful and perfect in every way to have so many grown men in such a tizzy.

I really like the ice house rescue—pretty unique and complicated, and one of those that might not be able to be rehearsed. That man's arm really did look like it was frozen to the ground. (Although I still say it's ridiculous that he was laid out on the floor so neatly.) One odd thing I noticed—in addition to the fact that some of the paramedics' equipment was lugged into the ice house and not used there; they couldn't treat him in there, so why bring it in, in the first place?—but what I find interesting is that we see Stoker take a hose out of the engine and unroll it, and he moves to hook it up to the hydrant. That leaves *Marco* to hook the other end up to The Beast (i.e., the engine). It just seems a little odd that the engineer is working with the hydrant, and allowing *someone else* to actually touch "his baby." Hmmm Meanwhile, back in the ice house, that definitely is an ice house, as I could see their breath when they talked. I also saw Johnny put an awful rag over his mouth—yuck, who knows where that's been! But getting the man out is complicated and not easy, but they manage and both J and R go to Rampart with him.

So Johnny finally sees Daisy, and fireworks explode. He gets introduced to her and immediately does his "Johnny thing," which includes smiling a lot and leaning in, invading the girl's personal space. (Ugh.) Back at the station, we also get a look at Dwyer with his ultra-cool sunglasses. Yeah, I'm sure those were all the rage at the time.

So Johnny's still thinking dreamily of Daisy when the tones go off again, and this leads us to Captain Larson, the old swabbie whose hands are glued to his (model) ship. This is a cute one, and the guys are very good with the old salt. Morton isn't quite as nostalgic, but he follows their suggestion of tipping the hands (and boat) up in order to get to the man's fingers. (What I wonder is, couldn't they at least have removed the masts and sails? I should think those would come out relatively easily and be just as easily replaced, and taking them off would definitely make transporting the ship a little (or a lot) less awkward.

May Fair

The next call is for a sick boy, three years old, who's unconscious. The mom says she wanted to take him to a doctor, but her husband "said no." *sigh* Needless to say, the kid does go to Rampart. Turns out the father has a reason (or thinks he has a reason) for not wanting the boy taken to a doctor, but still, a small kid is obviously sick, and the mother just does nothing when her husband says "no doctor"? Ugh!! I know, I shouldn't look at a '70s show through a modern lens, but I hate the thought that many women were taught to be complacent (and compliant) and not argue with their "men." (Funny scene: when the father drives up and we see the ambulance turn the corner behind him, the ambulance does a "slide" around the corner.

At the hospital with the boy, I got a little confused. They use the ambu-bag (sp?) on the kid... is there a reason they don't just hook him up to a ventilator? I thought the whole point of inserting an esophageal airway is to hook the patient up to a ventilator. (??) Anyway, about the Goldbergs... if I was the wife, I'd have had to have a serious think once I discovered my husband 'neglected' to tell me that he has a potentially fatal disease running in his family, ya know?? That doesn't mean she wouldn't have married him, but it's the kind of thing a woman might want to know when she's going to have a kid. Sheesh! Luckily, all's well that ends well for the Goldberg family, and little Jerry is going to be fine, although on a somewhat restricted diet.

So, back to Daisy.... Johnny runs into her in the hallway and asks if she'd like to go out. Not exactly a shrinking violet, she immediately says, "How about Friday? Here's the address, be there at 10am." (Really, Johnny? That doesn't set off alarm bells? A girl has cards made up and wants to go on a "date" at 10 in the morning, and you don't think that's odd?) Anyway, he does look a little surprised at her response, but apparently, because this is *Daisy* we're talking about, suddenly Johnny doesn't mind that a woman is being bold and practically asking him out. In another episode, that same behavior really turned him off, but not this time. Maybe it's the competition with the other paramedics that changes his mind, not to mention the $70 he stands to gain. Did anyone notice: during that one conversation with Daisy, two very attractive nurses walk past him, one blond and one brunette. I find that very ironic. Anyway, he's thrilled to have a date with Daisy, and doesn't see any problem on the horizon.

Last call is to a fire in a theatre. And of course there's someone who falls and is injured. A guy falls from a catwalk or something and lands on some pipes, so of course Johnny has to go down and get to him and secure him so they can get him out. It sort of reminds me of another rescue that's somewhat similar: I believe it's in a later season, but it's at a movie studio and someone has fallen across some wooden beams, one of which is about to break. And there's also another rescue of a man fallen on some pipes and they have to use foam in the building, but that was in the first season, and not quite the same kind of rescue. Anyway, in this particular case, the theatre is on fire while they're trying to rescue the victim, and they can't take him down to the ground, but they take him out another way to the roof and then get down via a snorkel. Oh, and at the start, the guys run into the burning building without air tanks. You'd think they'd know better!!

Final scene, we find out about the date with Daisy: a group effort doing volunteer work at an orphanage. And apparently these otherwise competent and proficient men are all thumbs and klutzes and incapable of performing simple tasks like pushing a wheelbarrow or hammering a nail. Not without hurting themselves, anyway. So they've all soured on Daisy. But Marco gets the prize when she visits the station: a quiet, one-on-one dinner at her place. Go Marco!!

4.8 Quicker Than the Eye

You've heard of the movie "There Will be Blood"? As far as I'm concerned, this episode's real title is "There *Should* be Blood." In general I find this one to be pretty ho-hum, and the unrealistic portrayal of the red stuff in two of the rescues is a large part of the reason why.

Not to mention the whole "let's fool Chet" thing. The episode starts out with him doing magic tricks, and Marco and Mike actually seem to be enjoying the show, so why does that merit having a prank pulled on him? I don't like practical jokes anyway, so I'm just gonna ignore all that cra—er, I mean, foolishness.

The first call is one of the reasons I don't care much for the episode. I guess Mark Spitz and his wife did an admirable job of 'acting,' but it's kind of hard to tell, since his character acted like he'd been underwater too long and practically all she did was roll her head back and forth (on the convenient halo of her hair) and murmur "Pete? Pete?" Plus, when she's lying on the kitchen floor she doesn't look *that* pregnant, but then she's in the treatment room at Rampart and, yowza! Looks like she has one of Kareem's basketballs under that top of hers. But the thing that really drives me buggy is... no blood. She's been shot, and there should be blood... but there isn't. Barely one ketchup packet, I'd guess, based on her shirt, and not a single, solitary drop on the kitchen floor. I know I sound like a broken record about blood, and I guess I've been watching Supernatural too long, what with their regular scenes of blood spattering the walls and floor, etc., but still. There should be blood. (And fair warning: the topic will come up again.)

Also, I had to chuckle: when Johnny is in the ambulance with the wife, and Angie (DeMeo) is in there also as the ambulance attendant, we see Angie mess with the IV drip gauge, as if he's adjusting it. You know, because that's his job, right?? (Not!!)

Watching EMERGENCY! Seasons 4-6

The next rescue is the workman at the movie studio. I love watching shows in which scenes are set on a movie/TV studio, because they always try to show us extras from different types of projects; usually there's an Indian/cowboy/saloon girl, sometimes an Egyptian goddess, or some other very easily-identifiable character from some bygone era. And they're usually all together, as if they're all working on the same project or something. Anyway, that's how TV shows let us know that we're looking at a movie lot.

The man-under-boat rescue is another one that bothers me, as supposedly the guy has a severed artery and is losing a lot of blood, but all we see is a one-packet amount of red stuff on his arm. Also, I'm not sure I'd equate Ringer's IV with a blood transfusion. The Ringer's is only to replenish fluids and obviously isn't blood, so if I were Johnny, I would have corrected the victim who thought he was getting a transfusion. It might not have made a difference to him, but then again, it might have. And I was surprised that Roy went in the ambulance with the victim, instead of Johnny, who'd been treating him up 'til then. (Without a helmet on, no less... Johnny's under a structure that failed, and is surrounded by boards that could come down on him at any time, and yet—no helmet.)

I do like the last rescue, with the paralyzed/catatonic man and the boy. It's a good example of the boys paying attention and taking note of things that may or may not end up being important. (In this case: may.) Transporting these patients to Rampart gives us two bloopers, one I've seen mentioned elsewhere, and one of my own discovery. First, as the ambulance backs in, it's an old hearse-style station wagon thing, but when the scene cuts to everyone piling out of the ambulance, it's the larger box-style. The second goof is more of a mystery. We see both Roy and Johnny get out of the ambulance, so that generally means that one of the FFs drove the squad to Rampart, right? Well, it couldn't have been Chet, since he was back at the station, sulking. Which means it must have been Marco.... except that we don't see him get out of the squad. When the squad returns to the station, we only see Roy and Johnny get out, and that's when Cap tells them that Chet is talking about quitting. So where is Marco? Was he even at Rampart?? Oh well, just a minor continuity goof, I guess.

Lastly, anyone ever notice how often the paramedics say something on the biophone that includes the phrase "at this location," or "at your location"? I heard it two or three times in this episode. It always sounds so stilted and formal and wordy. And unnecessary, if you ask me. If the boys say "at your location," they mean Rampart, so why not just say "Rampart"? Just sayin'.

4.9 Foreign Trade

So Johnny's thinking of selling his Rover. For such an active, outdoorsy guy, that seems kind of ironic. Where's he going to keep his mountaineering equipment and his fishing rod?? That first conversation the guys have is funny. Chet says, "Struck out again last night?" and Johnny replies, "That has nothing to do with it"... thereby confirming that he did, indeed, strike out again last night. (Poor Johnny!) But Chet is the instigator in this whole deal, as he's the one who kind of starts the whole "trading vehicles" ball rolling. Johnny wants something sporty, Roy wants something more practical. Ooh, ooh, did anyone else raise your eyebrows when Johnny mentions that Roy could "take the bed out of the back" of his Rover in order to fit the kids in there? Yeah, I know what he meant by "bed," but coming from a confirmed swingin' single like John Gage... it sounds a little suggestive, no?? Anyway, the two partners decide they might just want to switch vehicles. And then Chet gets in the middle of it—again—by mentioning money. Bad, bad Chet!

First call is to a nameless university and the frat house for the (fictional) fraternity of Kappa Kappa Omega. Johnny's doppelganger brother is a member of this frat and luckily he's not one of the diaper-wearers. But their victim is—and he's choking and unconscious from lack of oxygen. Johnny sticks his fingers deep into the man's throat (eww!) but has to call for the choke-saver, with which he successfully extracts the offending piece of raw liver. They get the guy stabilized on assisted breathing and take him into Rampart. (For those keeping count of these things, Johnny leaves the choke-saver behind—and the raw liver.) I love when Don and the other frat dude approach Roy about "not officially reporting" the incident, and Roy points to the approaching cop and says, "take it up with him." Ha, too funny!

At the hospital, Dixie deals with the Zimmermans, parents of Chokin' Charlie—oops, I mean Danny the frat pledge. Anyway, Mrs. Zimmerman gets upset and hysterical and Dixie has to calm her down. Personally I was hoping Dixie was going to slap the woman, but that doesn't happen, darn the luck. Oh, and did anyone recognize Mrs. Zimmerman? She's the same actress who plays (or is going to play, in a future episode) Millie, the former Rampart head nurse who tries to commit suicide.

Also at Rampart, we get Joe Early with a case of the hiccups (and, not surprisingly, there's a kid involved), and Dixie meets Mr. O'Brien, the all-important "Administrator" who offers her a new job. Yeah, just like that! They've never met each other, but within two minutes of meeting, he offers her a big promotion and has to have an answer in a few hours. (I've worked in HR for many years… that is *not* how it works.)

May Fair

Meanwhile, at the station, Johnny's suffering from Buyer's Remorse involving the car-swap, and the whole conversation at the table is awkward and a little painful to watch. For me, at least. Not surprisingly, Chet's provoking things and inciting trouble, but what *I* want to know is, why is Roy sitting quietly during the whole thing? Johnny's obviously feeling pressured, Chet's poking him with a stick, and Roy does nothing. Even when Chet implies that the sports car (*Roy's* sports car) is a piece of crap?? That just seems odd, especially Roy insisting that "a deal's a deal."

Speaking of cars, the next call is for Kareem Abdul-Jabbar, who is stuck in his. This is yet another sports star in a guest role, joining Mark Spitz, Larry Csonka, and Dick Butkus. (Three of these four appeared in the fourth season, for what that's worth.) Anyway, the Jabbar rescue isn't all that exciting or interesting, but I did notice that we never see the make of his car while he's in it. The way the scene is filmed, all the while he's stuck, we don't see the logo on the front of the car. It's not until Kareem is not only out of the car, but out of the scene entirely that we see it's a Mercedes. (Actually, to be truthful, there is a brief glimpse of half of the Mercedes logo as they work to get Kareem into the ambulance, but even so, he's *out* of the car.) In any case, this could be a total coincidence, and not unusual in the least. But the detail-oriented conspiracy theorist in me still wonders about it. Who knows, maybe at that time Jabbar had a contract with a particular carmaker, and couldn't be seen in any other type of car for any reason. (Eh, just spit-balling.)

At Rampart, Dixie's listening to everyone tell her she should take O'Brien's promotion, but all it takes is for Mrs. Zimmerman to quit crying and bake chocolate chip cookies for Dixie to realize where her heart is and she informs O'Brien personally that she's turning down the proffered job. As if to accentuate the rightness (?) of her decision, she rushes off to deal with two cops who bring in a cuffed and struggling ne'er-do-well with a head wound. Wipe hands; problem solved!

Start of next shift, Roy's on the phone with his wife (didn't he just leave home??) and we learn that he wants to trade back the Rover for his sports car (because it fits him so well, don'tcha know). But Johnny's telling Chet how a pretty girl waved at him that morning as he was in said sports car, so Roy thinks he's probably not getting his wheels back. Cue the alarm for their first call of the day, a car hanging off a drawbridge. Yes, another car rescue.

This rescue is interesting, if somewhat perplexing. First off, why does Marco shoot the line from the base of the drawbridge? Wouldn't it be better for him to go at least partway up so he could "aim" with a smidge of accuracy? Secondly, as soon as Marco shoots the thin wire ("safety line"), ropes magically appear on both sides of the drawbridge; Johnny's pulling one on his side, and Mike and Chet also have a rope on their side. Where did the ropes come from?? Okay, that's the first perplexing thing. The second also involves rope: why do they simply string a rope across the back of that ugly El Camino and "hold it down," literally? Far as I could tell, that rope does precious little to help secure the car. I'd have tried to get the rope through the open windows of the vehicle, which would have actually, you know, secured it in place. Anyway, I would also have used a shorter length of rope to secure Johnny as he unhooked from the "main" rope to get the woman out. Then both he and the woman could have been tied via the shorter rope to the main rope. That's how *I* would have done that rescue... because I'm such an expert at these things, y'know?? Anyway, Roy promises the woman they'll secure the car, but we don't see that or even see them discussing how to do that. That would have been interesting, too.

So back at Station 51 Roy thinks he's lost his car for good, but when he goes to sit in "her" one last time, he and Johnny decide to swap back. Chet tries to stir up more trouble, but they shut him down. All's well that ends well.

Stuff:

~ I wonder what movie Roy and Chet were discussing as they approach Johnny behind the station??

~ When we see the guys in the squad—side view, when they're actually moving—I wonder if the squad is being towed (like they did on Adam-12) or is riding on a flatbed. I don't know why that popped into my head as I watched this, but it did.

~ When Roy remarks to the basketball player (Jabbar) something about 'a heck of a way to make a living,' Kareem's response is almost inaudible, but it sounds to me like he says something like, "you're not jiving, man."

~ More crazy time distortion on the bridge rescue. The call came in first thing on the shift, but it looks like late afternoon when they're actually rescuing the woman. I know the voices of Roy, Johnny, and the woman were likely all dubbed in later, but as usual this show does a pretty good job of making it seem (sound) real.

~ Roy says he's had his car for ten years. If he's about 30 at the time, how did he, as a 20-year-old, afford to buy it to begin with? It would have been more expensive ten years earlier. And we know he spent time in the Army. (Related question... I wonder how long Kevin owned that car? I'm assuming *he* didn't own it for ten years.)

4.10 Camera Bug

So Johnny's on a new kick. Anyone surprised? And yes, he's gonna drive the guys crazy before the episode is over. And by the way, in that first scene, Roy *stinks* at pretending to stretch, as Johnny requests. Obviously he's hoping that if he 'poses' badly, his partner would quit asking him.

The first call is to a fire in a school. Cap tells Roy and Johnny to get their masks on, but he doesn't tell anyone else? Seems odd. So inside the school, who's actually manning the hoses? Anyway, as they drive up to the school, we see a neat camera angle, right over Cap's shoulder. Wonder how they got that, as I didn't think there's room in the cab for a third person (or even a camera). Guess it could be through the window to the jump seat. And at the scene, there are a couple of interesting things going on. First, Cap tells Engine 90 to "bring us a line." I take this to mean that Engine 90 will supply 51 with water, i.e., 90 stays closer to the nearest hydrant, so they can supply 51 with as much water as necessary. (That's my assumption, anyway.) I don't recall off the top of my head if I've heard one engine supplying another before—except in Inferno, when another engine resupplied 51 in the middle of a brushfire. But there weren't any hydrants handy in *that* episode, so once the water was gone, it was gone.

Anyway, another odd thing about this school fire: Cap told Johnny and Roy to put their air masks on, but he didn't tell anyone else to. And he tells Chet to pull a line and, "Roy and John can take it in" to the school. Why them?? He's got probably eight other FFs there, and yet he sends the paramedics—alone—into the school with a single line. ??? Far as I know, they didn't know of anyone being in the building, so why was Roy even looking for someone? Cap does order some FFs up onto the roof to open it up, which leads to a third funny thing. We see Stoker at 51's engine controls, then in the very next scene we see him and Marco setting up a ladder for someone to get up on the roof, and in the very next scene, Stoker is back at the controls. Makes it look like he has a twin! (Hmmm, interesting thought….)

May Fair

In any case, Roy does find a victim, and he and Johnny bring him out. They estimate him to be about 15 years old, yet Rampart orders a D5W IV and nobody bats an eye. I think we've debated before that there might be an age below 18 when the paramedics can administer IVs without parental consent (although it's a tricky topic).

At Rampart, Deputy Vince goes into the coffee room and has a somewhat forced conversation with Dr. Morton. Not that the convo between the two is forced, but it seems odd to the viewer that these two particular characters would end up having any conversation at all, when I don't think we've ever seen them say two words to each other before. But it's a sort of a PSA scene, and it also sets up the next scene, in which Morton talks to the young school-fire victim, sort of "brother to brother." Morton gives a little of his jive talk and demonstrates that he knows where the kid is "coming from," etc. He barks at Dixie when she sticks her head in the door, but this heralds the arrival of the boy's mother and soon everyone's crying and calm and the crisis is past.

The paramedics get a call to Station 68 for an apparent heart attack of a fellow FF. (It's Mort Metzger, before he hangs up his hose and becomes a sheriff in Cabot Cove, Maine.) We see the front of the real station 68 (just like yesterday we saw the back of the "real" station 51—er, I mean 127), but I wonder if the inside was real or a studio set. (My money is on a set.) In any case, turns out that Fireman Bob isn't having a heart attack, he just made his chili a little too spicy. Don't you just love the footage we see of the boiling, bubbling, bloopy stuff that's supposed to be the chili? I think we see that same scene at station 51 a time or two.

At Rampart, Dixie's having a heck of a bad day, including the man (who used to be choirmaster in Mayberry) who complains about the hospital ripping off his $12 shirt in order to save his life while he was in cardiac arrest. (That $12 shirt then would be about $60-plus today. Still not worth getting all het up about, considering.) But because Dixie's having a "no good, very bad day," Kel offers to treat her to lunch at someplace called The Velvet Slipper. Hmm, maybe it's just me, but I'd kind of expect a place with a name like The Velvet Slipper to be a very different kind of place, rather than a fancy restaurant, y'know? (Yeah, probably just me....) At the restaurant, no sooner to Doc and Dix start into their salads when the owner tells them about a woman who collapsed and is in their (empty) banquet room. Of course they go to help, of course she's eight months pregnant, and of course she's going into labor. Brackett whips a handy-dandy cloth off a nearby table, Dixie brings him his doctor's kit, and bing-bang-boom we get a nice, quick delivery with just enough drama to make it interesting. And, of course, no blood. This *is* Emergency!, after all; there's never any blood or goo or icky stuff in childbirth in Emergency!-land.

Meanwhile, the boys are busy responding to a woman down, who's a stewardess back from her Acapulco run. They take her to Rampart and everyone's mystified as to why she's out cold—until Morton notices a mark under her arm, at the same time that Dr. Early comments that it sounds like a scorpion bite. Roy and Johnny race back to the apartment and find the offending critter, which means that now they can safely treat her appropriately. (Related tangent: the two stewardess' names are Trudy and Rachel. Sound familiar to anyone??*)

Johnny's still annoying everyone with his camera, including Cap, who calls him a twit when Johnny blinds him with the flash (although there was no flash when he took other photos). And then he (Johnny) inadvertently hits Roy in the head with the camera. That's when next call comes in, for a truck over a cliff, and off they go.

A good rescue. Angelo DeMeo is pressed into service as the truck driver who's wedged in his cab, and he suffers quite a blow when Johnny uses the K12 to cut the steering column to get him out. Yikes, I hope Angie has a good dental plan! But the truck is carrying dynamite (of course!), and Cap says it's better to "let it burn so it won't explode." Funny, your first instinct is that something that explodes would, well, explode when it's in a fire, but instead it sounds here more like running a hose on the dynamite is the dangerous thing. Go figure!! Ah, well, they get Angie/driver out of his cab and haul him awkwardly up the embankment. Left the K12 down there, though, so that's not good.

Finally, we learn that while they were hauling the driver up the embankment, Chet used Johnny's camera to take a picture, and the newspaper bought the picture, for $25. That's more than $100 today... definitely nothing to sneeze at. Of course, Johnny's livid when he realizes that Chet took the pic, and the episode ends with the squabbling brothers going at it again. *sigh*

* Did anyone ever read the Coffee, Tea, or Me books? They came out in the early '70s and were (supposedly) memoirs of a couple of stewardesses and their carefree sexcapades. The book's 'authors' were two stewardesses named Trudy and Rachel... the very names of the two stews in this episode. Coincidence? Not likely.

4.11 Firehouse Four

I think this one aired on Christmas Day (or maybe Christmas Eve?) so I didn't watch. Even though I can watch on Netflix at any time, I've been watching along with MeTV's schedule, and with the holiday hoopla last week, I missed a couple of episodes.

But yeah, The Firehouse Four (and Firehouse Quintet) are some of the weaker episodes, in my book. Just like Parade, I find those particular storylines silly and almost embarrassing to watch.

I do agree about Mr. Gibson's recurring catastrophes, though. He definitely wasn't as grateful as he should have been (at least at first). But it got to be kind of funny how he knew all the guys (squad and engine) by name after the second rescue. Now that I'm thinking about it, what other episodes did the guys respond to the same place/person more than once? That we *see*, I mean, not just hear about. There's the lady cooking dinner for her boyfriend.... the woman from Séance.... and this guy Gibson. Is that it?

We *hear* about other cases in which they get called out on a recurring basis: there's Edna Self, the woman who kept calling the paramedics for trivial stuff because she was lonely (and Johnny gave her the little dog); and an old lady apparently calls the fire department when her cat gets outside and won't come in. And of course Molly, the fireman's widow who kept calling the guys as if they were the local handyman service.

Are there other instances where we see them respond to the same victim more than once? I'm not counting Larry Storch, the disgusting diner owner. The first time we see him/his place, he's not the victim. (The second time, he is, though.)

~ ~ ~

Okay, let me just reiterate that this is not one of my favorite episodes. In fact, I admit I almost had to force myself to watch it this time. Maybe I lose a little patience when I know what's coming and don't particularly care for it.

At a station meeting, Cap mentions that the upcoming Fireman's Picnic is going to have a barbershop quartet competition. Everyone scoffs, Johnny most loudly. Until Cap mentions a trophy for the winner, then he's all ears. Heaven knows why a trophy would suddenly change things; is Johnny now a kitten who's easily distracted by shiny things?? Anyway, in the blink of an eye Gage suddenly wants to discuss it and talk the other guys into it. Come to find out, the only one of the group with any actual singing experience (Roy, in—of all things—a barbershop quartet) isn't interested. (Also, did I detect a hint of mustache on Mr. Gage in this scene?)

First call is for a biker over a cliff. If the general location of this rescue looks familiar it's because the nearby waterfall was the scene of a rescue in a season 2 episode. Anyway, the biker is Mr. Gibson, who is *not* happy that Johnny had to drop his expensive new bicycle, and in general is just grumpy and annoyed. He's not hurt too badly (though he does faint) and at the hospital he tells Brackett that his wife wants him to quit smoking and get some exercise, which is why he was riding the bike. Kel suggests he find a safer form of exercise. "How about jogging? On a nice, quiet, safe, level street." Yeah, we all know foreshadowing when we see it, right? *wink*

Meanwhile, Johnny's trying to get some advice from Dixie on how to get "the guys" on board with the quartet idea. (And we all see the "big wink" when he asks Dixie if she knows anything about singing, and Julie London shrugs and says, "a little.") Also at Rampart, a man brings in a woman he says overdosed on some pills. He apparently thinks the emergency department is nothing more than a convenience provider that will gladly pump the woman's stomach and send her on her way. He thinks it's all a great joke, and even laughs when he says, "whenever she tries suicide, she calls me." Yeah, that's a real hoot, buddy.

Back to Mr. Gibson… he obviously took Brackett's suggestion about jogging—sort of. Except instead of a "nice, quiet, level street," he chooses to jog in a construction zone with open excavation holes, and guess what happens? Yeah, Station 51 has to come out, get into the pit with him, and deflate his "sauna pants" so he can be pulled out. He doesn't go to Rampart this time, but he does get another piece of exercise advice, this time from the garrulous John Gage. "Why don't you take up gardening? All you need for gardening is a shovel, and you can't get in trouble with a shovel." The words are already out of his (helpful) mouth by the time he sees Roy's "stop talking!" face.

I suppose I have to mention the barbershop quartet thing again. Roy doesn't want to participate but Johnny scolds, guilts, and even shames his partner into agreeing to "coach" the others. This is a new low for Johnny, I hate to say; I really don't like him much at that moment. To make matters worse, he immediately talks about future plans for fame and stardom. That "thinking big" thing isn't new for Johnny, and that's silly and not unexpected, but not nearly as unpleasant as trying to guilt and browbeat Roy into doing something he obviously doesn't want to do. Bad Johnny!! So the guys practice once or twice and we see them playing their act using table clothes and fake mustaches, and they're not that bad, but according to Roy, they pretty much stink.

Back at Rampart, the OD woman gives the staff trouble and doesn't seem to want to get better. This is the episode (and the scene) with the infamous X-rated error when a nurse on the near side of the woman's bed steps away unexpectedly for a few seconds, giving the camera (and us) a view that we likely weren't meant to see. But, ultimately, the woman dies; her friend tells Dr. Brackett, "I never thought she'd do it," and Kel replies, "neither did she." (Yeah, it's a really uplifting storyline.)

So the final call is for a "man trapped," and at the scene a woman says her husband had an accident while building a wine cellar in the basement. She says it seemed like a good way to get exercise. (Antennae on alert!) Johnny asks her husband's name and yes, wouldn't ya know, it's Gibson. Ol' Fred got himself into some trouble and has a water heater on top of him, and water flooding the basement. Needless to say, Roy and Johnny do what needs to be done, while Cap and the guy work from topside, opening up a hole in the living room floor. Gibson's wife hands her husband a cigar and says, "Here, take up smoking again, don't get any exercise, sit in your chair where you're safe!" Well, obviously those aren't her exact words, but it's pretty much what she says. Then Fred says maybe he'll put in a swimming pool in the back yard, and in a nice meta reference, says, "Mark Spitz, eat your heart out!" (Spitz was a guest-star just a few episodes ago.)

Finally, another scene at the station lets us know that Roy's getting over a cold and he missed the fireman's picnic (very convenient), and he's stunned when Johnny tells him that they (the barbershop quintet) won a trophy. Roy's all impressed until he reads the trophy (over Johnny's objections, of course): Best Comedy Act. That pretty much sums up most of Johnny's schemes, don'tcha think??

.

4.12 Details

Thank heavens Netflix had this episode!!! Watching them on **site name deleted** was awful. I'm sure Hulu is probably better, but it takes me long enough to watch an episode as it is, without having to worry about watching %$#@ ads.

So, show of hands—who thinks that Valerie was trolling for a husband from the get-go? She made a sly remark to the driver of the car that hit her, about his wife, to see if he said "I'm not married." He didn't say that, so she switched her batting eyelashes to Johnny and um...... "Roy."

Watching EMERGENCY! Seasons 4-6

This ep was written by Mike Norell, so I'm glad to say it wasn't unreasonably derogatory toward women. Johnny seemed to be smitten with Valerie, although personally I don't think she was as beautiful as he described her. She was pretty, but he's dated (or been dumped by) better-looking women. Plus, she probably also lied about her age: 23, and has an 8- or 9- or 10-year-old kid?? (Not sure how old the "biter" was.)

Speaking of ages, was Roy just trying to be polite when he gave the "exotic" dancer's age as 35?? Even 48 might have been stretching it. But that's okay, I know day-care centers just love to hire former strippers. So many possibilities for the kids on Activity Day.

~ Did we all see Johnny's little head-shake to shake his helmet off into the cab of the squad?? Too cute! I think it was at the belly-dancer place.

~ Also, back at the station after Chet and Marco teased him about "striking out with his own wife," Johnny tossed a plate in the air, which Chet caught.

~ One of the first door-lock scenes with the squad that I recall. Johnny's rushing away from Valerie and the kids and the squad door is locked.

~ Right after that scene, Roy and John in the locker room talking, Roy mouths a line or two of Randy's lines. (I remember this being brought up before.)

~ Inside the burning building, there was some re-used footage of the guys with their equipment on. I'm not even sure what the heck they were supposed to be doing in that building to begin with. Incidentally, when they were jumping onto the Life-Net, where did their helmets and O2 tanks go?

~ Odd scenery: We see a scene of the squad passing the granary (a **commercial** area), and LA pages them for a call. As we see

May Fair

an inside-the-cab view, listening to the call, out of the passenger-side window we see lots of trees and greenery, as if they're driving past **a park** or a rural area. Then we see an external view of the squad, and they're driving down a tree-lined wo-lane **suburban street**, with houses and fences on either side. Johnny acknowledges the call with "squad 51, 10-4", and the **park** is outside his window. Then another external shot of the squad, and they're in a **commercial** area again. That's *three* different locations in about 25 seconds in what is supposedly the *same scene.*

~ ~ ~

Or, the one where Johnny thinks about getting married. In general, I do like this episode, although the topic of Johnny getting married still pushes my buttons a little. (But not out of jealousy or anything, of course!) This episode was written by Mike Norell. Also, I think I noticed some things that I hadn't noticed in previous viewings.

So, on the way to a call, Roy and Johnny witness a pedestrian get struck by a vehicle. Yeah, it was her fault, and she was a ditz, but it introduces us to Valerie. Who, by the way, does *not* look 23. I think it's kind of funny that as the engine drives off, Cap calls dispatch and requests another squad for their call, and Roy is talking to LA at the exact same time from the squad. But I like the way the guys handle the call: Johnny kind of checks each arm and leg before moving them so they can do their job, and Roy introduces himself and Johnny to her. (Although we don't usually see them do that, I don't think.) Meanwhile, Vince shows up (and he has a partner with him for a change) and takes the driver's information. Valerie is sweet as sugar to the driver, and says something along the lines of, "if your wife is ever hit by a car, I hope it's by someone as nice as you." But since the guy doesn't immediately say, "I'm not married," she loses interest right away. And later apparently decides to sue the "nice man."

Then there's the story of the man who stored gasoline next to his water heater and a person dies and his wife is badly burned in the resulting explosion and fire. It's a serious matter, and is pretty thoroughly explored.... Right up until it isn't, and the storyline disappears completely. I would have actually liked to hear a follow-up on it. Is the man charged with involuntary manslaughter or something? Does he have to go to jail?? (And I think we've seen that house before. Almost looked like the tumbleweed house, or maybe the house with the blind grandpa. Also, did anyone notice that when the ambulance is getting ready to leave, Angie the attendant closes the ambulance door and goes back around toward the front; Johnny reopens and recloses the ambulance door. Wonder what that was about???)

Speaking of our resident Romeo, has he seen Nurse Juanita? I thought she was every bit as pretty as Valerie... and much more Johnny's type.

At the station, when Johnny's talking about Valerie and that he's serious about her, etc., Marco teases that Johnny has "those veins popping out of his forehead when he's 'really in love.'" Uh, Marco, the veins that pop when Johnny's in love are *not* in his forehead, ifyouknowwhatImean. *wink* Oh, and there's a mention of someone named Barbara, with whom he was madly in love just a few scant weeks ago. Proof that Johnny tends to think he's in love relatively often. (And of course he pronounces women "incredible" on practically a daily basis.) But the whole notion of him marrying Valerie is sketchy from the get-go. First he talks to Roy about how nice it must be to come home to a warm, loving family atmosphere, not to mention a home-cooked meal. (Don't get me started on *those* as reasons to get married!) But, after knowing her for only two or three days, he tells the guys "I'm thinking of getting married." Not one minute later Cap comes around and Johnny says, "I'm getting married." Is it odd that he goes from "*thinking* about getting married" straight to "*getting* married" in about thirty seconds?? Seems to me that being engaged is like being pregnant—you either are or you aren't. A woman doesn't announce a pregnancy when she's only "thinking about" having a baby, and once she's actually pregnant, she doesn't say she's "thinking about it." It's only semantics, I know, but in this particular context it almost seems like Johnny is looking for the shock value of his statement more than anything else.

In the end, it doesn't matter, as Valerie found a better provider—er, rather a better prospect—than Johnny. Lawyer trumps firefighter any day in the paycheck department, I guess. And no way is she 23 if her oldest kid (!!!) is about nine years old.

The call at the restaurant with the belly dancer is good. I wonder if Chet ever goes back to see Big Red? He couldn't go that same evening, since he was on duty, but it would have been nice to hear a follow-up on that, as well. Anyway, I noticed the paramedics report to Rampart that the woman is showing normal sinus rhythm. I guess they hooked her up to the scope, but we don't see that, do we? And in addition to Drs. Early and Brackett being the only doctors at Rampart, they're apparently in charge of *everything* there as well, including who gets hired in the day-care center. Dixie tells the dancer she could put in a good word with them for a recommendation for Ginger to work in the daycare center. You know, because all parents want former strippers teaching their kids, right??

I also like the last call, the structure fire that eventually flashes. But I admit to being stumped on this one. We see John and Roy go into the building, to the third floor, with a hose, per Cap's orders. But as soon as they get to the stairwell, the hose runs out (not long enough to go further?), so they just... drop it on the floor and leave it. Does that make *any* sense at all?? (I think we also see this same scene in a different episode, as well.) Then a moment later, they're upstairs (and hmmm, I see a rope already up there, too) and Johnny says "Hmm, this place might flash." So they immediately go out on the window ledge, and voila! there are explosions conveniently placed in two of the windows. (Thanks for warning the guys on the other floors, by the way.) Once the explosions happened, why don't they just go back inside the building?? I realize there might be fires inside, but that's nothing new and doesn't mean they wouldn't have any way to get out—at least, ways that are worse than having to jump. I think the situation is really just an excuse to show us the life-net. Which nobody had ever used, apparently. Seriously, though, wouldn't you think they'd practice and train on those things???

P.S.:

~ One of the FFs from Station 98 slips and almost falls when he was running to grab some hose.

~ Roy and Johnny both left their helmets up in the building.

* * *

Somewhere I read an interesting point about this episode. Johnny had spent time with Valerie over three days and was head-over-heels for her (ha!)... until he found out she had kids. Not only did he not know *that*, but, until the call for the dog-bite to the boy (and the boy-bite to the dog), he also didn't know where she lived. Maybe she drove to meet him for their date(s), or went to his place, because after all, she couldn't have him see/meet her kids. Unless that house we see for the dog-bite call was the home of a friend or relative where the kids stayed during the day.

Anyway, I thought that was an interesting point.

4.13 Parade

Another episode that doesn't do a lot for me.

May Fair

~ Johnny's owie. Did we all see his forehead boo-boo? I think the Exalted Book tells the story of how that happened, and that Randy "hit the wall" and got the nickname Crash. And of course his cut had to be written into the script. His neck looks a little red, also, but that could just be bad lighting or something.

~ That heart-victim guy in the parking lot at the Italian restaurant... what a head of hair on him! Also, Roy didn't get him to sign the waiver that people who refuse treatment have to sign.

~ The driver of the car he hit, I don't think Early ordered an IV for her. All he said was "keep her head and neck immobilized and bring her in." Not even the usual D5W-TKO.

~ The guy who came in and had a "hypertensive crisis"... where'd he get a robe so quickly?

~ Behind the station, we see leggy Johnny arrive with his aviator glasses. **(Yum!)** And then Roy comes in (driving a Chevy truck) looking just as hunky (although I think he could use a visit from the "wear this, not that" people).

~ At the final fire, I think Roy should have slugged the guy who pushed him away and climbed up the ladder without being tied off. Yeah, I know, Roy would never do that, but he should have at least threatened to bring him up on assault charges, just so the guy was clear about how stupid he was.

~ All sorts of continuity errors in that final set of scenes... the fire was apparently extinguished in record time, by the time Cap and Chet got to the roof. ... When Roy and Johnny got back to their engine, the street was dry, not to mention empty. Did all the other fire personnel leave already? Engine 36, engine 19, and truck 8, they couldn't have *all* left so quickly ... The brick of the building fell apart—right into the middle of the street, where the engine was. Riiiiight. (First of all, I'm sure Roy would've known better than to park in the middle of the street, with all the other trucks and engines that would be responding. Second of all, brick doesn't jump when it falls; it just falls.)

~ ~ ~

Believe it or not, I don't care for this episode all that much. Mainly the day of the actual parade, with Roy and Johnny dressed in the old-timey uniforms and riding the old engine around. To me it's all just too silly. (Yeah, go ahead, call me a fuddy-duddy.) Plus the inconsistencies at that fire they responded to and stuff that happened there—totally unrealistic and unbelievable.

I do like some parts of the episode, though, like the guy at the pizza place who refuses treatment and then causes an accident and dies. I like that one. But I have to admit, the woman whose car he hit, after the guys inflate that thing around her neck and tape her head down, it still doesn't look like the woman's head/neck is either straight or immobilized. So, good job there. Also, Johnny tells Rampart the ambulance hasn't arrived yet, but we very distinctly hear a siren as they're putting that neck brace thing on. I guess it could have been the cops arriving, but we never see any cops at the scene. So either way, it's odd that we hear it and not see it. (In real life it wouldn't be odd, but on a TV show it is.)

And I like the guy who, it turns out, was going to slip his date the 1974 version of Rohypnol... or, as they say in the movies, slip her a Mickey. That was interesting. And disappointing for the girl he had dinner with. And yet funny, since he got the drug himself. Dude, meet Karma (and you know what they say about Karma).

At Rampart, Mr. Carmody is interesting, how one minute he has a terrible headache, then it disappears and he's feeling 'better,' and then suddenly he has a seizure. But when we see him in the treatment room a while later, he's wearing a..... (wait for it!)...

a *robe*. Not even a simple hospital gown, but an actual robe. I didn't think that much time had passed, and he *was* still in the treatment room, so where did he get a dang robe?

There was a nurse Sally in this episode. Did we determine that Sally is the female equivalent of Charlie?

* * *

I too noticed that the guys didn't get the pizza parlor heart-attack-waiting-to-happen guy to sign the waiver refusing treatment. Maybe Roy figured the guy was already upset enough so he didn't press it. And if push came to shove, the lady from the restaurant could be their witness that they attempted to treat him. Legally, probably not as good as a signed waiver, but I think it would work. And she wasn't related to the man, so that would probably be more reliable than relying on a spouse or girl/boyfriend as a witness.

4.14 The Bash

~ I wonder if they even had to do any "prep" work for that scene at the studio, with the bear. Who knows, the interior of one of the houses where Squad 51 has answered a call might have been in that very building!

~ For the "Stuff Left Behind" file… Roy left the drug box behind as he and Johnny tried to get "Batman" out of the soundstage (or whatever it's called).

~ If that's a pack of smokes that Randy keeps in his uniform shirt pocket (and I used to think it was a mic-pack; silly me!), then he must have been smoking pretty heavily during this time period, as the pack is visible in most of his on-duty scenes in this episode.

~ I'd be curious to know what Randy and Kevin thought about the "bash" storyline. They weren't huge stars (not on the level of, say, Burt Reynolds or Lee Majors or Peter Falk, etc.), but they were well known. I wonder if they actually went to parties like that. (Hopefully any actual Hollywood parties they went to would be more interesting, though, y'know?)

~ Sometimes I think the writers go out of their way to make Roy look like a doofus. Who doesn't know how to pronounce "soiree"? I can probably understand the 'creative' pronunciation of beef bourguignon, but really... soiree?? Usually they hint toward him being sort of a nerd/intellectual—always reading, not wanting firefighters to be depicted as simply gung-ho thrill-seekers, etc. (In his locker in later seasons is a poster for some art or literary magazine... a *French* art or literary magazine; that's not a typical pin-up for a doofus.)

~ The editor or whoever puts these eps together made a crazy boo-boo. While Johnny and Roy are in the *locker room* talking about "the bash," the tones go off. A piece of stock footage is used to show the guys responding, and we see all the guys—*including* Roy and Johnny—come out of the *day-room.* And Johnny's hair is significantly shorter than it had been just a second ago. (The footage must have been from early season 3, because the Ward-LaFrance was there, and Chet had his mustache. Not sure about Marco, though.)

~ Was it just me, or did Monique Morris look like Geena Davis?? Even more so since Monique wasn't a dumb ditz, and Geena is a member of Mensa.

* * *

Re Johnny's "object" in pocket... I have a hard time thinking that anyone would be carrying a pack of cigarettes in their costume during filming, no matter how much they smoked, especially as the set was surely loaded with smokers and cigarettes anyhow.

This is why for a long time I was *sure* it must be a mic-pack... after all, it's easy enough to keep ciggies nearby, and the producer or wardrobe/continuity people wouldn't allow an actor to have something on him that the character wouldn't have, right?? I even tried to convince other people that it wasn't cigarettes. But then I noticed that he even had the "thing" in his pocket in scenes on a closed set (like this ep), where mic-packs weren't needed. And someone pointed out an instance (can't remember which ep) in which the brand logo was barely visible through his shirt pocket... might have been Vantage, with the concentric circles like a bulls-eye. In any case, I still feel (and I feel bad for saying it, even though it's true), but I find it unprofessional for an actor to constantly have on him a personal object, that takes him "out of character." If the character doesn't have it on him, the actor shouldn't either.

~ ~ ~

I agree, this is not the best episode either. This season seems to have a number of mediocre-at-best episodes clumped more or less together. Luckily, each episode usually has at least one rescue in it that sort of saves the day.

In any case, every time I see The Bash I always end up asking, "Why does Roy *ever* listen to Johnny??" I'm thinking mainly about the tuxedo business, but that same question can apply in so many other circumstances, too, amIright??. Among other issues I find silly: I find it hard to believe that Joanne would not be interested in going to a "thing" or bash or whatever, and also that little scene in which Roy butchers the word "soiree." Roy must be schizophrenic, as sometimes he comes across as being serious and well-educated, and other times they write him as some sort of simple country bumpkin. I would like to think that most 30-something-year-olds would know how to pronounce soiree.

Back to the episode.... The opening scene is interesting. Not only is it not at the station, which is odd in itself, but we have an unusual angle/view of the squad. Then dispatch calls and they get sent to another call. I do like the rescue at the movie lot. Kind of funny on a number of different levels. For one thing, Roy leaves his helmet in the soundstage; in fact, I'm kind of surprised he wore it in there to begin with, as he usually gets rid of it upon arrival unless it's a dangerous rescue. Also, the drug box gets left behind too. (Next time we see Charlene the bear, she's drugged up and wearing the helmet, looking for a pole to slide down.) Also, it's too funny when Johnny's in the studio while they're looking for the victim, and he's trying to whisper, "Roy? Roy?" And then he jumps when Roy opens a door nearby; does Johnny really think bears can open doors?? I wonder how many scenes from this show were filmed in that same soundstage... maybe one of those living rooms they passed through were ones we've seen before.

The trichinosis thing at Rampart is kind of interesting. Maybe a little too much like the botulism storyline, though. By the way, in the past we've heard them mention St. Francis hospital before, but in this episode Brackett says someone was taken to St. David's. Was or is there a St. David's hospital in LA County? Never heard it mentioned before on this show. Anyway, the health department guy says that one victim has been "a big help" in their investigation. Never mind the fact that the whole outbreak is that man's fault to begin with!

The 'rescue' of the guy holed up in his house is a little hokey. This is another scene that was similar to another one, in this case similar to the sniper in the abandoned building. This guy has guns and hostages and explosives, etc., but mainly I think the house (in real life) was probably scheduled for demolition so the Powers That Be just found a way to fit it into a script and blow it up. But what I find silly is that there are police officers flitting around in a disorganized fashion and there seems to be only two SWAT members (yay, Angie!) on the scene, and, what's worse still, nobody seems to really be in charge. And then after the house blows up, you know the cops wouldn't let too many people inside (firefighters or not) before they clear the place of further guns and/or explosives. That was just shoddy police work.

Now, the bash. I don't like their tuxedo bow-ties. They're too big or something; I can't put my finger on what was wrong with them, I just don't like them (yeah, I realize they were stylish at the time, so I shouldn't judge by today's standards). Anyway, when they first arrive at the man's house, it's funny to see Roy sort of hiding behind the front gate of the house like he doesn't want to go in. But once he's there, he wises up and heads straight for the bar. Who can blame him?? Also funny how Monique Morris says "here, sit down"... and Roy sits down next to her before Johnny could. Something about that actress always reminds me of someone else, can't put my finger on exactly who, though. She does look a little like Geena Davis, but there's someone else she reminds me of, too, though for the life of me I don't know who.

Anyway, this isn't one of the most stellar episodes in the lineup

4.15 Transition

I had a hard time with the first rescue. The wife was talking about sulfuric acid and caustic soda crystals.... when it comes to stuff I have in my house, I wouldn't want anything with the words "acid" or "caustic" in the name, much less would I combine the two. But apparently that's what people did to unclog their sinks before Drano and Mr. Plumber came along.

Watching EMERGENCY! Seasons 4-6

Anyway, that might have been obvious in 1975, but she didn't explain why they were using two nasty-sounding ingredients, so I had no clue. *Then,* this was all made worse by the fact that I couldn't tell what the heck was going on in the kitchen... couldn't see a thing most of the time.

When John and Roy and Gil were helping the doctors (who were conveniently all in the same treatment room), is that the first time we ever see (and hear) Johnny doing the "countdown" (or actually "count-up") for defib? I honestly don't recall seeing him do it before, but he could have.

This must have been "film for free at Beach Ave Amusement Park" day. Two calls there at Queen's Park in the same episode (though not on the same "day" on the show)... can't be a coincidence.

Continuity alert: on the first call they go on with Gil, when the squad is pulling out of the station, we see that the old Crown engine is in the bay, and not the Ward-LaFrance. (oopsie!!)

In the final scene at Rampart, after the amusement park, when J and R are there, and Gil, etc., and the little heart-tugging transplant patient kid is being checked out.... they get a call on the Handy-Talkie. "Man down... time out 1:05." Um, Sam, I think you mean 13:05, right?? I really doubt it was 1:00 in the morning when that kid was being discharged, especially since it was broad daylight outside.

~ ~ ~

Or, "The One With the Trainee who Went to High School with Johnny." In the capability and likability spectrum for paramedic trainees, Gil falls somewhere in the middle, or actually a little more toward likable/capable. Sort of. Ever notice that they never have a trainee who's just a normal, average person? They always lack either likability (Marlow, Karen), competence (also Karen, and maybe Gil), or confidence (Gil and Billy).

May Fair

Anyway, I remember this being mentioned last time around, but right after Cap tells John and Roy they'd be getting a new trainee, Cap walks away, but it looks like Roy wants to ask him something. I wonder what that was all about?

The first call is to some sort of chemical reaction and sink malfunction in a house. These crazy kids with their sulfuric acid and caustic soda.... how many times do we have to tell them not to mix acid and soda?? Worse than diet Coke and Mentos. But I like that rescue, even though it's kind of hard to see what's what in that smoky, fume-y kitchen. When they get the victim outside on the porch, Roy calls Rampart and tells Joe Early the guy's pulse and respiration... even though I don't think he ever checked either one. And later we see Johnny check out another nurse at Rampart. Randy must have liked playing that part of his character, as I bet that wasn't in the script.

Last week we had a kid named Harold, and now in this episode is a boy named Larry. Probably not that unusual for a kid to be named Lawrence, but I always associate the name Larry (and Harold too) with an adult, not a little kid.

When we meet Gil, does anyone else get the impression that the casting director for this show (or maybe it's the PTB at LACoFD) had a definite "type"? Gil looks like Dwyer who looks like some of the 'real' firefighters I've seen on this show, right down to the side-parted hair and mustache.

Speaking of Gil, I like the rescue with the cobra. He doesn't hesitate taking care of Roy and his baby blues, and even though he doesn't check the other victim in the room, he makes an assumption based on available information and looks for a snakebite. The fact that he didn't find one doesn't mean it wasn't the right thing to do. And he was very clever to use that glass ashtray as a shield to protect his own eyes from snake venom. (Lastly, that scene gives Johnny the chance to say again those famous words: "What the hell happened?")

This being a "trainee" episode, we get to see Senior Paramedic Roy and his patented pep-talk/chat, complete with the always-comforting statement that "If you haven't got it, we'll let you know."

The amusement park rescue is a good one. Kind of complicated, but good. All in all, I like this episode, even with the shmaltzy ending with Gil and Larry and then Larry and Dixie. That scene is so full of saccharine that it gives me a toothache.

* * *

I forgot to mention that at the first rescue, at the poison kitchen, Marco got some stuff on his hands, under his gloves. Roy checked him out while they were in the house, but later on they just forgot about him. He should have at least had his hands rinsed off, like the wife did. Poor guy, he was sitting there with two paramedics, and they didn't even remember that their 'brother' might have sustained an injury, even if it was minor.

4.16 Smoke-Eater

I so totally agree about wearing safety equipment and other processes or policies that are meant to keep FFs safe. I certainly hope that in this day and age, people (firefighters and civilians) accept these practices as a matter of course, and don't think they're for "sissies." To paraphrase the title of an Adam-12 episode, "A dead firefighter can't help anyone."

Other than that... I definitely noticed a couple of stock shots of the squad leaving the station, with old footage (based on

Johnny's hair length). Also, the old Crown engine is visible when Roy is backing the squad in toward the end.

~ The wife of the heart attack patient is an actress we've seen before in a number of episodes. And yes, I agree that she seemed the "right amount" of upset: not hysterical, and not repeating the same stupid line over and over. ("My boy! My boy!")

~ I wonder what the other FFs do in those cases when they're not needed inside. Stoker probably kept a book under his seat in the engine, since he's left behind so often, so maybe he was reading aloud to Marco and Chet until Cap called for them.

~ Apparently, in Emergency-land, salt = ketchup. During the lunch scene Chet asks for salt, Marco hands him the red stuff. And Chet uses it!! Talk about not breaking character.

~ Don'tcha just love when Roy Gets Righteous?? We all love Johnny, and we know he always flares up quickly, but Roy's not like that. Takes a lot to get our senior paramedic going, but when he gets there—watch out. (He wasn't really angry here, though, as he was talking to a Captain; gotta watch the job security!) Kevin was born and raised in California, but it's so funny how he has the Brooklyn-style accent on his short "a" sounds: "all," for example.

~ One of their calls was on Willis Ave. My sister and bro-in-law live on Willis Ave. Not in LA County, of course, but it's still odd to hear the street named on national TV.

~ Can't believe Dixie tolerated "Spike" calling one of her nurses a broad. Now, in real life, I'm sure Julie wouldn't have a problem calling herself a broad, but Dixie wouldn't tolerate it.

~ In the final fire, it was funny when that man hiding in his lab said "I'm afraid of fire," and the Captain said "so am I." Ha!

~ When we see Roy carrying the woman out of the building, you can see Johnny coming out behind him with the captain. But then a second later they show Johnny from another angle exiting the building again.

~ Speaking of that last call, Roy and John are in the Captain's office when the alarm sounds. The clock there is easily visible and says 6:30. But a moment later when the call comes in, the "time out" is 16:05 (4:05).

* * *

> I don't know why they put wall clocks on the set. We'd never notice if they weren't there.

I agree about the clocks. If you're gonna insist on having them on the set, be sure they match the time involved!! (Although I'd bet $100 that nobody on set knew which rescue was gonna be called next, or what time Sam was going to use for it. I'm not even sure the actors 'hear' the tones and call-out at the time of filming.)

~ ~ ~

In a way this could be considered a variation of an "issues episode," as Roy and Johnny have to deal with doubts and skepticism about their profession and their skills. Bad enough when they get that attitude from the general public, but this time it comes from someone within their own department. Ouch!

So Captain Roberts is filling in for Cap for a day or three (??). Apparently he's somewhat of a legend, going back to some big fire a few years ago, but he's also part of—get this—a two-man station. I know that a captain is a captain, but being captain at a two-man station has got to be weird, you know? In any case, it's obvious pretty early on that this guy is an old-school hard-a$s. So old-school, in fact, that he scoffs at how firefighters "nowadays" rely on their air masks and safety equipment.

May Fair

Apparently "he-men firefighters no need new-fangled sissy equipment. *grunt*"

Meanwhile, at Rampart, Joe Early is playing apples-and-oranges with the vending machine in the coffee room. I think most of us can relate to something along those lines: you choose one thing and get another. But it is funny and of course Dixie comes out smelling like a rose. Or, an apple, as the case may be. (I wonder, though: is this the scene in which she got pranked in the blooper reel??)

The next call is a possible cardiac case, and even though it's a squad call, Captain Roberts decides the engine will go along for the ride. (He wants to watch the paramedics in action, even though he apparently already has his mind made up about them—and it ain't a positive opinion.) It's just as well the engine does tag along, as Roy and Johnny can definitely use another set (or sets) of hands on this one. The victim goes into cardiac arrest, and it's 'all hands on deck' as our boys work on him with everything in their arsenal. In the end, defibbing doesn't work, so it's manual CPR all the way to Rampart. The final glimpse of the scene is very telling, with debris from the rescue scattered all over the floor. Usually the guys try to clean up after themselves, but this time their attention was focused elsewhere.

After getting the victim to Rampart, and losing him there, even though everyone worked on him for over an hour, Johnny and Roy go back to the station while the others are eating lunch. The guys express their condolences that the guy didn't make it, and Cap Roberts makes some comments that rub Roy and Johnny the wrong way. On one hand, the Captain was right: there was nothing else to be done, under the circumstances. I guess it must have been the "under the circumstances" part that sets Johnny (and Roy) off, and Johnny asks Cap exactly what he means. This is where the Cap says he doesn't think the FD should be in the paramedic business, which is simply his opinion, to which he's entitled. He also says "you guys aren't doctors; nobody expects any more out of you." Also true. Then he says, "It's not your fault." Again, true. So on one hand, we know he doesn't approve of the paramedic program, but on the other hand, he doesn't hold the guys responsible for the man dying. He does ask if they could tell him, "flat out," if, had the man gone directly to the hospital right away, he would still have died. And of course Roy has to say "No"; they can't tell him that. Which is probably a question Roy and Johnny ask themselves on a regular basis, I'd bet. But the Cap does step in it and show his disdain when he says, "What is it these guys are supposedly so good at? Because I haven't seen it yet." (Oooh, burn! Yeah, that had to hurt!!)

There *is* one funny bit in this scene: Chet asks Marco to pass the salt, and Marco hands him the ketchup. So Chet just uses the ketchup as if that's what he wanted all along. Way to not break the scene, Tim! Also, Roy does his Staten Island impression when he says "It's not okay... it's not okay at awwwl."

Later there is another rescue, of a young boy stuck under a fence and suffering severe asthma. Of course the guys from Station 51 get the boy out, and Roy and Johnny are treating him for his issues. They're about to administer some epi when Cap says they should take him directly to the hospital. They just look at him for a minute and it almost seems as if they're debating whether to do what he asks, but instead they finally go about their business, making the boy feel much better almost immediately. I would have liked for Roy to tell him, "We don't answer to you. On medical calls we answer to the doctors at Rampart, and we're going to do exactly what they prescribe." Come on, Roy, next time I watch this episode, that's definitely what you should say!

(Interestingly, when they're treating the asthmatic boy, we see Dr. Early OK the epinephrine that Roy suggests, but Early's words don't match what we see his mouth saying. It *looks* like he's saying to administer it IV or intravenously (?), but what we *hear* is him telling them to administer it IM.)

Once back at the station, Captain Roberts seems like he might be thawing. He asks Roy and Johnny to come into the office, and they just sigh and shrug in resignation. But Cap doesn't harangue them again or belittle their job; instead he asks about epinephrine and how it works, etc. Definitely a good sign. But the tones sound right in the middle of Roy's explanation.

At Rampart, a guy named Spike—big dude with a bad wig—comes in and asks for a bandage. He gets nasty with a nurse and Dixie springs into action. (She should have told him, "don't talk to my nurses that way." I'm surprised she doesn't.) When Dixie tries to explain to Spike that he needs stitches, Spike takes exception to that and raises his voice. This catches Brackett's attention as he's passing by and he goes in to investigate. Spike swings at Brackett and knocks him down, and you can tell that Kelly Brackett is just spoiling for a good bout, and I think he enjoys it when he decks Spike without a problem. Luckily the guy's wig doesn't fall off (that we can see), but Spike seems to have gotten the message. And I bet Robert Fuller enjoyed being able to let his inner cowboy come out for a change.

The last call of the episode is a structure fire to a building where—surprise!—there are dangerous chemicals in the building. And of course—double surprise!—there are people stuck in there somewhere. Although our guys don't know it for sure when they arrive. Anyway, Captain Roberts does his "smoke eater" thing and runs into the building without an air mask as he looks for people in the building, and of course by the time he finds a fallen victim, he ends up passed out due to the fumes. Roy finds them and takes the scientist out of the building while Johnny gets to carry the Cap. And of course they have to treat him as well as the other victim and this time

Cap really sees the paramedics in action, up close as well as first-hand. As a result, back at the station later he shows an interest, a *real* interest, in the squad and the equipment it carries, and you can tell that Johnny and Roy are more than happy to show him how it all works.

When responding to that last fire, it looks like they're driving in a commercial area, but when they bring out the victims, it looks more like an office park area. Also, the engine rolls in first, ahead of the squad. That doesn't happen very often.

4.17 Kidding

Re the soldier with PTSD... the actress who played his wife was in a bunch of things during the '70s. She'd been in a number of Happy Days episodes, as Richie's girlfriend, I think, and also had a role in the original Battlestar Galactica. She also was in a couple other E! episodes.

I think it's funny how this ep opened with the guy thinking about opening a "hamburger stand" down the street, but we never hear anything more about that, in this ep or any other. But I guess that's how things go in real life, so... whaddaya gonna do?? (And when was the last time you heard the phrase "hamburger stand"?? Kind of reminds me of a shack at the beach, literally, a wooden stand where bad burgers are sold to hungry swimmers and surfers.

~ Johnny says "I remember when I was 10 years old. I wasn't very smart." Chet's reply: "You're not very smart now." Hahaha! If that scene had been written today, Johnny would have said, "Man, I walked right into that one."

~ The hallucinating soldier: Roy was on the right track, by pretending to 'surrender' to him. But I wonder why it didn't occur to him to take the illusion farther. Roy could have said "Private, I'm Lt. DeSoto, and I'm giving you an order to release that woman." Or something along those lines. (Hey, it worked in an old episode of Hawaii Five-O.) And we never heard anyone say "Vietnam." We've heard references to "the war," or "overseas," etc., but other than that one episode with the trainee, the word Vietnam has never been mentioned... every reference to that years-long boondoggle has been very vague.

~ Johnny got a little overeager with the soldier's wife. If I had a quarter for every time he said "Come on" to her, I could take all of us and all of station 51 to that hamburger stand for dinner.

~ Still on the subject of the soldier... I wonder why nobody mentioned the VA hospital, or getting his records from the military? I would think his medical records would be pretty thorough while he'd been serving, so they could at least rule out some stuff. Also, someone may have already mentioned this, but I love watching Joe Early examine someone's eyes. I love how close he gets, which is very realistic, as I recall. But geez, talk about getting in someone's face....

~ The wife... she may be pretty, but she's also kind of stupid. She's just been told that surgery is her husband's "only chance" to live, and she says.... "I have to think." Um, what?? Whiskey tango foxtrot, woman!! What's there to think about? Surgery = husband probably lives. No surgery = husband will die. Yeah, lady, take all the time you need. And then... and then, she turns to Dixie and says, "You understand how I feel. You're a woman." !!! Oh, major barf!! Seriously, *is it just me???* WTF does being a woman have to do with anything?? Is she worried about making a "big decision" on her own because she's just a helpless female and she's incapable of it? If I didn't know better, I'd have thought she was just stalling and waiting for the situation to solve itself.

deep breath Okay, rant over. Whew!

~ Why did Roy kick the door down in the garage? It took him a few tries. By that time they could have gotten a pry-bar and forced the thing open.

~ I love the bus rescue. When they first get to the airfield, as the engine passes we see the photographer's arm or something on the screen. Later, when they're getting the "dead" pilot out of the plane, he miraculously moves his foot to give them a heavenly assist in their efforts. Lastly, I thought Roy, John, and the other captain were the only ones in the bus with the driver. But when they were all climbing out (once Chet said it was gonna blow), it was like a friggin' clown car, as firefighters just kept climbing out one after another.

~ ~ ~

There's a lot to like about this episode, so I have to say I mostly like it. Or maybe I like most of it. Either way, it gets a passing grade from me. The thing I do not like about it is probably obvious and I'm sure I'm not the only one: once again, Johnny is made out to be an idiot—in this case for totally underestimating 10-11 year old kids. I'm aware that Randy had no problem playing his character for laughs at times (obviously never while Johnny was 'on the job,' though), but many of us who appreciate the show *do* have a problem with the way the some writers purposely (and repeatedly) make him look like a fool. I know from comments on this forum that I'm not the only one who feels that way. (Right? *Right??*) Anyway, on with the show....

I'm not sure why there was the scene with the man who was thinking about opening a hamburger stand "down the street." I guess it was just one of those random scenes of things that happen at the station from time to time, like when those little kids came in because they lost their handcuff key, and Johnny scared the #$%& out of them by getting out the K-12. (Cute scene!) But in that case, the scene came to a natural conclusion (with a pair of pliers) and everyone went home happy. In *this* case, though, there was still an open-ended question that was left hanging: would the guy open the burger joint, and would it be successful?

Then Chet lets the guys know that coffee was on. I don't recall there ever being a general announcement about coffee before, but hey, Chet can be kind of weird sometimes. Also, this gave us two examples of Johnny (Randy) doing something he does quite often: repeat himself. When Chet repeats his announcement more insistently, Johnny says, "we heard you, we heard you!" Chet replies like a fishwife that the guys never acknowledge him and Johnny does it again: "We're acknowledging, we're acknowledging." As we all know, there are numerous other examples of Johnny repeating a line like that.

Speaking of Johnny and Chet (always a lively combination), Johnny asks how old fifth-graders are. He's told they're about ten, and, after Roy suggests that kids are pretty smart, Johnny snorts and says "When I was ten, I wasn't very smart." And of course Chet can't let that pass, so he brings it home: "You're not very smart now." Yeah, Gage, you did walk right into that one.

I do like the first rescue, of the military vet and his hallucination. I think they handle it quite well, for the most part. I do think that Johnny is not only invading the wife's personal space—he looms over her, more or less holding her in place with his hand on her shoulder, as she sits on the bumper of the squad—but he also talks to her like *she's* one of the fifth-graders. But, I totally get that she was on the verge of hysteria and he's trying to talk sense into her so she doesn't inadvertently make things worse, so I give him a pass on that for the most part. Also, I'd have liked to hear Roy talk to the guy, soldier to soldier, like ask his rank, give him an order to stand down, etc. It would have been natural for another military vet to do something like that and would have been interesting to see; after all, these guys are supposed to be able to improvise when necessary, right?? Additionally, this is another instance of the writers finding a medical excuse for someone who has behaved badly. We've seen it with the woman who hit her kid and turns out she'd hit her head a few months ago and that caused some sort of injury to her brain, blah-blah-blah. Now we have a guy who gone nuts and is threatening people, and he has a tumor that needs to be removed. I guess they didn't want to have the pretty military wife be told, "We're sorry, your husband is simply crazy."

And that brings me to the topic that I know we discussed last time. Twenty lashes with an inch-and-a-half to the writer of this episode. Brackett and Early tell the wife about the tumor and say that if her husband is going to have *any* chance of recovery, they need her to sign off on the surgery, immediately. So what does she say? "I need time to think." Whiskey tango foxtrot!! What's to think about?? Surgery = chance of success and healing. No surgery = hubby plays Private Crazy-Pants in the insane clown posse. Then the woman looks at Dixie and says, "You're a woman, you can understand how I feel." If I were Dixie I'd say, "what does being a woman have to do with it?? You're an adult, and your spouse needs immediate surgery. Put on your big-girl pants and sign the d@mn paper." Sheesh, that scene really burns my incense.

Next is the lady stuck in the doggie-door, and while this isn't a serious rescue, it isn't as silly a scene as some others we've seen (like the clowns-on-ice call). I thought the guys were polite and professional throughout that situation, so it was OK.

I was thinking today that in a way it's a little unusual that this show has dealt with a number of attempted suicides. Obviously those things do happen and the calls are based on real incidents, but for a show that can't bring itself to show realistic blood in instances in which blood would be expected, and seems to be sensible about the "family" aspect of the show and the young viewers, it has a surprising number of mentions of *suicide* or *kill myself*, etc. Anyway, I do like the rescue of the novelist who tried to off himself. It's touching (though, again, unrealistic) that the kids at the hospital know him and have read his books. However, glitch alert: at the scene of the rescue, when Roy goes to get the biophone and other equipment, Johnny and Cap are with the victim, and there's some sort of low-voiced exchange. Cap says something indistinct and then "don't need to." To which Johnny replies "yeah, you do." I wonder what that was all about?? Related to the rescue, or just a remark about the acting or props or set?

And I think it's funny that at the hospital the writer, Maxwell Hart, refers to Joe Early as "that young doctor." Too cute!

So we see Johnny with his six smart kids as he gives them bubble-gum and balloons. (Apparently they don't want either, as Johnny later distributes them to the guys at the station—who, ironically, *do* want them.) Anyway, of the six kids....*four* of them have red hair. Considering the fact that only about 5% or 6% of Americans are redheads, I find the two-thirds number quite mystifying.

In the next scene, Dixie and Mr. Hart are in the elevator, and it sounds like he's being taken to Psychiatric, as he asks her what he should tell the doctor. They start off on the 4th floor, at least, and end up on the 1st floor. This is mystifying as well, since, as far as I know, the emergency department is on the first floor, so they should have been going *from* there, not *to* there.

After these events of the afternoon, Roy beats Johnny at chess (big surprise) and there's a call for a plane in trouble. The airfield looks like the same one from the rescue where Roy talks the boy through landing the plane when his father's sick, and the plane looks a little like it could have been "Charter 220." In any case, I do like this rescue. It's busy, it's complicated, and it ends up being dangerous. We do see the "dead" pilot move his leg to assist in his own extrication, but otherwise it's a good rescue all the way around. I always like how, when a fire is going to explode, the FFs drop their hoses and run, but as soon as the explosion goes up, they automatically run back and pick up their hoses again and go on about their business. Now *that's* a hero.

4.18 Prestidigitation

First off, a severe frowny-face for Roy's hair. Looks like he got his bangs cut and someone got a little too snip-happy.

Okay, on to new business...

~ Saw a number of stock shots, which I'll enumerate in the appropriate thread. (But at least they're getting their money's worth out of them.)

~ Ever notice how Johnny seems to repeat himself quite a bit? I wonder if that's in the script, or if it's just Randy getting into character. "I'm working on it, I'm working on it!" Etc.

~ The skier with (now) two broken legs... I had to freeze the scene of his head-board and all the books on there. They're obviously real books, and the ones I could actually read were published in the '60s. The Piano Sport, Another Helen, Big John's Secret (which was republished in 2010)... and I think one was called simply Move, although I couldn't find out anything about it. Wonder if they were bought wholesale for the prop department. *Fun fact: there were two copies of the book The Piano Sport.*

~ In the final rescue, with the gas-fueled fire-jet, I know Cap was trying to knock down the fire enough for him and Roy to get close with the "dry powder." But I'd think that a more concentrated jet from the hoses would have been better than the wide spray they were using. Just a thought.

~ Also, I found it ironic that, at the same scene, Johnny did all that work in using the Jaws to try to extricate the woman from the car. And just when he's about done Roy shows up and helps her get out.

~ Similarly (or should I say parallel-y) Johnny spends all that time with the "magic globe" with few results, and Roy picks it up and... *voila,* it comes apart for him. Not sure exactly what that says, but... maybe John should take note.

~ ~ ~

Before I watched this episode today, I was thinking I was going to have to start off my comments with "not one of my favorite episodes," but actually for the most part I don't mind this one. It's not as exciting or interesting as some others, but it's still pretty good. However, like yesterday's Kidding episode, I don't care for the running theme indicated by the title. The whole "secret sphere" thing is a little much, and of course it's a Gage Obsession, so right there it falls down the list for me. Luckily they don't make Johnny into a doofus or a complete idiot, but still, an obsession is an obsession. How many times can the writers go to that particular well? (Obviously, quite a lot.)

The guys are grousing about an aborted rescue for a "man trapped under a house with an alligator." That does sound intriguing, but if the call was cancelled I guess it's safe to say the man got out on his own. Either that or the gator ate him and solved the problem that way. But I have to wonder: why is there an alligator in California? Unless maybe it was a pet gone rogue, as I don't think they're native to the Golden State.

The "rescue" of Lorenzo the Magnificent is good, especially watching Johnny up on the crane. By this point I'm sure TPTB knew to not even ask Kevin if he wanted to do a high rescue like that one. Anyway, back at the station, Roy tells Johnny the 'secret' of Lorenzo's amazing escape from the trunk: he wasn't in it; he's lurking under the pier while Johnny does his high-wire act. So Johnny (the supposed idiot?) asks the next logical question: How did Lorenzo get out of the trunk in the first place? Which of course Roy doesn't know. *My* question is a bit different: why did Roy look under the pier to begin with?? To scope out a possible rescue of the trunk? That doesn't seem like it would be necessary, as the trunk wouldn't have landed near the pier. So why did he go down there? (Note: in the closed-captioning, Netflix credits the wrong character for a line in the Lorenzo rescue. It's not important in any way to the story, but I just found it interesting. Especially since I don't really use the CC feature much and just happened to turn it on at that point.)

Another note: Roy got his haircut, unfortunately where he could least afford it.

At Rampart, Brackett is shocked to see who the ambulance brings in: his father. (Query: was Brackett senior given a first name? He's listed on IMDB only as "Brackett's father." So I guess he's only known as Mr. Brackett.) The doc mentions that dad wanted him to be a lawyer, so I wonder if that's what Senior is. Probably not, though, since Kel says something about his father "toughing it out" a number of times over the years. I took that to mean adversity in some way: business failures, job loss, etc. That wouldn't really apply if he was a lawyer, most likely. Anyway, we know neither his first name nor his occupation. (I do that in my writing sometimes, and not always consciously.)

May Fair

Anyway, one thing I'm very, very glad about is that the writers didn't give us a father/son tension storyline. You know: father appears in the hospital, tension crackles in the air and when they're in private conversation they talk about past grievances and childhood hurts, etc. Bleah, I'm *so* glad they didn't do that. And now I guess we know where Brackett gets his deep, gravelly voice.

So the paramedics are called to the house of a man who blew up his chimney. I like that rescue, even though it's not really complicated. I was curious as to why the guys automatically put the O2 mask on him—before they figured out he was having trouble breathing, before they checked the vitals, before they even confirmed he was still alive. (Isn't there a movie like that: Dead Men Don't Wear Masks? Yeah, I know, I'm booing myself for that one.) Also, I like when Roy checked how many fingers the man saw, etc. They don't often do that, so it's always interesting to see. Also, I giggle every time I hear Johnny on the biophone saying, "He's been unconscious for about several minutes." Ha!

I also like the rescue of the skier who now has two broken legs. It's an interesting problem and all the guys are involved. I do wonder, though, when Roy and John first go up to the second floor in the building, Johnny is first up the stairs, but he pauses at the top of the stairs and lets Roy go first. I wonder if there was a reason for that??

Brackett's father gets operated on, and—news flash!!—there are other doctors at Rampart! We know that two of them did surgery on Early a while back, and now yet another surgeon operates on Mr. Brackett. So we know there are at least three other doctors who work there. Good news!

The final rescue is interesting too. Roy works with Cap, Chet, and Marco to try to contain the gas fire while Johnny handles the Jaws to try and free a girl trapped in a smashed car. I do wonder why Chet and Marco's water stream wasn't more concentrated and aimed at the base of the fire. Meanwhile the truck driver and Johnny protect the girl while they work on the hood of her car to get her out. Once the reinforcements arrive (and the other captain walks all the way around two engines, apparently) and they get the fire taken care of, Roy goes to help Johnny out. By that time Johnny has crunched the car hood and Roy is able to simply lift the girl out and walk away as Johnny is busy retrieving some of the equipment.

Finally, at the station, Roy is merely toying with the magic sphere when it literally falls apart in his hands. (If that scene had been filmed today I think we would have seen the sphere fall open, but unfortunately we *don't* see that.) Johnny's ticked off at that, especially since the "secret of the universe" ends up being "made in Japan." He's definitely not happy that the thing fell apart so easily for Roy, saying, "I do all the preceding work and you take the credit." Ha, that's exactly what happened at the last rescue scene, too: Johnny did all the work with the Jaws and made it so the girl could get out, and Roy just shows up at the last minute and hands the girl out and walks away with her.

Additional notes: Dixie is hardly in this episode, maybe just two or three brief scenes. You'd think we'd have seen her more, giving Brackett moral support, but it's actually Joe who's mostly there for him. On a similar note, Mike Stoker in this episode is like a little kid in a rich family: seen but not heard. We see him in a couple of scenes at the two big accident rescues, but I don't think he spoke a word in this episode. Yesterday, in Kidding, I don't think we even saw him, except maybe in stock footage. If we did, he was once again silent.

4.19 It's How You Play the Game

First off, I find it very unlikely that not only had Chet never played baseball (even just pick-up games with friends?) but that he supposedly didn't even know much about the game. Same goes with Johnny suddenly being an expert and being able to 'train' Chet. (Gage never struck me as a team-sports athlete, either. Except I *could* see him as a track athlete.) Ah well, as we all know from TV shows of that era, anything worth doing is worth *overdoing*.

Behind the station (when it's clearly evening, and not lunchtime), I mainly see a lot of 'beater' type vehicles. No sign of Johnny's Rover or Roy's foreign job, although I do see the blue Chevy pick-up that Roy drove in The Parade. (Keep an eye on that truck; we'll see plenty of it, going forward.)

At the first rescue (accident with the drunk guy), when J and R get out of the squad, Vince tells them what's going on. Immediately after that, you can hear Cap say "Right in the water, you dunce!" As the camera pans out, we see Cap, Chet, and Marco walking through or around a big puddle, and Stoker is backing up the engine. I wonder if Mike missed his driving mark and sent Cap into the drink.

Also, once they got that accident victim in the ambulance and Roy went with him (maybe Johnny was afraid of being assaulted again?), Johnny took the biophone and put it in the squad. Wasn't that supposed to go with Roy in the ambulance??

Speaking of the biophone, Johnny had it in the ambulance when he took "Trader Jack" to Rampart, but when he and Roy left the hospital, no sign of the orange box. He had the drug box, but no biophone.

After the waterbed 'rescue,' Johnny's gobsmacked when the girl gives Roy a kiss. Roy says, "she was just saying thank you." I could just see Johnny's thought bubble: "Hey, I was there, too!"

Lastly, in the final scene, it looks like Johnny showed up for work already dressed in uniform. What's up with that??

~ ~ ~

Another episode in which I don't like the title-related storyline that runs throughout the hour. This one doesn't make sense to me for a number of reasons. For one thing, none of the guys at Station 51 strike me as (nor ever acted like they were) guys who had ever played sports. (Team sports, that is; we know that Roy was a swimmer and Johnny did track, but those don't count as they don't involve team play.) Johnny never really expressed any interest (or proficiency) in baseball, and yet suddenly he's the coach. Worse, Chet says he never played baseball (really? not even in an empty lot or behind the school?), and while he says he's "seen it on TV," that would lead me to believe that he doesn't watch regularly, much less follow it. He probably watches baseball the way I watch golf—only when I can't leave the room or change the channel. As a result, I don't know all the rules or terms, and certainly not any intelligent golf strategy (other than to get the ball in the cup, of course). And yet next thing you know Chet's acting like an expert and trying to call plays and deal with runners who take too big a lead, etc. Totally unbelievable. And of course once again Johnny messes things up for everyone. Seriously, the way these writers portray him, it's amazing he's competent enough to rent an apartment and get a driver's license, much less be trusted to administer drugs to the unsuspecting public. Come on, writers, Randy's a professional actor... give him something meaty to work with.

Okay, rant over. On with the show!

The first accident is funny for a variety of reasons. First, when they arrive on scene, our guys are all in full sun. By the time they get the guy out of his truck, the scene is in total shade. Seriously, it didn't take *that* long to extricate him. Also, put your ears on and rewatch when they first arrive on the scene.

May Fair

Roy gets out of the squad and Vince first tells him about the accident. Offscreen we hear Cap say something like, "right in the water, you dunce." As the camera pans over, we see Cap skirting a broken hydrant and Stoker is moving the engine back, away from the hydrant's geyser. I guess he parked a little too close, eh? Or maybe the production people told Mike to park there, not realizing the hydrant would be "live"?? Anyway, I thought it was funny. Additionally, Roy either mispronounces *pedal pulse*, or he thinks the victim—a guy—is pregnant, because I'm pretty sure that Kevin said "fedal/fetal pulse." Maybe he merged the words *foot* and *pedal*. And of course this is the scene in which Johnny gets punched in the nose, and then he takes the biophone in the squad instead of Roy having it in the ambulance with the victim. Good thing nothing went wrong on the drive in to Rampart, right? I guess when stuff like that gets mixed up, the actors just do their best to roll with it and play it off, so they don't have to reshoot the whole scene. I'm assuming, of course, that Randy even realized he shouldn't have the phone.

*Didja ever notice... at most car accident sites, a lot of times the vehicles are old beaters? And look like they just came from the junkyard?? Hmmm, I wonder why???

I like the Trader Jack rescue. It's definitely different and again the guys use their ingenuity to solve a problem: in this case, keeping the tiger calm while they get the driver out of the car. For the record, for those keeping score at home, in this one season our guys have dealt with "lions and tigers and bears." (Okay, I'll say it: Oh, my!!) Yes, there was the lady who fell in the *lion* exhibit at the zoo, Charlene the *bear* in The Bash, and here's Willy the *tiger*.

In this episode we also see another example of Roy's charisma, as the waterbed lady gives him a kiss once her husband (?) is safely put in the ambulance. In that scene we see both stunt doubles (Hal and Angie) as ambulance attendants.

I also sort of like the ongoing story at Rampart, as the doctors are trying to figure out what's the matter with Gus, the accident victim who was Johnny's face-puncher. And of course they manage to tie that in with the final scene which was a house fire on some horrible studio back lot. I have to wonder about that last scene, though. Vince (who, like Brackett and Dixie, seems to work 24 hours a day) says they tried to serve a search warrant, and the guy set fire to the place. And yet, the guy was still in the house, in the basement. That doesn't make any sense to me—if I'm going to set fire to a building, I'd make darn sure to vacate the premises, ASAP. In any case, upon first arrival, Cap orders air masks on everyone, but when Roy and Johnny go into the basement, neither one is wearing their masks. They have the tanks on, but not the masks. Additionally, I don't know why Johnny wore that rope harness thingy. Roy just climbed into the basement without any rope, but Johnny wore the kind of rope that's tied into a harness that goes around the crotch. What's the point of that?? It was a small basement, not the Grand Canyon.

Lastly, final scene. When Johnny arrives for his shift, Roy is in the locker room getting dressed, but.... Johnny's already in uniform. That's just plain strange, even for this show. Maybe Randy didn't want what he wore to work that day seen on camera...?? Honestly, I can't think why he would already be in uniform upon arrival at the station.

4.20 The Mouse

~ Not sure how Chet or anyone would have seen that mouse so often... mice are nocturnal, so they wouldn't have seen it during the day; in the middle of the night is when someone could have seen "Herbert" running around the kitchen.

May Fair

~ As the station is leaving on the first call, we plainly see Cap sitting in the cab of the engine as we 'hear' him acknowledge "KMG-365." He's quite a ventriloquist—never saw his mouth move once!

~ At the house fire (with the barred windows) a whole bunch of engines got called out to it, but I only saw 51. Also, when Johnny was working on the man they got out of the house, and Mike had the O2 on him, Mike kept looking at his watch. I half-expected him to say "pulse is 55," or something like that.

~ While transporting the guy from the laundromat who was in cardiac arrest—no, he wasn't—yes, he was, etc. How did Johnny, who was in the squad, hear the ambulance driver call to dispatch—the *ambulance* dispatch, not LACoFD dispatch?? They're totally different systems (I assume). Just another case of creative license for TV, methinks. Also, you'll notice that Roy did *not* have the ambulance pull over.

~ In the bar scene, Roy and John were literally backed against a wall by the tough guys, until Vince came in. Then suddenly Johnny presses his luck and gets all cocky with the two thugs; meanwhile, Roy's just thanking his stars that Vince showed up.

~ After that run, when they get back to the station, Roy and Johnny didn't get their bunker gear set up for any night runs. They more or less jumble their blue uni's on the mystery shelf (except that Roy nicely lays out his blue pants at the foot of his bed). Speaking of pants and bunkers... in the morning Chet puts his bunker pants on *over* his uniform pants. Wonder how uncomfortable that would be??

~ I have to say, I really like the fighter jet/apartment collision rescue. I like the danger, the teamwork, and the uniqueness.

~ Pasadena FD doesn't have truck #s on the front of their trucks/engines.

Watching EMERGENCY! Seasons 4-6

~ Did we notice how Johnny 'helped' the Pasadena guy rescue him? He sort of stood himself up once the guy pulled him. He's so helpful!

~ I use headphones when I watch the show, so maybe nobody else heard it, but I kept thinking during that jet crash/apartment house rescue: "will someone *please* find that woman who keeps screaming???" No, not the one Roy and Johnny went to help, but in the audio files of the background sounds there was a woman who was just screaming. And of course they looped the audio so I heard it over and over and over.

~ ~ ~

So I actually like this episode—yay!—there's no particular storyline that I don't like, and there are a number that I do like. I feel like I've been such a Negative Nelly lately by not liking this or that about recent episodes (usually the episode-long storyline that usually involves a certain brown-eyed fireman who usually is written to be a doofus). Anyway, I can safely say that I don't have such reservations about this one.

The ep opens with a tense situation as Chet, Marco, and Mike are ministering to a victim with a fractured femur, among other ills, as Roy and John supervise. But suddenly—and surprisingly—the tones sound and the guys all jump up to respond to the call, and we see that they're at the station practicing some first aid on a dummy. (Or "Buster," for those of you who know who Buster is. *wink*) Anyway, it's nice to see the other guys learning a little more to help them be more effective in the field. (Random useless thought: I wonder if there were stated, explicit limits to what the paramedics could teach or advise the other guys about?)

I do like the first rescue, of the fire at the house with bars on the windows. Personally I think they just wanted a reason to show Johnny looking tough and using the K-12, starting with a quick head-shake to get his protective visor in place. I do wonder why Chet resorted to kicking in the door… why have we never again seen them break down doors the way Johnny did that one time, by throwing himself into it backward, O2 tank first? (Fun fact: I saw a firefighter do that in another show recently.) But I did like seeing Chet and Marco get blown off their feet. I think that was Stoker who helped get them back up, probably thanking heavens once again he passed that engineer's exam and doesn't have to deal with explosions and backdraft anymore. Also, show of hands: who thought the neighbor guy was probably going to go in and rob the victim blind as soon as the ambulance disappeared? (By the way, a certain interesting gold Mustang was seen at this, er, scene. Extra points for anyone who knows the significance of that car.)

By the way, when the man is brought into the treatment room at Rampart, he's apparently holding the little rubber squeeze thingy they use to pump up the BP cuff. Then as soon as he's on the bed, a nurse with stethoscope walks up to him and starts squeezing the thingy. I can only assume that he was already wearing the BP cuff, even though we didn't see it?? I've never seen that before, I don't think; do the paramedics regularly leave the cuff on the victim? That would be a PITA to have to keep retrieving it.

At the station, Chet discovers "Herbert," a mouse who's come to visit. Where's that alley cat, or even Boot, when you need them?? I find it interesting that Chet references the mouse's reproduction prowess when he says something about how they multiply, "once they start hitting the sack." Even though he's talking about a mouse, was that risqué' for prime-time TV in the mid-70s??

I like the rescue of the Ronnie Schell character, who keeps going into full arrest for brief moments and then recovering. He always seems to play such interesting characters on this show. Anyway, I like that Morton gets a little comeuppance when he witnesses first-hand Harold's little medical oddity. Although I find it highly suspect that Johnny, who's in the squad, would have been able to hear the ambulance driver calling his company's dispatcher. Just a little creative license, don'tcha know.

This is also the episode with J. Pat O'Malley, who brings in his wife of 48 years when she has trouble breathing. He tells Dixie about their kids and grandkids... one of whom must be a boy who likes to go with Gramps to shoot off model rockets in the park (*wink*). But I find it interesting that in the treatment room, Dixie seems to perform the same service that Cap does at a rescue scene: get concerned family members out of the way and comfort them as best they can.

The paramedics get called out to a bar, although it's not a very crowded bar, apparently. This might, for me, be the weakest scene of the episode, but it's still OK. I just don't like how Johnny acts once Vince gets there, like he's the cock of the walk. If he'd drop that attitude, it would be a much better scene. (Although, arguably, not as interesting for some fans.) But what would have happened if Vince had to leave before Johnny was through treating that bar-fly??

Back at the station, the paramedics get in late and go right to the dorm. Meanwhile we hear some sort of strange ding-ing sound through that whole scene. It almost sounds like some sort of notification or alarm bell, but of course it's not, it's just some sort of strange "background noise." I find it annoying and distracting. Also, I know most people (women-people) have eyes glued to the screen as a certain dark-haired paramedic disrobes... didja notice how he just crumbles his clothes and puts them on that ledge, while Roy takes the trouble to nicely fold his pants? And shouldn't Johnny have left his t-shirt on in case they get a run in the middle of the night??

In the morning Chet's afraid to look in the kitchen, but the other guys go in with him and they discover that Herbert has somehow eluded the trap and yet managed to make off with the cheese. (I know the feeling; I've seen that happen, and it's very frustrating.) Anyway, the alarm goes off and there's a call: fighter jet crashes into apartment building.

We know that Dispatch gave them their wake-up call, and Chet mentioned that C-shift would be there in about an hour. So by the time they get that apartment fire under control, their shift (B-shift?) is working overtime. Do the C-shift guys just hang out at the station until the engine and squad return? That would be weird, as you know they can't get called out, so they literally have nothing to do. And get paid for it, too.

Anyway, I do like that last rescue, a lot of interesting stuff going on. There are other engine companies responding, interesting-looking vehicles, and even a truck from Pasadena. Am I correct in remembering that this apartment building was slated to be destroyed, so the show was able to use it for that purpose? I wonder what "real" firefighters thought about being involved in these scenes; they were used as training exercises, but still, I wonder if some guys liked it, or thought it was silly, or what.

P.S., at one time we discussed Johnny and his holster, how he was wearing it on his left side. Recently (season 4) he's now wearing it on his right side, which makes sense as he's right-handed. Roy still wears his on his left side.

4.21 Back-Up

I do like this episode, for a number of reasons. One of which is that it's an "Issues" episode, although not as serious or personal as some of the other Issues episodes. And also, I might totally skip the next one, 905-Wild, since that one is almost unwatchable for me.

~ When John and Roy arrive at Wild Bill's place, Engine 10 is there... with a First Aid kit. I could just imagine them putting on a band-aid or applying merthiolate to a scrape. (Bonus points if you remember merthiolate—or mercurochrome—and *don't* have to look them up!)

~ When they left Wild Bill, the deputy was still there, chiding the old geezer. On their way back, they get called to the football guy's house and... *voila!*, the *same* deputy is there giving mouth-to-mouth, and got there *before* them. Did Scotty beam him from one place to the other??

~ Speaking of Football Guy, Dixie tells Roy to start an IV of D5W and asks where the electrical contact was made. Roy answers the ankle and Dixie tells them to put on a dressing, and literally in the *next breath* Roy says "we administered the IV and dressed the ankle." Boy, is that the quickest medical service in LA County, or what???

~ At the hospital, did anyone notice how crowded the treatment rooms are? When Dixie agrees to take a kid from Pediatrics, she tells the other nurse to take the kid to Dr. Morton in Treatment 3. A moment later Roy asks Dixie where Johnny is, and she says "Treatment Room 3," and not two seconds later is a page that says "Dr. Reid, Treatment Room 3." (!!!) So, Roy goes into #3, and there's Johnny and Dr. Morton... with Wild Bill. No sign of the kid from Pediatrics—or Dr. Reid!

~ Chet's fill-in, Bill, was cooking cherry-filled stew (!!) at the station. Roy "KMG-365'd" the next call, and as the squad pulled out, there was no engine in the bay. (So why was Bill still there??) But a while later, when the squad caught up with

51 at the heart-attack house, Bill was there with the other Engine 51 guys. Hmmm.

Lightning round:

~ On that heart-attack call, I think Dr. Early said "lidograin" instead of lidocaine.

~ On that bogus call with the squabbling couple (guy was watching TV), the couple reminded me of those married hicks on Hee-Haw. (More bonus points if you've remember watching Hee-Haw.)

~ Marco got to drive the squad! That doesn't happen all that often, bet he was glad Chet was out.

~ At the hospital, Johnny mentions the "MIC" unit and how it's designed to help people in emergencies. MIC is Mobile Intensive Care unit. I don't think the paramedic program has ever been referred to by that name on the show before, has it? Or since?? (Although that *is* what their name-tags say.)

~ When Marco pulled up to the scene of the ambulance accident, we can clearly see he pulled next to a dark blue pick-up truck. (Yeah, we've seen that truck before, right?) Yet when the camera angle changed, there was no pick-up truck next to the squad.

~ In the treatment room at Rampart, after Brackett defibs the heart-attack guy the second time, watch Johnny try to disentangle the stethoscope from the wires of the datascope.

~ Maybe Chet and Vince went to a Dodger game together, since neither one was on duty this day, and thus we got Bill and Officer Cutie.

~ Anyone notice that Bill, Dwyer, and Johnny's friend Gil all have the same 'look' about them? Same hair, same '70s 'stache, etc. Did Universal have them all cloned or something??

Last, but definitely not least: treating and defibbing a patient on the top of the engine as it runs down the streets.... that has got to be about the most bad-ass thing these guys have done on the show. Rappelling, climbing, jumping in water, those are all fine, but *that*... that was COOL.

~ ~ ~

As I mentioned last time, I like this episode, so that's two in a row. Yay, I'm on a hot streak!! Oops, the hot streak is already over, considering what the next episode is. (**Note:** some of this is pretty much the same, even copied, from the previous time.)

This is one of the few episodes (before the final season) that opens somewhere *other than* the fire station, or with characters *other than* Roy and Johnny. Two guys wheel in an unconscious girl on a gurney and then take off, ditching her there. Nice friends, huh? Turns out they injected milk into her, to try to help bring her around from her high. (Brackett fills her in on how dangerous that is.) Apparently this was common enough that the PTB felt they should mention it in a mini-PSA, but I admit I'd never heard of that milk thing before. Of course, since I was just a young'un when this show was on, there's no reason why I *would* have heard of it, and since I've also never heard of it as an adult, it must mean that the practice has probably gone the way of the dodo. So maybe the PSA worked—all the junkies watched Emergency! on Saturday night and decided they wouldn't inject milk into their high addict friends any more. Hurray, problem solved.

So the squad isn't there when John and Roy start their shift, and they have to wait for Dwyer and partner come back. Once they do, shouldn't the new shift do that whole calibrating the biophone thing that we've seen once or twice? I realize that the other paramedics have used it and it must work fine, but I bet that every shift is supposed to do certain things, like check supplies, test equipment, etc., when they first come on duty. Of course, the alarm goes off before they can do much of anything, so I guess that absolves them... in this case.

The first call (a long drive) is to Wild Bill, who pretty much just needs someone to talk to and fuss over him a little. Maybe the guys should set him up with Edna Self—she can keep herself busy by looking after Bill, and they can both keep each other company.

When they leave Wild Bill, the deputy (Scotty) is still there, chiding the old geezer. On their way back, they get called to the football guy's house and... *voila!* Scotty is already there giving mouth-to-mouth to the old coot; he got there *before* the paramedics. Did Star Trek's Scotty beam his namesake from one place to the other??

Speaking of Football Guy, Dixie tells Roy to start an IV of D5W and asks where the electrical contact was made. Roy answers the ankle and Dixie tells them to put on a dressing, and literally in the *next breath* Roy says "we administered the IV and dressed the ankle." Boy, is that the quickest medical service in LA County, or what???

At the hospital, did anyone notice how crowded the treatment rooms are? When Dixie agrees to take a kid from Pediatrics, she tells the other nurse to take the kid to Dr. Morton in Treatment 3. A moment later Roy asks Dixie where Johnny is, and she says "Treatment Room 3"; and not two seconds later is a page that says "Dr. Reid, Treatment Room 3." (!!!) So, Roy goes into #3, and there's Johnny and Dr. Morton... with Wild Bill. No sign of the kid from Pediatrics—or Dr. Reid!

So, is "Bill" the new "Charlie"? In this episode there's Wild Bill, and also paramedic Bill. Another episode has Old Bill.

Back at the station, Chet's fill-in, Bill, is making cherry-filled stew (!!) from Chet's recipe. Luckily for the guys, they get a call before they have to eat it (yuck!), and as the squad pulls out, there's no engine in the bay. So why was Bill still there?? Then, a while later, when the squad catches up with engine 51 at the heart-attack house, there was Bill with the other Engine 51 guys.

So the guys get called out to the hovel—er, I mean house—of a run-down squabbling couple, which turns out to be a bogus waste of time. From there they pick up a call they should have had to begin with, and where Engine 51 is. It's a guy apparently having a heart attack. The paramedics do what they can and his situation is so severe that they both get in the ambulance for transport. And of course there's an accident and the ambulance is toast, out of commission. (Question: why was Marco driving so far behind? The squad doesn't get to the accident site until after the guys check everyone out and call for assistance, and Captain Stanley responds that the engine would be there in one minute. Not that Marco could have done anything at the scene, but usually the squad is right behind the ambulance.)

So then we see the famous (and uber-cool) scene of the two paramedics treating a patient on the top of the engine. That's twice that Mike drove with 'passengers' like that. I wonder if that was filmed on closed city streets? And I assume that the 'traffic' behind the engine was actually production vehicles, whose drivers could keep an eye out and be ready to stop on a dime if anyone fell off the engine. And again, where was the squad?? No wonder Chet usually drives the squad if Marco's such a slow-poke.

May Fair

Too bad they don't show the engine at the emergency entrance at Rampart. That would be an interesting sight, to say the least.

In the treatment room at Rampart, after Brackett defibs the heart-attack guy the second time, watch Johnny struggle with the stethoscope, trying to disentangle it from the wires of the datascope. Then once he finally gets the stethoscope, he has trouble getting the BP cuff in order. LOL, if I were him, I'd have just given up and faked it.

By the way, there was not one, not two, but *three* different sightings of the blue pick-up in this one episode. It's not really even challenging anymore. I've been getting screen pics but I think it's kind of boring to post them, at this point.

* * *

You're right, it makes no sense at all to look at your watch and say "ETA is XX minutes." Perhaps the looking-at-the-watch thing is purely an acting exercise, an action that gives the impression of something (perhaps intangible) being done. Like in old movies when someone was on the phone and we suddenly hear a dial tone, the person always looks at the phone in his hand, as if by looking at it he could divine some useful information. (Nowadays, with cell phones, that would make total sense, to see if there's a "call ended" signal, but back in the day, TV or movies would show people looking at their phone handsets. Because they had to do *something* to indicate the character's confusion.) In any case, maybe Randy looked at his watch as an indication to the audience that he's calculating the ETA, even though it didn't make sense, and in real life it wouldn't happen. After all, TV is a visual medium, and it's all about perception; they show us an action to indicate something that doesn't normally require action.

* * *

That's because they have to open up the patient's shirt to do CPR and defib, so if it's a woman they have to strategically locate something or someone for obvious reasons!

Yes, there are a couple of cases in which they "patch in" female victims. One is the high-school student on the roof-top gym class who ended up dying, and another is the mother of the pregnant woman (who of course went into labor while they were there). They don't show us the patching-in process for the women, for obvious reasons... we simply see the result: the victim with the wires already sticking out from under her blouse (and yes, her blouse is kept on, as opposed to ripping the shirt open as they do with the men). Suffice it to say, there are far fewer instances of defibbing women on this show.

And yes, as has been mentioned, there is that one infamous case of the woman who ended up dying—she took a bunch of pills but probably didn't really want to die. She's in Rampart with doctors and nurses working feverishly to save her, and a strategically-placed nurse moves out of position briefly, giving the camera a brief view of the woman, who is (apparently) nude above the waist.

4.22 905-Wild

This episode of Emergency! is... well, perhaps "universally disliked by fans" is a little too strong, but I think it's safe to say that many, many people (perhaps a majority?) don't care for it.

It's well known that this was a backdoor pilot for a new show from Mark VII, to be called (surprise!) 905-Wild, dealing with the LA County Animal Control services. I'm sure it would have been about more than rescuing cats stuck in trees, or picking up stray dogs; the "wild" part of the title would probably show up with some regularity.

To be fair, I don't believe the concept of the show was necessarily awful; after all, there have been other shows about animals that were successful, and with the increasing urbanization of the LA area at that time, encounters with wildlife were certainly a real issue, and still are in a lot of areas (including where I live).

But, I think there were a number of reasons why this pilot didn't work. For one, it was just plain terrible in the execution. The focus on the goat and the improbable surgery at a busy hospital really stretched things too far, imho. And the writing didn't help, either. If it hadn't been so cheesy, in that rat-a-tat-tat Webb style, it might have been easier to bear. But also I think the public's taste in TV shows had evolved. Those of us of *ahem!* a certain age might remember the Sunday night Wonderful World of Disney, or Wonderful World of Color, or whatever it was called. Those were kid-friendly, heartwarming stories for the most part, many of which included animals. But even the mighty Disney machine began to fade in popularity by the mid-seventies. So, if even Disney shows were losing ground among families and kids, what chance did a poorly-written Webb-isode have??

Disclaimer: I realize that 905-Wild probably wasn't written specifically to appeal to kids (although with that stereotyped gap-toothed little girl and the $%@! goat, it's a natural assumption), but under different circumstances, I think maybe it *could* have worked as a kid-centric show. Think Flipper with paws.

In any case, for kids or adults, the 905-Wild pilot episode didn't have what it took to get on the air. I'm just glad it didn't reflect badly on Emergency! in the long run.

Watching EMERGENCY! Seasons 4-6

~ ~ ~

So I made myself watch this again. While I still don't like the episode—and probably never will—I think this additional viewing put me somewhat at peace with it. But, big-picture stuff later. Now is for the nitty-gritty.

As the episode begins we see the squad rolling out on a night call—or very early morning, actually—to a small mom-and-pop grocery store. Man injured with some gashes. Johnny, thinking the "maniac with a knife" could still be nearby, goes in the backroom to check. After closing the back door—which was open—he looks up to see a tiger on top of a freezer, gnawing on some raw meat. Don't bother thinking about details or logic regarding this situation, because there isn't any. Just go with it: tiger loose in the store. Needless to say, Johnny and Roy get the victim (and his friend, the reliable Virginia Gregg) out of the store in a flash, and Roy calls in to LA request Animal Control respond as soon as possible.

Cut to said Animal Control officers, who are removing a family of kittens (a *large* family of them) from a woman's attic. (Funny, when Mark Harmon's character asks the deputy on the ground to "turn the spotlight to the left," the man adjusts it slightly to the *right*.) Anyway, once they get the little furballs out of the attic, the officers stow the little darlings in their truck (squad) and rush off to answer the call at the mom-and-pop store. I just hope the kittens won't be used for tiger-bait.

When one of the officers goes into the store after the tiger, the store sound system is playing some horrible generic, tuneless music. Which is odd, because it hadn't been playing 15 minutes earlier when Roy and Johnny were in there. (And I doubt the music would be on a timer.) But one thing I find quite notable, even unavoidable, in the store scenes: the prominence of Pepsi products. The backroom has cardboard boxes with the Pepsi-Cola name, and the store itself has a noticeable display case of Pepsi cans (although the text on the familiar blue-and-red logo at the top of the case says "soda"). There are other product names visible as well: Hawaiian Punch, Carnation, Hi-C, and Minute Maid, among the most prominent. Some of the cardboard boxes even had IBM on them; I wonder what came in those? And I'm not sure if Mrs. Cubbison's Stuffing is/was real, but that even has its own sign on the wall. (Update: I just looked it up, and apparently yes, it *is* a real brand of stuffing. Who knew?)

Anyway, the tiger eventually goes up through a conveniently-open skylight and onto the roof (I told you not to bother with logic or common sense), and both control officers end up there. The tiger wanders around the rooftops a little, and is actually kind of cute when it plays with the pigeons; I'm just glad we didn't see her catch one. Finally, the lead Animal Control officer gets a decent shot and shoots the animal with a tranquilizer, causing her to soon stumble and fall over, helpless and harmless. I do wonder how they got a tiger to stumble around like that and finally lie down; I sort of hope the animal was trained to do that, but on the other hand, I have mixed feelings about wild animals being trained to perform. (On yet another, I don't even want to entertain the possibility—however unlikely—that they actually tranquilized a wild tiger at that location and filmed the animal as it got knocked out.) In any case, all's well that ends well for this big Bengal baby.

This is when the pilot show actually begins, as we now meet the other characters of the series: the gruff but kindly older veterinarian who works at Animal Control; the sharp and efficient director who deals with the myriad pesky administrative details (played by Gary Crosby, who moved on from his roles as an LAPD cop, LACoFD fireman and LACoFD paramedic), and the perky female office assistant. We even have what's known in some circles as an info-dump, but we E!-fans are more familiar with them as PSAs—Public Service Announcements. We're told, through character exposition, that

Animal Control isn't just for picking up stray dogs and cats, but serves a bigger purpose as well. And when ol' Doc Whatever-his-name-is introduces a visitor to the clinic's current residents, we get a glimpse of a number of different types of wild animals (fox, coyote, mountain lion, raccoon, etc.) who live in LA County, and who somehow try to coexist with the humans who are forever encroaching on their turf. Yes, it's a bit tedious and obvious as a PSA, but I guess it serves a purpose.

The officers are sent to the compound of a local private zoo, the owner of which has been a thorn in the side of the good people at Animal Control. This is where I really have to fast-forward. Call me a coward, but I don't want to see or hear about animals that have been neglected or abused, as the creatures in that place definitely have been. Long story short, the tiger Johnny and Roy encountered escaped from this so-called animal compound because it was hungry and hadn't been fed for days. (It's not spoken aloud, but I guess the implication is that it's lucky she only broke into a meat market and didn't go after human prey.)

Next is a wildfire to which the officers respond, and of course en route they have the sort of in-car conversations that we all know and love... and which are apparently a staple of Mark VII shows (Adam-12 and Emergency!, at least; not sure about Dragnet.) Anyway, at the fire's command post, these officers once again cross paths with our favorite paramedics. John and Roy have apparently been at the scene for a while, as they're all sooty and dirty—in other words, just the way we like 'em! They're ministering to a man and his very young granddaughter, both straight out of central casting: feeble old timer played by Burt Mustin, who might be recognized from Adam-12, The Andy Griffith Show, or just about any other 1960s TV show you can think of. And the little girl... well, I will admit, she is cute as a button, honestly; really adorable. And yet between her missing front tooth and the fact that she's lame (leg in a brace for some unexplained reason), she's a walking cliché. In any case, just as the tiger is the four-legged star of the first half of this episode, the girl's pygmy goat William is in the spotlight for the second.

The Animal Control officers take off into the burning countryside to look for the little goat (and they do not wear any sort of mask or air tank, believe it or not; yeah, I'm rolling my eyes here), and when they find him, poor William is in a bad way. Back at the command post, Johnny puts an air mask on the animal, which is cute, and they even use the paddles to look at his heart (although how Roy knew where to place the paddles is a little baffling; I'd have thought one would need to be on the animal's belly). Then Johnny does something really odd—he calls Rampart and simply says, "We're sending you an EKG." Huh. That is *not* how those conversations usually begin, so that's bizarre from the get-go. And of course Brackett responds while assuming the "victim" is a human, and then learns it's a.... goat. I do find it odd also that others at Rampart make Kel feel like an ogre for trying to play by the rules and refuse to assist in treating a goat. You'd think he'd at least have stodgy, stick-in-the-mud Morton in his corner on this one, he who wanted to cut a man's prized model ship right out of his hands—literally. But to me, the *really* crazy thing about this (aside from Dixie smoking a cigarette, *right there in the ED*) is that Rampart isn't even busy. If they'd been slammed with patients, it would have been easy for Brackett to say, "Sorry, 51, there's no room at the inn for a goat." But that's not the case.

Poor little William is taken by the Animal Control guys from the scene of the fire to the nearest vet, yet along the way the plan changes and they head for Rampart instead. Leaving the little bleating baby in the truck, they go in to talk to the doctors, and run across the same brick wall as before: and this wall is named Dr. Kelly Brackett. Luckily for the little girl—and William, of course—the "brick wall" crumbles as Dixie stands there holding a pitiful-looking animal. That is when we get another unfortunate burst of Webb-speak, as Brackett rattles off things he'll need in order to treat the goat.

"Somebody set up an EKG monitor—thoracotomy airway—all the hardware!"

"By the time you count to ten," Morton replies.

"By the time I count to *nine*."

Ugh.

So yeah, they operate on William the goat. And everyone gets in on the act. The Animal Control guys look on, Roy and Johnny look on, and the firefighter with the injured hand that our guys brought in looks on too. He even gives Dixie the equivalent of that dramatic line we hear in war movies, "My bleeding hand can wait; save the goat first." *Major eyeroll* This total dedication of every resource makes me wonder what would have happened if Rampart had suddenly gotten busy? I can imagine Brackett's reaction now: "A woman with severe chest pains? She'll have to wait. He cut his leg with a chainsaw and is bleeding out? Sorry, we're in the middle of goat surgery here." And apparently it takes all three highly-trained doctors and a head nurse—not to mention a million dollars' worth of technology—to do the job. Yeah, *that's* the best use of hospital resources!

Well, I don't need a spoiler warning to say that everything turned out fine. Johnny and Roy grin at the heartwarming sight of a recovering William. The two Animal Control guys actually each wipe a tear away. Brackett gets to meet the "busy" but amiable veterinarian, and Doc Coolidge gets to meet the "busy" and heart-of-gold Chief of Emergency Medicine. Best yet, William goes home with Cutest Girl Ever, complete with a new bell from Dixie for him to wear around his neck. A happy ending all around.

Well, not so much, since the network didn't pick up the show. Mark Harmon would have to find another way to stay on our TV screen, as his two attempts with Mark VII didn't quite work out (Emergency! and Adam-12; his episodes of both shows aired about a month apart, ironically enough).

Now, back to the "big-picture stuff." It occurred to me this time around that this episode (for me, at least; I don't claim this is universal), anyway, the episode seems to be split into two separate and distinct parts, or components. The first is the tiger capture, the Intro to Animal Control 101 at the clinic, the situation at the so-called zoo, and even brush fire scene, up to and including the fire itself and the rescue of that little scamp, William. The second part (yin to the yang?) is the rest of the episode, with William the Rampart VIP (Very Important Patient), implausibly requiring the services of every member of the hospital's staff.

To be honest, I don't like either of these two halves, or segments, or whatever you want to call them. But... I dislike them for different reasons, and I think that's an important distinction. The first half of the show, the Tiger Terror part, is bad (imo) in part because of the awkward PSA info-dump at the clinic that I mentioned earlier. It's not a fatal flaw, however, as it's a "one and done" thing: once the information and characters are introduced to the viewer, it's over and done with and we can all get on with our viewing. The zoo and brush fire scenes are unpleasant too; I don't want to see or think about neglected and starving animals, forced to live in unnatural and tiny cages. And I also don't want to see rabbits running through a fire. (Or deer, skunks, chipmunks, etc.) Those things are sad and depressing, and I don't want to see that sort of thing. But... again, not a fatal flaw. Those scenes were in *one* episode; if this show had been picked up by the network, I assume every single episode wouldn't have such distressing, depressing scenarios. For that reason I might (*might*) have given the show a chance.

The goat-surgery part, though.... That was just plain silly. If that's the sort of story the writers would have given the viewer every week—and the sort of dialogue—I'm not sure anyone over the age of 12 would have watched, since it's so hokey and unbelievable. (Again, just my opinion. Yours may vary.)

If the first part of this ep hadn't included the sad and depressing scenes at the zoo and wildfire, more people might have actually enjoyed it. And if the cheesy dialogue and treacly, stereotyped characters weren't involved, maybe the network would have actually picked up the show.

Season Five

Here's the new season's thread. Reminder: some of the comments on the second pass may be the same as the first go-round, and some specific points may even be repeated. In Season 5 we see some changes at Rampart:

1) The new base station, enclosed in a dedicated alcove, and

2) Painted lines of various colors on the floor, leading to different areas of the hospital.

I can't think of any other changes this season off the top of my head, but these two were noticeable in the first episode, so they spring to mind.

5.1 The Stewardess

Okay, first things first—about the plane/flight.

~ Remember when people used to dress up to fly? (Yeah, me, either.) But nowadays you see people dressed more like it's a rainy Saturday spent in front of the TV.

~ As people walk through the plane, we see the overhead bins, but there's nothing in them! Which could be because...

~ ...all the luggage was tossed into the hold. (And I do mean *tossed;* bet the airlines wouldn't want anyone to see what that looks like these days.)

~ The flight was from San Francisco and going through to San Diego, so it was an inter-state flight. And yet... it had a lounge. A *lounge,* people!! I've flown quite a bit in the

Watching EMERGENCY! Seasons 4-6

continental US in the past 20 years, and I've never been on a plane with a lounge. Do they even still have them on overseas flights??

Now onto more usual E!-type stuff:

~ I know Roy and Johnny said otherwise, but doesn't it seem as if you'd want to have a heart patient lie down, rather than be sitting up? It seemed awkward.

~ The other paramedic who came with Dwyer, I think he was referred to as Carlson... didn't he look like the firefighter in San Francisco, from the two movies? I can't find a credit for him on this episode, so I don't know for sure, but I thought it looked like him.

~ Roy was all bummed out because no girl ever asked for his phone number. But what about that episode in which he had an admirer who kept calling him, both at home and at the station? (And now that I think about it, how did she get his home number, I wonder?)

~ I know this is fictional TV and all, but it just seems odd that six grown men are all sound asleep at 12:20 in the morning. As if they had an 11pm bedtime or something.

~ Dr. Early did this week's Public Service Announcement, reminding the viewing public that people who have epilepsy are not "mentally deficient." I guess it's easy for me to giggle and think that's silly, but obviously some people did think that, and possibly some still do. But what seizures could possibly have to do with a person's mental capacity is beyond me.

~ ~ ~

So this one begins with Roy and Johnny on a plane, and whoa, let me count the ways in which this whole scenario is odd. Planes that have lounges... passengers who actually dress up to fly (rather than dressing down)... overhead bins that are empty... those funky headphone sets... "stewardesses" walking down the aisle carrying coffee pots... and—drum roll, please!—simply knocking to get admittance into the cockpit.... It's crazy, right?? Also, is it really so easy to access the cargo hold? And yeah, TransCalifornia Airways probably didn't appreciate the whole world seeing how luggage was just jumbled all over the place and tossed helter-skelter. (That was an actual airline at one time. No idea when it went out of business, though.)

Anyhoo, Johnny's relentless, in-your-face pick-up style finally pays off as Stew Sue realizes that as a medical man, the guy who'd been chatting her up for the past half-hour might actually be able to help in an emergency. It's funny/sad that she had to be dubious and question his credentials, as some people (i.e., men) exaggerate their skills. But in this case, obviously Johnny hasn't just been blowing smoke, and at Stew Sue's request he and Roy check on their fellow passenger who is apparently in the midst of having a heart attack. And all they have available is a first-aid kit.

In mid-flight, the captain helps them establish contact with Rampart, and Roy and a crewman go in search of the paramedics' equipment. Meanwhile Johnny does the best he can with little to no equipment, including applying rotating tourniquets (ties, scarves, whatever's around), and listening to the man's chest by laying his ear directly on it. (I bet *that* was a fun scene to film! Even without the well-known blooper, it was probably odd and took a number of takes due to one or the other of the guys busting out laughing.)

Once Johnny explains to Rampart what's going on, Brackett requests a squad and ambulance be sent to the airport to meet the plane when it lands. Oddly enough, guess which squad is dispatched? You guessed it--squad 51. Now, I don't know where all the various paramedic teams are stationed, but what are the odds that squad 51 is the closest one to LAX? Two minutes on Google tells me that 14 is probably closer. (Yeah, I know, maybe the closest unit wasn't available at that time, or squad assignments changed over the years.) Plus, it doesn't even matter which other squad responds, because "our guys" are already on screen.

Anyway, one thing I noticed here... I know the paramedics usually repeat Rampart's orders, to be sure they "read" correctly, but when Johnny is repeating Brackett's orders about D5W TKO, Lidocaine bolus, etc., I could almost see him doing that to impress Sue the Stew.

Did anyone notice the other paramedic, Dwyer's partner? I think Johnny referred to him as Carlson, although the character is uncredited. He looks like the same guy who played the firefighter in the San Francisco movies. No way to confirm or deny, though. Or maybe he was one of Randy's doubles? He sure does look familiar, though, in the couple brief glances we get of him.

The scene of the plane actually landing: is that the same clip of footage we see in the opening segment of the original Hawaii Five-0? Maybe not... I assume one plane landing looks pretty much like another, for the most part. As for the ambulance ride... they sure drive through some strange neighborhoods to get to Rampart, don't they? Of course from the strangely short and curving streets in one or two scenes (see screen pics) it's obvious they were driving on a studio lot.

One odd thing I noticed in this ep... both at the hospital, while standing at the base station, and again at the station in the next scene, Kevin's mic pack is visible both times.

May Fair

Which I find odd, because I assumed that when filming on a studio set like those are, they wouldn't need body mics, they'd have boom mics.

Back to the rescues: The motorcycle accident rescue is good, has enough elements to make it interesting. I like watching the guys determine injuries and rule things out. Also, upon first arrival, watch Cap "shoo" away the neighborhood kids. I've mentioned before that it's fun to watch Cap gesture this or that with his hands, and he does it here with the kids. In any case, I felt bad for the victim, David, when he's told he probably has epilepsy. I did think that Dr. Early gave him the news before sufficient testing had been done for a definite diagnosis, but maybe not, maybe I misjudged the timing. And yeah, also, I'm not a doctor.

So Johnny and Sue have been talking on the phone a lot, just like a couple of 15-year-olds. He was thrilled that *she* asked *him* for his number... unlike that other episode when he was appalled that a girl was calling him. I'd like to think that John Gage has matured a little, but maybe it's just that he likes Sue better than he liked that other girl. However it may be, Johnny can't help but gloat and glow at how compatible the two of them are and how much they have in common. And the kicker? "She *bowls*." A high bar, indeed, for any potential Gage Girl to meet. Finally, after hours of conversation by phone—often in the middle of the night—Johnny's going to take her out on an actual date. Maybe then the guys in the dorm can get some uninterrupted sleep!

However... when something sounds too good to be true, it usually is, and friend John finds this out the hard way. As their next shift begins, he's just started to tell Roy the sad story of his terrible, horrible, no-good, very bad date, but the tones go off and away they go.

The call is for a structure fire at some sort of "plant." Nothing toxic or poisonous, apparently, just fire and flammable materials. (Yeah, "just" that.) And, for a change, nobody's missing in the building! But Cap calls for the foam mixture and we see some nice 'group shots' of everyone working together, both station 51 as well as station 8 and whatever other units were called out.

The excitement comes when Cap attempts to turn off some leaking valve, and even though Chet is hosing him down, the material ignites and explodes and Cap takes a header into a sea of foam. John and Roy go in and fish him out, and Roy manages to get the valve shut off and he and Johnny accompany Cap back out to relative safety and calmness. I wonder if the paramedics have authority to 'order' Cap to get checked out at Rampart? (If *they* don't, I'm sure the Chief does!) In any case, I bet that scene was fun to film, with all that foam and everyone getting soaked. Or maybe it's like a lot of things that look like they might be fun, but really aren't; heck if I know!

Last scene: Johnny finishes telling Roy about his date with Sue. The "perfect" girl with whom he's "so compatible" turns out to be a nightmare, and not someone he wants to see again. Of course, there's a lot of vague talk and stammering and not really saying anything as Johnny implies he told Sue he wasn't interested in her anymore, but we, knowing Johnny, know that just because he *thinks* he got the point across, in reality he probably didn't and he's in as much trouble as he ever was. Poor John... when he gets what he wants, he realizes he doesn't want it anymore. Maybe he should try getting to know women he *doesn't* think he'd like. After all, "if you do what you've always done, you'll get what you've always gotten."

5.2 The Old Engine Cram

I wonder why it's called The Old Engine *Cram?* That doesn't seem to make any sense. And apparently director Dennis Donnelly agreed; he once said he thought the episode title should be The Old Engine *Scam*.

~ A lot of people think the scenes of John and Roy in the show's opening sequence are from this episode. They're not. They were filmed at the same time and location, but are obviously not what we see in the episode.

~ I often times find the writers' choice of words funny. I've previously mentioned how they refer to someone "fouling up" when they make a mistake. In this episode Roy said he hoped the guys at 116s wouldn't "be sore at us." Honestly, I can't remember the last time I heard anyone in real life use the word *sore* to mean *angry*. Hey, maybe it was in 1975.

~ Had to laugh at the dirt-bike rescue, when the guy who led the ambulance in came to see how his buddy was doing. He stood right over the victim, and Roy kind of pushed him away and just flat-out said "You wanna get out of here? Thank you." You tell 'im, Roy!!

~ Those mic packs must be pretty high quality to work in the water like they did. Also, Roy really did look comfortable in the water as he made his way over to the victim. And did you see him being raised back into the chopper? He looked like a kid on a ride at Disney World! It was too cute!

~ Speaking of that rescue, I'm sure they did a lot of takes and took a lot of video, but there were two distinct times that they say, "We'll splint him in the chopper."

~ Johnny told Roy to keep an eye on the incoming waves, but then Johnny was the one who kept saying "watch out, watch out!" A little of Randy's own discomfort in some water situations coming to the fore, perhaps??

~ And, finally, I think Johnny left the Handy-Talkie on the rocks.

~ ~ ~

Aside from the crazy title that doesn't make sense, I do like this episode. At least, I like the rescues in it. Again, not too keen on the running gag storyline. I don't like practical jokes, so maybe that's one reason for my antipathy.

So this one starts at a training site, with a little bit of trash-talk between the guys of 51 and 116s. (Note: once again, Marco rides tailboard as Mike backs up the engine upon arrival.) Then we hear about the dangers of sulfur trioxide, which will apparently burn through clothing and presumably disintegrate human flesh. Good times! Anyway, Station 51 tries to tackle the bad stuff with light water, which has no positive effect, so the training coordinator moves on to something else. Meantime, we see Roy, Johnny, Chet talking with one of the guys from 116s about a prank. Is it just me, or does that fireman, Joe, look like he's older than Cap? Anyway, the next thing to try against the sulfur trioxide is hyex (sp?). It seems to be working okay until one guy carelessly falls into the bone-melting stuff and everything grinds to a halt. How inconsiderate! (By the way, I loved the evil-sounding bubbling noises that we hear from the toxic concoction. Also, what happened to the sulfur trioxide that Station 51 tried to deal with? The chief had more of the stuff released for station 18.) In any case, Roy and Johnny spring into action, and after the victim is practically stripped naked, they get him off to Rampart. This is the part which is similar to the scene in the opening sequence.

May Fair

Next we see Roy and Johnny at Rampart, checking to be sure they didn't get exposed to the sulf-tri themselves. At first I was wondering why Roy was wearing his blue uniform pants instead of the bunkers, but apparently he had the blues on under the bunker pants because we get a glorious pic of him with the bunkers on, but totally unsnapped. (And yes, did you think I *wouldn't* get a pic of *that??*)

I like the rescue of the dirt biker, although I'm not sure the first kid's directions were correct. He said, "Go down to the dirt and turn right." It was *all* dirt, if you ask me, and what do we see Roy do then but turn left, not right. (!!) But luckily they found the injured kid and it was a good rescue. And Roy must have heard our comments about dealing with bystanders, because he told that one guy, "You wanna get out of here? Thanks." (Note that even when telling someone to move, Roy is always polite.)

At Rampart, Dr. Morton checks out a little boy who has flu-like symptoms. The kid's mother wants Morton to just hand over some antibiotics, but the good doctor tells her that antibiotics are ineffective on viral infections. In any case, a few days later the boy is back with some other symptoms, which point to paralytic polio. Of course, Morton feels badly that he didn't pick up on that, and apologizes to Brackett for his lapse, but Brackett says (correctly) that a couple of days' delay couldn't make any difference in the boy's condition, and the fault instead lies at the feet of the mother, who never got her son vaccinated against polio. As Brackett says, the vaccine is "free, painless, and abundant." Call this storyline a micro-PSA.

Meantime, it's evening and a girl and her father stop in at Station 51. The dad wasn't feeling well and instead of driving all the way home, the daughter stops in at the station. Roy escorts the man to the "washroom" (really? it's the second time in a couple days they used that word), anyway, in the midst of the slowest walk ever across the apparatus bay, the man collapses and Roy calls out for 'a little help here.'

I really do like this rescue. Cap immediately calls in a still alarm at the station and Mike, Marco, and Chet immediately go to the squad for equipment and even open and set up some of the stuff. All of this is done without a word, without being asked. Professionalism and brotherhood. One thing does confuse me, though.... After the guys successfully get the dad back in sinus rhythm we see the girl on the phone with her mother, telling her to meet them at Rampart. Then Cap hands her a leisurely cup of coffee and they walk out of the room to... where?? Has the ambulance not arrived yet? And if not, why not, and why is she stopping to drink coffee? Or has the ambulance already been and gone, in which case *why* is the girl still at the station?

Next is the call to meet up with the Coast Guard chopper. This one has me wondering: I always thought—no, actually, I've always *known*—that one of the Coast Guard's primary duties is search and rescue? Surely they have their own people who could have gotten that victim off the rocks? Maybe our Squad 51 guys would need to be on hand to render medical assistance in the chopper, but I refuse to believe the CG doesn't have people who are specifically trained to do exactly what Roy and Johnny did. Anyway, as we mentioned last time around, the water at the rescue site is choppy and rough, Johnny leaves the handy-talkie on the rocks, and Roy looks positively gleeful as he's lifted back into the helicopter. Aside from that, the whole rescue was pretty poorly edited.

Okay, a show of hands: who wouldn't love to be lying on your back, looking up at Roy and Johnny above you saying, "let us do all the work"?? I know I woul3cidoiur doiueotoihbj djfhjherkkmt5522 Oops, sorry, I got distracted there for a minute. *wink*

* * *

> I was always under the impression that the girl and her father were out walking when he became ill. I'm assuming she was waiting for a cab or a friend to take her to the hospital.

Ha, I was under the impression that father and daughter were driving. Especially since the station isn't exactly adjacent to any convenient neighborhoods for an evening stroll. Regardless, there's no reason she couldn't have ridden to Rampart in the ambulance. Or maybe even the squad, which would have followed the ambulance to Rampart.

But I agree that she looked and sounded so calm and casual talking to Cap while the guys were working on her father. You'd think she'd have been a little more agitated or frantic or whatever. I'm pretty sure I wouldn't have been able to sit still in that situation. Especially when seeing two guys send high voltage through my loved one's body, and hearing phrases like "flat-lined" or "no conversion." (Even if you don't know exactly what those phrases mean, you know they don't sound like good things.)

5.3 Election

Well, we have the requisite scene of Johnny talking with food in his mouth. And we also have the requisite stock footage of the guys getting into the squad/engine. In fact, one second Johnny's in the rec room talking to Chet, and he has his usual long, uncombed hair. But the sound of the tones must do something to his hair, like those Barbie dolls of the '70s, whose hair could magically change length, because a second later as he goes out to the squad, Johnny's hair is short and parted on the side. To be precise, it's early-3rd-season short. And then it's long again. (Also, the numbers on their helmets are the old white as they got into the squad, instead of teal.) Another stock footage masterpiece.

The guy who was choking on the beer tab... why didn't they use the Choke Saver, which they utilized in the rescue of the choking frat boy? Instead they tried the forceps, which obviously weren't long enough.

When Dixie, Brackett, and Morton were in Brackett's office, Kel suggested finding the boy Tommy's father and Dixie goes off to do that. Where did she go? She went off-screen to the right, and the office door is to the left.

I do like the final rescue of the injured man on a crane—difficult, complicated and dangerous—but a couple of things about it bother me....

1) I know John Gage is fearless and brave, but why wasn't he tied off up on that crane?? Only two times did I see him clamp his hook/carabiner to secure himself, but most of the time he was crawling around up on that crane—including on the *outside* of it—without any safety measures at all. More proof (to me) that they were really filming only 15-20 feet up, and had a six-inch pad underneath them in case anyone fell, but still....

2) In the season 1 episode Cook's Tour, when a guy threatened suicide by jumping off the crane (and then changed his mind but was too afraid to come back), Roy and Johnny got to him by walking on the *outside* of the crane. The camera-man was obviously inside the triangular part, on the metal-mesh walkway, but the guys were outside. And I

wondered at the time why they didn't just walk to him from inside. Well, they must've learned that lesson, because *this time,* that's what they did: walked to the trapped man on the inside.

3) This crane rescue is an example of something I've wondered about before: why did it have to be the paramedics who rescued that guy on the crane? There's no way they could do anything for him medically while he was up there, and all the firefighters know enough basic medical stuff to secure an injured victim until they can get to more help, so Chet and Marco could probably have done exactly what the paramedics did. So why risk the highly-trained guys on a dangerous rescue that (most likely) any firefighter could do?

(Yeah, yeah, someone's going to say that Roy and Johnny can assess the injuries, but there's nothing they could do about it up there, so the assessment could just as easily be done on the ground, I would think. Plus, if something happened to one of them, they'd be one paramedic short.)

~ ~ ~

Alternate title for this episode: "Good Man." (Get it?)

Another day, another scene of Johnny talking with his mouth full. Twice, I think. So the guys are thinking about someone from Station 51 running for a spot on the County Firemen Benefit and Welfare Association. Before he knows it, Roy's been nominated... to which he responds, "But— but— but." (And he needs his wife's permission to do this... why??) The guys mention that the suitable candidate has to have enthusiasm, drive, imagination, a strong sense of responsibility, and ability to communicate with people, etc. It's possible that Johnny thinks they're describing *him*, which is why it's funny to see his balloon deflate when

Marco nominates Roy for the opening. Eventually, goaded by Chet (really, Johnny, when will you learn not to listen to Chester B??), Johnny decides to run also. He's afraid Roy will be upset at this news, but Roy gladly offers to drop out and let Johnny run unopposed, but Gage doesn't want that, so apparently they both stay in the race. (Hmmm, I think there's an episode of Andy Griffith with a very similar storyline when Barney decides to run for Sheriff.) In any case, the two guys spend a good part of the episode telling each other that this silly election (to a supposedly very important role, which we've never heard a single word about—ever) is not going to come between them and affect their friendship or partnership. Yeah, heard that one before!

First rescue is to the guy whose arm is stuck in the pipe from his washing machine. The guys come up with a good idea, to insert a small tube and blow air in to break the suction, but why didn't they just put the wire (unbent clothes hanger) *inside* the tube? The tube looked like it was wide enough to accommodate the hanger as well as 'air.' Am I missing some piece of information that makes that plan a bad idea? Anyway, after that "rescue," the big dude, Clyde, accidentally aspirates a beer-can tab and has trouble breathing. When Cap returns to the kitchen and is apprised of the situation, he gets on the HT and tells the guys of the engine to bring in the O2, "on the double." And guess what? We never see them bring it. The scene in the kitchen continues for a full minute, including a conversation with Rampart, and still no O2. (Also, it looks like Cap speaks into different parts of the HT to talk to the Engine and to LA. What's up with that?)

Last time around, I wondered why they didn't use the same tool on Clyde that they used on the frat boy choking on the raw liver, because the forceps they try obviously don't cut it. Also, at the hospital, I found two things to note, one is interesting and the other just plain funny. Interesting: you know how they sometimes put the O2 canister between the victim's legs during transport? This time they put it on a pillow that was between Clyde's legs. Not sure I've seen that before. Funny: watch when Joe is putting in the scope to look down Clyde's throat... it looks like he's putting it into his shoulder, because obviously in real life it is *not* going in his throat.

Elsewhere at Rampart, there's another instance of E!-magic time distortion. Dixie takes a phone call asking if Pediatrics can send some of their "overflow" patients to the ED; she consults Morton and the two of them decide it's OK, so she says "we'll find room," and hangs up. As she does so, Morton says "I'll go over and see what they have." He walks to the end of the hall (the admitting desk) and ¡voila!, the kids from Peds are already there! I wish I could get things to work like that for me.

Speaking of time distortion... we see the squad back into the station, next to the *Crown* engine. It's not just a quick glance, but quite an extended scene, with the old engine clearly visible. No sooner do the guys get out of the squad and have a 10-second conversation than the tones go off and they're off again. Except when they drive out of the station, it's the Ward-LaFrance in the bay next to them. Hey, more E! magic!! (More about stock footage in a bit.)

So a lot of people love the sculpting rescue. I think it's OK, mainly I love the dirty and/or disgusted looks that Roy and Johnny give the artist. (Maybe Johnny doesn't like her because she reminds him of a certain deputy he once dated. *wink*) Anyway, I bet cutting that plaster-y stuff really ruined their scissors. I wonder if they have to buy their own instruments, or if the County or Rampart provides them? By the way, I think the "victim" was wearing two pairs of boxers. For modesty's sake, I'm sure.

At Rampart, Morton takes charge of a boy who's in the (crowded) waiting area and who suddenly breaks out in hysterical yelling. This is further proof, by the way, that the squeaky wheel does get the grease at Rampart. Anyway, Brackett suggests that Dixie track down the boy's father, since the mother is acting squirrelly and being somewhat evasive. "Alert the authorities, see if you can find the father." Okay, and she's supposed to do that *how??* Just call the cops and say, "Hey, I'm looking for Tommy Lawson's father. All I know about him is that he and his wife are probably divorced." Interesting how that works, huh? Also, I know I mentioned this last time, but how does Dixie leave Brackett's office? She doesn't go out the office door that leads into the Rampart hallway. I think Julie just walks right off the set, stage right.

The final rescue, on the crane, was good. A few things about it bother me, though. (**Note:** this part is more or less copied from my last comment on this episode.)

1) I know John Gage is fearless and brave, but why wasn't he tied off up on that crane?? Only two times did I see him clamp his hook/carabiner to secure himself, but most of the time he was crawling around up on that crane—including on the *outside* of it—without any safety measures at all. More proof (to me) that they were really filming only 15-20 feet up, and had a six-inch pad underneath them in case anyone fell, but still....

2) In the season 1 episode Cook's Tour, when a guy threatened suicide by jumping off the crane (and then changed his mind but was too afraid to come back), Roy and Johnny got to him by walking on the *outside* of the crane. The camera-man was obviously inside the triangular part, on the metal-mesh walkway, but the guys were outside. And I wondered at the time why they didn't just walk to him from inside. Well, they must've learned that lesson, because *this*

time, that's what they did: walked to the trapped man on the inside.

3) This crane rescue is an example of something I've wondered about before: why did it have to be the paramedics who rescued that guy on the crane? There's no way they could do anything for him medically while he was up there, and all the firefighters know enough basic medical stuff to secure an injured victim until they can get to more help, so Chet and Marco could probably have done exactly what the paramedics did. So why risk the highly-trained guys on a dangerous rescue that (most likely) any firefighter could do?

Yeah, yeah, someone's going to say that Roy and Johnny can assess the injuries, but there's nothing they could do about it up there, so the assessment could just as easily be done on the ground, I would think. Plus, if something happened to one of them, they'd be one paramedic short. **End of repeated section.**

Also, I noticed that Cap put on a safety belt as they were going up in the elevator. Did he know he'd have to go help? And again, why not Chet and/or Marco?

Oh yeah, about the stock footage. I'm repeating what I said last time:

We have the requisite stock footage of the guys getting into the squad/engine. In fact, one second Johnny's in the rec room talking to Chet, and he has his usual long, uncombed hair. But the sound of the tones must do something to his hair, like those Barbie dolls of the '70s, whose hair could magically change length, because a second later as he went out to the squad, Johnny's hair was short and parted on the side. To be precise, it was early-3rd-season short. And then it was long again. (Also, the numbers on their helmets were the old white as they got into the squad, instead of teal.)

* * *

> but why didn't they just put the wire (unbent clothes hanger) inside the tube? The tube looked like it was wide enough to accommodate the hanger

It would impede airflow -- that's my assumption.

Oops, I guess I misspoke, I meant to say that the tube looked like it was wide enough for the hanger and also airflow around it. Or they could have just conveniently found some tubing with a little wider diameter. After all, with that old wire coat hanger on the outside, they could have inadvertently given that guy a nice long arm-scrape that could get infected. Heck, who knows, the following week Arnie might have shown up at Rampart with a nasty case of tetanus.

> I get what the writers were doing with the surprise twist at the end, but are the boys really so dumb that they never considered that other stations were putting forward candidates too?

Yeah, this is another example of stupid television (il)logic: acting as if these characters are not only the stars of the show, but the only people of significance in the universe. *Other* candidates? Pshaw! Irrelevant. People to run the unseen 90% of Rampart, a large county hospital? Insignificant, and totally inconsequential. Paramedics other than those at Station 51? Competent enough, but hardly worthy enough to rate a mention, much less compare to the blindingly stellar guys of squad 51. Heck, other firemen? Paltry substitutes who only exist to complement and serve alongside our intrepid heroes of Station 51. So *of course* it didn't occur to John or Roy that someone else could win. Especially by a landslide.

> I think Julie just walked right off the set, stage right.

> Dixie is a woman of great power. Doors? She doesn't need no stinkin' doors!

Ha, I forgot, she's Dixie Friggin' McCall. Before there was MacGyver, before there was Walker, before there was Jack Bauer, there was Dixie McCall. You're right, she don't need no stinkin' door.

5.4 Equipment

Another minor "issues" episode. I wish the theme had been carried out farther into the episode instead of just relating to that first call. But that rescue and scene was good.

~ Episode directed by Kevin Tighe. Interestingly, a couple of the episodes he directed (the ones we've seen so far) have specifically filmed scenes at "real" stations--Station 127 filling in for Station 51, and this time Station 8. These "real locations" could be totally coincidental, and those decisions made above Kevin's pay-grade, or they could be decisions he specifically arranged; obviously I have no way of knowing which is true. But I find the use of real stations to be both interesting and admirable.

~ I like Stoney. He's a good character, and I wish we'd seen him again in other episodes. Hmm, I wonder... if a paramedic (John) can sub at another station as a firefighter, I wonder if a captain (Stone) can sub somewhere as a paramedic?? I don't see why not.

~ I wonder how the other LACoFD paramedics would feel if they heard Brackett refer to Gage and "Stoney" as "two of the best paramedics we ever trained." Kind of like chopped liver, I bet, huh??

~ After that first rescue, as the heart victim was being transported to Rampart, I had to chuckle--we saw the ambulance rushing to the hospital, being followed by a squad, and yet neither one was carrying anyone we know.

~ Neither Squad 8 nor Squad 39 are listed on the Rescue Squad Status Board at Rampart. And yet 39s took the heart attack victim there.

~ When the ambulance delivers the guy to the hospital, we hear someone (sounds like Roy, but can't be) say "Number 4," as in Treatment 4, maybe?? But after working on the guy, Brackett comes out of Treatment 1. So I don't know what that Number 4 business was all about.

~ At the "water flow alarm," when the door next to Chet blew out, all I could think was, "stunt guys must thank heaven that so many empty cardboard boxes are always around for them to land on." Not just on this show, but on TV in general, anytime someone gets thrown off a building or blown across a warehouse, there's always a convenient pile of cardboard boxes conveniently stacked in just the right place.

~ Also, as soon as that one door explodes, Cap calls the building "fully involved." We only saw a few flames come out the door, and yet... fully involved. Good thing Marco was there to wash down poor Chet. Er, I mean "stunt-Chet," as the real Chet was bone dry when he was carried out to the street.

~ Speaking of Chet, I thought it seemed odd that they were thinking of having a "dinner or something" for him when he got back from being in the hospital. Not that it's a bad idea, or even it being odd that Johnny suggested it, but Chet wasn't really even hurt in the first place. Also, since Kevin was directing, I wonder if that was really him under the squad, or someone else to give the impression of being him? (Yeah, I know, I think tooooo much!!)

~ ~ ~

(Full disclosure: this incorporates some of my comments from last time... plus new ones.)

I like this episode, it's another minor "issues" episode. I wish the theme had been carried out farther into the episode instead of just relating to that first call. At the very end, Stoney again references having more paramedic equipment available, but it would only be helpful to *him*, who's already certified as a paramedic and authorized to use it. Other FFs wouldn't be able to do anything with most of that equipment.

This episode was directed by Kevin, and once again we see some interesting camera angles. Also, a couple of the episodes he's directed have specifically filmed scenes at "real" stations—Station 127, when we see the parking area behind 'Station 51,' and this time Station 8. Filming at these "real locations" could be totally coincidental, and not Kevin's doing (I don't know), but I find the use of real stations to be both interesting and admirable.

So Stoney mentions that "five weeks from Tuesday I'll be married." Does that mean that he's going to get married on a Tuesday? That seems weird. Anyway, I like that we see Stoney both at the beginning and at the end of this episode. But now I'm wondering... if a paramedic (John) can sub at another station as a firefighter, I wonder if a captain (Stone) can sub somewhere as a paramedic?? I don't see why not.

Watching EMERGENCY! Seasons 4-6

Anyone notice that Brackett refers to Gage and Stoney as "two of the best paramedics we ever trained"? Hmm, how does that make the other paramedics feel, if they maybe overheard that comment?? At the construction site scene, I think Stoney responds to Brackett "10-4, LA," instead of "10-4, Rampart." That doesn't seem right; I wonder why he does that? Also, I think this first rescue is kind of disjointed in the time department. I don't know why these things strike me, but sun and shadows we see tell me that they took quite a bit of time filming this sequence, and not always in the order in which we saw it.

As we saw the ambulance rushing this guy to the hospital, being followed by a squad, it occurred to me that neither vehicle was carrying anyone we know. Also, I noticed that neither Squad 8 nor Squad 39 are listed on the Rescue Squad Status Board at Rampart, and yet 39s took the heart attack victim there. I assume Squad 8 would as well.

Did anyone notice this?? When the ambulance delivers the guy to the hospital, we hear someone (sounds like Roy, but can't be) say "Number 4," as in Treatment 4?? It sure does sound like Kevin/Roy; maybe he dubbed in a voice. Anyway, after working on the guy, Brackett comes out of Treatment 1. So I don't know what that Number 4 was all about.

On the next call for 51, after driving through a horrible back-lot scene, we see a building that shows no outward sign of fire, but suddenly blows poor Chet off his feet and into the requisite pile of cardboard boxes. And even though there aren't any flames—anywhere—I love how Mike comes rushing over and hoses Chet down. Oddly, Chet's bone-dry when they get him out to the street. (And I hope someone retrieved his helmet, which flew off his head and landed on the stairs of the building.)

May Fair

Speaking of Chet, I still think it's odd that they're thinking of having a "dinner or something" to welcome him back to work after being in the hospital. Not that the idea is bad, or that it's odd that Johnny suggests it, but Chet wasn't really even hurt in the first place; they probably only kept him at Rampart overnight for observation, so dinner seems like overkill.

At Rampart, Brackett says they're expecting one of the squads to bring in a man with collapsed lung, and "ETA is five minutes." More E! time distortion here, because less than *twenty seconds later,* the man is brought in. So on this show, not only does one ketchup-packet of blood equal a severed artery, but twenty seconds is the equivalent of five or more minutes.

Also, for those who now notice clothing and ties (and you know who you are!), note what Brackett is wearing when he treats the full arrest. Then note what he's wearing the next day, when he tells Johnny that the guy died. Yep, same shirt and tie. Maybe it was a busy night and he didn't get a chance to go home and change? Heaven knows that can happen if you're one of only three doctors who work at such a large hospital.

By the way, a few episodes ago Johnny had trouble with his stethoscope in the treatment room. This time, with the collapsed lung guy, Morton has trouble with his rubber gloves.

We do see Stoney again in the middle of this episode, with the boy who fell and couldn't move his legs, and again at the fireworks-factory fire. One thing that occurred to me during this scene with the boy: I know the boy's mother is right there, but shouldn't the paramedics ask her if they can treat the boy (IV, etc.)? I realize her permission is implied, but for legal reasons, I'd think they would have to actually ask the parent or guardian.

The fire at the fireworks factory is a mass of stock footage and awkward moments, including a blink-and-you'll-miss-it glimpse of the Kiddy Time Toy Factory. And Roy gets hurt in an explosion and ends up at Rampart. Hmm, this seems to be sort of a trend when Randy or Kevin direct an episode: their characters end up in the hospital.

A few quick notes:

~ It's odd (for me, anyway) to see some random oil pumps at work as Station 51 arrives at the scene of the final fire. I always think of most oil as coming from Texas, and being in the middle of nowhere rather than in populated industrial areas.

~ At the end when Johnny visits Roy in the hospital and brings him a box, does anyone find it unusual that Roy has Johnny unwrap the box in the hospital? And that Johnny does it while it's in Roy's lap?? That's scene is nothing but a certain kind of fanfic waiting to happen, if you ask me.

~ We've noticed the stalker blue Chevy truck before, but now there's another vehicle to add to the list: in this episode, at least three times, there's a wood-paneled station wagon that seems to lurk and make its presence felt. I think I got one or two screen-pics of it.

~ **Edit:** I noticed that while subbing at 8s, Johnny's wearing his paramedic holster, even though he's subbing as a fireman. Interestingly, Stoney, however, is *not* wearing a holster.

5.5 The Inspection

First things first (dun-dun-*dun*): Roy's hair. (Extremely sad/unhappy face here)

Thank you. We now return you to your regularly-scheduled commentary.

~ When Squad 51 calls Rampart and the buzzer sounds at the base station, Brackett is leaning over a nurse at the nurse's station... and he has his hand on her back. Maybe that was okay back in the day, but I doubt too many male bosses do that anymore.

~ Okay, we have another nominee for the Stupid Wife award. A while back it was the PTSD military guy's wife who hesitated to make a life-or-death decision for her husband to have necessary surgery because, you know, "I'm just a woman." ***Grrr*** Well, in this episode the heart transplant guy's wife is right up there (or down there?). Apparently his wife was "against" him having the transplant, and he and the doctor had to "talk her into it." Whiskey tango foxtrot!!! Again, the hubby is going to **D.I.E.** without the procedure, and the woman has to be talked into it?? I'm not sure which is more stupid: the wife as she was written, or that the writer actually wrote her that way. *head/desk*

~ Brackett tells the wife that the heart is a pump, "nothing more, nothing less." In the very next scene, Roy tells Johnny that the Chief's visit is nothing but a simple inspection, "no more, no less." Methinks the writer got that phrase stuck in his head and it got put into two scenes (which ran back-to-back).

~ I got a kick out of them being called out to "114 East Western." Yeah, I've been there, passed it on my way to 513 North Southern.

Watching EMERGENCY! Seasons 4-6

~ I always chuckle when the squad and engine turn onto that winding dirt road, like they did in this ep (and they'll do it again), and the engine supposedly hits the air-horn. Why would they need the air-horn on lonely country dirt roads? The siren or sounds of the diesel engines aren't enough to alert bystanders?

~ "Lucky" the parachutist didn't want them to cut his expensive harness, so they didn't. But they also didn't retrieve the harness, either, but left it up there. So what was the point of "saving" it??

~ At the scene of the accident in the dry riverbed (is that what it is?), did anyone think that scene of Johnny cutting himself was suspicious?? It seemed very odd. We see Johnny very plainly using the Ajax tool on the crashed car and helping to get the car door open. Suddenly the focus moves to Roy and we see "Johnny" (note the quotes) only from the back. Or rather, we see someone with dark hair and wearing a Gage turnout coat, from the back. A sudden cry of pain, and we see two hands, one of which is bloody. Roy calls for the Cap, Cap makes some comment about wearing gloves, and we see the dark-haired person (from behind) being led away out of sight. Then Roy and the others extract the victim, and with Mike's help, and Chet's, Roy takes care of him. I wonder if maybe Randy might have gotten slightly injured during filming, and they hurriedly re-worked the script to film around his being gone. They could have added that one scene, of Cap 'bandaging' Johnny's hand, later (shadows were different).

Anyway, I thought it was odd that we didn't actually "see" Johnny once he supposedly cut his hand.

~ ~ ~

May Fair

The Roypadour!! Too funny!! Here's what I said last time about it:

"First things first (dun-dun-dun): Roy's hair."

I think that pretty much says it all. Especially after he looked so good in Equipment.

Anyhoo. Other than Roy's hair, I too like this one. And it's worth noting that it was Boot's last appearance. He died a few months after this episode aired. (Maybe that's why he was whining and hiding under the engine??)

Interesting note: The heart-transplant patient's name was Fenady (Fenaday?). The episode was directed by George Fenady. Coincidence? Discuss.

Speaking of that heart transplant storyline.... it provides us with another nominee for the Stupid Wife award. A while back it was the army vet's wife who hesitated to make a life-or-death decision for her husband to have necessary surgery because, you know, "I'm just a woman." Well, in this episode Mrs. Fenady is giving the army wife a run for her money. Apparently the wife was "against" him having the transplant to begin with, and he and the doctor had to "talk her into it." Whiskey tango foxtrot, what kind of a wife is that!!! Again, the hubby is 100% guaranteed to **DIE** without the surgery, and the woman has to be *talked into it*?? Personally I think Brackett showed great restraint in not literally smacking some sense into her.

Oh and yes, Mr. Fenady's pants could probably cause anyone's heart to stop. Yikes!

Later, after the guys take such pains to keep the squad clean because they're expecting an inspection, we see Roy and Johnny start out on a call and get splashed with some muddy water. Anyone notice that Roy's window was suddenly closed? It's rolled down *every. other. time* we see them in the squad, but in this one scene it's closed and you can see the water that gets splashed on it as he looks in the rear-view mirror. (Also, there's another glimpse of the blue Chevy truck right before they hit the waterworks. The Wily Wagon might be there too, but I couldn't tell if that's what it was.)

Next comes the parachutist on the transformer, and Wolfman Jack to boot. I remember hearing about him way back in the day. It's a good rescue, but obviously it's not Randy and Kevin way up there (look carefully). Also, Lucky made a big deal about not cutting his expensive harness, yet once they unhook him and bring him down, they left his precious harness hanging on the tower—way to "save" the equipment, right? By the way, when Chet was getting ready to ride in Wolfman Jack's radio station van, they left the tripod on the roof.

At Rampart, Brackett is treating a man who was bitten by a dog. Kel voices his concerned that they be able to locate the dog so the man won't have to get rabies shots, and as it turns out, the patient is a veterinarian, and knows the dog—and its health—very well. It's a very pleasant and friendly conversation between the vet and Dr. Brackett (and Dixie, too), and for some reason—maybe the change of pace—it just really sits well with me. Nice to get a break from the heavy drama we usually see in the treatment rooms.

Finally we get to the last rescue, the car overturned in the waterway. This is where Johnny cuts his hand... probably because I'm betting that *Randy* cut *his* hand. Here's what I wrote last time: We see Johnny very plainly using the Ajax tool and helping to get the car door open. Suddenly the focus moves to Roy and we see "Johnny" (note the quotes) only from the back. Or rather, we see someone with dark hair and wearing a Gage turnout coat, from the back. A sudden cry of pain, and we see two hands, one of which is bloody. Roy calls for the Cap, Cap makes some comment about gloves, and we see the dark-haired person (from behind) being led away out of sight. Then Roy and the others extract the victim, and with Mike's help, and Chet's, Roy takes care of him. I wonder if maybe Randy might have gotten slightly injured during filming, and they hurriedly re-worked the script to film around his being gone. They could have added that one scene, of Cap 'bandaging' Johnny's hand, later (shadows were different).

Anyway, as for the victim, it was interesting to see the doctors keep the anti-shock pants on him during a lot of his testing. But I have to wonder: when Brackett begins letting the air out of the trousers, he warns Paul that some of the pain might return. And yet it looks like he lets the air out at a pretty fast clip. Why doesn't he do it very gradually?

* * *

Or is it Georg Fenady?

Yikes, I think you're right. Apologies to Mr. Fenady for misspelling his first name. But I thought the same/similar name for the character was interesting, especially after the episode The Promise which has a woman named Edna Self. People usually note the similarity of her name and that of show producer Edwin Self. Maybe just some writerly humor? Implying that Edwin Self needs to make friends, like Edna, and Georg Fenady needs to have more heart?? (Just kidding, of course!)

Interesting about the multiple mentions of "pictures" in that one scene at Rampart, some of which meant X-rays and some didn't; I hadn't noticed that. (Do hospital personnel still refer to X-rays as pictures??) One thing I did notice in this episode is that Brackett tells Mrs. Fenady that the heart is simply a pump, "nothing more, nothing less." In the very next scene, Roy tells Johnny that the Chief's impending visit is nothing but a standard inspection, "no more, no less." Kind of unusual to have such a phrase used twice in such quick succession like that, I thought.

> The guy racing against Paul looked about twenty years older than he was. Also he was apparently racing some sort of motor trike against Paul's muscle car.

Yeah, I thought the different types of vehicles being raced was pretty odd. I confess I know nothing about drag-racing or the types of vehicles used, but that just didn't seem probable or likely to me. In one scene I was kind of distracted by the older guy's tattoo(s). One on his arm looked a little like the shape of Australia, but I finally figured out it was of a whale of some sort. Not really as macho as I'd expect, but then, he had plenty of other ink to prove his machismo.

5.6 The Indirect Method

I sort of dreaded watching this episode because of, well, you know—*her*. But I forced myself to watch, and you know what? At first I kind of liked her. She came in in a no-nonsense way, very reasonable, etc. I understand the quibble the paramedics had with her about her handling the old lady with the gun, but their "talking" method didn't seem to be having much effect, either. In the "call review" scene at the day-room table, I even liked how she started out. She said, "I don't expect any special treatment, but I'd also appreciate no special obstacles." (Or words to that effect.) I thought that was very rational and reasonable. Okay, so far, so good. But then she pushed it a little... asking with a little huff if she could act on her own initiative. That's when Roy puts on his Senior Paramedic hat and tells her, in no uncertain terms, **"NO."** (Really, does she not know the meaning of the word *trainee*??)

~ Had to laugh, when Karen talked the old woman down, Roy opened the door and called the ambulance attendants in.... but nobody took the woman's gun away from her. Wouldn't you want to do that *first??*

~ This ep was written by Mike Norell, but I kind of cringed at the heart-attack scene on the sidewalk. There was almost an implication that women were too weak to give CPR for an extended period of time, and also that they might simply lose interest and give up.

~ When Roy was talking to Karen next to the squad and the tones went off, the driver's side door was locked and he had to reach in to unlock it.

~ Am I imagining things or did Johnny/Randy get his bangs trimmed? He doesn't have to 'part the curtain' in order to see anymore.

~ The house fire (final big scene)... I feel like this whole rescue scene was poorly done from start to finish. I don't think a firefighter would ever step out a window directly onto an unsecured ladder (and not even a FD ladder, at that). Roy would have stepped out onto the lower-floor roof first and seen to it that the ladder was secure before anything else happened. Especially with that power line being so close. Then after he's electrocuted it's funny because you can visibly see Kevin breathing when he's supposed to be not breathing, non-responsive, etc. And as Karen is getting ready to defibrillate him, Marco is making a mess of trying to get the oxygen mask hooked up (he finally drops it in disgust, only to pick it up again a moment later).

~ Meanwhile, in the upstairs bedroom, Johnny's still holding Aunt Tilly. Another engine arrives and he calls to them, "over here, bring a ladder," etc. The problem here is that he looks to the *right* when he yells this, and then the guys with the ladder approach from his *left*. And Cap... when have we ever known Cap to be so clueless about what was going on with his own crew? I mean, this was a two-story house, not the Taj Mahal. I know he was the 'officer in charge' and directing all the action, but how hard is it to keep up with five other guys? Especially when two of them are right in the front yard, in full view??

~ ~ ~

Okay, so another airing of the episode that probably is on a lot of peoples' "least favorite" lists. Here's what I said last time around:

> I sort of dreaded watching this episode because of, well, you know--*her*. But I forced myself to watch, and you know what? At first I kind of liked her. She came in in a no-nonsense way, very reasonable, etc. I understand the quibble the guys had with her about her handling the old lady with the gun, but their "talking" method didn't seem to be having much effect, either. In the "call review" scene at the rec-room table, I even liked how she started out. She said "I don't expect any special treatment, but I'd also appreciate no special obstacles." (Or words to that effect.) I thought that was very rational and reasonable. Okay, so far, so good. But then she pushed it a little... asking with a little huff if she could act on her own initiative. That's when Roy puts on his Senior Paramedic hat and tells her, in no uncertain terms, **"NO."** (Really, does she not know the meaning of the word *trainee*??)

May Fair

Yeah, I still feel that way, except this time when I watched it I felt less *indignation* and more... *resignation.* The sort of feeling that's indicated by a slumping your shoulders, letting your head drop, and saying "Uggggggghhhhhh." You know, like every thirteen-year-old everywhere does when told they have to take the trash out or look after their younger sibling for an hour. Anyway, not only was I less bothered by Karen (maybe I'm getting immune to it), but I was also, I hate to admit, more annoyed with Mike Norell, who wrote this one. Seriously, has this show ever featured a "major" female guest character who was *not* totally annoying or just plain stupid? Mike, Mike, I had hoped you were better than that.

One part of the episode I did skip entirely was Chet's idiotic fake aneurysm act. I do agree with Karen that it was stupid and demeaning. Later on, when she asks Johnny and Roy if that's the standard initiation for a new guy, Johnny starts to say something about, "when a new guy arrives at the station...," but Roy cuts him off. "No," he says simply. "It's not our standard initiation." Thank you, Roy, for not treating her like an idiot. I know firehouses are known for their pranks and perhaps many do have an initiation for a "new guy," but lying to her and telling her that that's what this was... that would not have been smart.

On the plus side.... anyone else get a kick out of hearing Roy tell Cap "we're cool now." Have Johnny say that? Sure. Chet? Absolutely. But to hear it from Roy is just funny. I wonder if Norell wrote that line for him?? Also, when they arrive back at the station after that first run and the engine's gone, I wonder if those were (supposedly) skin-mags on the table, and that's why Johnny cleans them up and put them aside so hurriedly? I doubt that was the intent of that scene, but it's always the vibe I get when I see it.

The rescue of the guy who jumped out the window after changing his mind about suicide... I don't really feel that what Karen did (the observation about the man's pupils) was totally her fault. I wouldn't be surprised if that difference in dilation would be easy to miss, for anyone. When she tells the pupil status to Roy, Johnny gets a look on his face like he already knows that's not right, but I don't know how he could possibly know that off the top of his head. Later, Dr. Early calls it a "mix-up" on the pupillary reaction, when it was actually more of a correction. (But again, I'm not a doctor, nor do I play one on TV.)

After that we see everyone eating (or have just finished) lunch at the station. At the sink, Chet again acts like an idiot, and Johnny, thankfully, doesn't want to get into that conversation right at that moment because I bet Karen could hear them if she put her mind to it. Usually Chet is written as being goofy but funny, and deep down he has a good heart, but again, in this episode, Mike Norell sort of butchered Chet's character to make him out to be pretty much insufferable. (Incidentally, the background audio behind the Chet-and-Johnny convo is interesting; based on that audio, you'd think they were in a huge cafeteria with 100 people instead of a fire station with just four other guys. I'm not counting Karen in that number because she wasn't talking to anyone at all.)

Back at Rampart, the gun-totin' grandma finally gets to visit with her hubby, and after mildly flirting with Dr. Brackett, she asks the good doctor if she can be alone with her husband so they can hold hands, which was kind of sweet. But I'm not sure: does the man himself say more than five words of dialogue in the entire episode? Oh, another thought about this rescue: back at the gun-totin' grandma's house, after Karen asks the wife if he has a history of heart trouble, Johnny shoots her one of Those Looks. I know they try not to stress out victims or their families, but how can they learn if the man has a history of heart trouble if they don't, you know, *ask* if he has a history of heart trouble?

From here the episode really goes downhill, fast. First is the heart attack guy on the street. After doing chest compressions for a while, Karen seems to just sort of gives up, and there's a definite implication that a woman can't effectively do CPR for extended periods of time. Also, it looks like she's doing the compressions awfully fast; when Johnny takes over for her, he doesn't do them as fast as she did.

And that leaves us with the final rescue, the house fire with "someone left inside!" First, at the station, Roy gives Karen the standard Senior Paramedic pep-talk. Usually that talk ends with him saying, "we'll keep an eye on you, and we'll let you know when you're ready to do it on your own." But this time she asks Roy when she'll know she can do it on her own. His response: "When you have to." A little foreshadowing there, perhaps???

In any case, there's so much that's wrong with the final rescue that I don't want to rehash it at the moment. Characters acting out-of-character, poor editing, things that just don't make sense.... not gonna go there right now. But I do wonder if Cap's method of firefighting actually worked: go into a fully-engulfed room, spray around for five seconds, then close the door and let the steam put out the fire. It sounds good in theory, but I have the feeling it's not quite as successful in real life.

Quick bits:

~ They didn't give Karen a helmet to wear in the squad. If she was going to eventually ride as a paramedic in an LACoFD squad, she'd need one when she begins doing that.

~ At the final house fire, as Roy and Johnny are getting their air masks on, Johnny bends down and picks something up and gives it to Roy (he has to poke him a couple of times to get his attention). It looks like Roy's watch.

~ When the guys have to go out a window with a victim, *why* don't they just tear down the curtains first, instead of getting tangled in them??

~ Stoker told the captain of another engine that the hydrant was dry and he'd have to go to another hydrant. How is that possible? I thought hydrants were all connected to the main water system. To me, that's the point of a fire hydrant: to have access to water in the city system.

~ ETA: we all know how often we see Johnny with food in his mouth (actually, we see the *food* in his *mouth*--ugh). But we rarely see Roy eat, and even when he 'eats,' it's rarely more than a bite.

5.7 Pressure 165

Kind of a so-so episode, all the way around. Nothing to write home about, I don't think.

At the pressure chamber thing, I wish more had been explained. Yeah, I understand the basics of "the bends," but what are the tables they were talking about? Is the table based on the patient's weight? Shouldn't the change in pressure have been drawn out longer, to allow those inside the chamber to adjust gradually? (Note: I'm *not* looking for answers here; I'm just giving examples of questions that viewers might have.)

I didn't see a credit for that Doctor Scott, who was with Johnny in the chamber. He didn't look like an actor playing a doctor... he sort of really looked and acted like a doctor.

May Fair

I wonder if there was any particular reason that Randy (Johnny) went into the chamber. It wasn't a heights-related thing (favoring Randy) and it wasn't a water thing (favoring Kevin), so I wonder if either one had strong feelings one way or the other about doing it. Or not doing it.

Did anyone notice the two orderlies who wheeled Freddie the drug-boy to surgery? A black guy and a small blond guy with scruffy beard. In the very next scene, as surgery on Freddie is about to start, we see some medical types in the surgical viewing room. The *same two* guys are there, dressed as residents/interns, or whoever it is who watches surgeries. (I honestly doubt that orderlies would be allowed to do that.) I guess this show was determined to get its money's worth out of their extras.

~ ~ ~

So, whereas in the first season there was an episode in which Roy was given grief about his so-called "cooking," this time Johnny's the one in the culinary hot-seat. Apparently his repertoire consists of only hot dogs or hamburgers. Hmmm, let's do the math: if Johnny cooks only every fifth (or sixth?) shift, and they work only two or three shifts per week, then it's likely at least two weeks between his meals. I don't think too many people would complain about having hot dogs or hamburgers every couple of weeks, do you?? (Assuming, of course, that none of the other guys on the shift also make burgers 'n' dogs, though.)

First call is to the hyperbaric chamber. For what it's worth, the footage of Roy and Johnny getting into the chopper, taking off, and flying over the water to Catalina is all the same footage from The Old Engine Cram, when they had to rescue the guy off Catalina. Anyway, they meet up with Dr. Scott, who was supposedly at some seminar conveniently nearby. (Although it looked more like he'd been playing squash or tennis, if you ask me.) Anyhoo, does anyone know why the doctor and Johnny have to take off their shoes when they entered the chamber? I get why they took off their shirts, as it got very warm in there, but did that apply to the feet, as well?? I rather doubt it, but.... Maybe it's for comfort, in case their feet swell a little when it gets really warm.

I did notice the victim had quite a Carpet of Virility going on. Also, I looked up "bottom time." No, it's nothing kinky, S&M-related... just means time spent at depth, not including any time during ascent or descent.

Meanwhile, back at the ranch.... er, I mean the station: the squad had gotten called out before Johnny could make his burgers for lunch. Upon their return to the station, Chet informs Johnny that "Squad 116 came over" and picked up Johnny's lunch duty, the result of which was some sort of yummy meatloaf. (Pardon a moment, I had to check to be sure there's not an injunction against using the words "yummy" and "meatloaf" in the same sentence.) Now really, how often do guys of one squad "stop by" another station and just volunteer to cook?? How often did John and Roy ever do that, do you think??? (Yeah, me, either.) Anyway, in the ensuing jibe-fest, Mike says something that Johnny declares 'profound,' and Cap comes up with a line worthy of MASH: "Let's not have any profundity around here; it'll ruin our image." Ha-ha, good one, Cap!!

Next Cap sends the squad guys (who probably missed lunch altogether, by the way) out to test some new hydrants, and possibly come up with some footage to add to a future blooper reel. *wink* On their travels they see what they believe is a structure fire, but it's only Chef Michel, trying out a new recipe. Out of gratitude for their assistance in dealing with a small kitchen fire, the chef gives Roy and Johnny each a copy of his cookbook, and you can practically see the light bulb as it appears over Johnny's shaggy-haired head. "Hey," he says, "why don't I take the most complicated, over-the-top recipe in this book, and make it for the average Joes at the station?? Without any practice or training? That sounds reasonable, right??" So that's what he does. Next shift, he comes back from the store with all sorts of fancy ingredients and tells the guys he's going to fix *Bordure de soles a la Normandie.* As he said when he was reading the names of some of the cookbook dishes, "I hope they taste better than they pronounce." (That doesn't even make sense. And it's also very similar to what he told Roy in Cook's Tour when Roy mentioned Beef Bourguignon.)

For those keeping score at home, here's what Johnny's going to make for dinner:

A ring of creamed fish is poached and turned out onto a plate surrounding a shellfish ragoût mixed with Normandy sauce. Fried smelts are then added. Finally, some poached fillets of sole are laid on the top, garnished with poached oysters and slices of truffle.

For more specific info on the ingredients, here's the shopping list: sole ~ double cream (?) ~ oysters~ shrimp ~ fish stock ~smelts ~ shellfish ~ cream ~ egg yolks

(Ugh, none for me, thanks.)

I did find it odd that when he has all the ingredients on the table and someone asks "what is *that?*", Johnny replies, "I don't know." How can he not know what one of the ingredients is? He's the one who bought it!

While all this is going on, the doctors at Rampart (except Morton, who I don't believe was in this episode) are dealing with a boy who was shot in the neck and is (at least temporarily) paralyzed. The father is so worried about his son that his beard has grown out of control, and he has apparently donned a leisure suit paired with a shirt that has a crossword-puzzle motif. Luckily he's not an Egyptian parent (that is, not in de-Nile) but reacts reasonably when Brackett talks to him about his son's drugginess. We even see the surgery on this kid, but oddly, never hear any follow-up other than Kel telling the dad that he's "optimistic" about Freddy's recovery.

Fun fact: in addition to being Morton-less, this episode doesn't include a single scene of Roy and Johnny at Rampart. That's odd, isn't it?

* * *

> were there no after-effects of that [chamber] like martinis would? Do they just come out of the chamber and feel absolutely fine?

That's a good question. My take on it is that once they get out of the chamber they're fine. After all, the pressure is decreased to simulate them ascending from the deep, and the lower the pressure, the less effect on the body, so that by the time they're at "surface level," they should be fine. (I'm assuming.)

> And as they got in the helicopter, is that little strap they put across that WIDE door supposed to be a safety mechanism?

When we saw them get in the chopper, I did wonder why the Coast Guard guy didn't just close the chopper door but only put that strap across it. Then Johnny stood there—nay, *posed* there, deliberately—and I realized it was only for a photo op for you-know-who.

5.8 One of Those Days

The good news is... Roy's hair was good again!! The bad news is... I think we have at least one more "bad hair day" for him coming up.

Anyhoo...

~ The pins in the map in the apparatus bay—I wonder what they denoted? It was shown in the first scene, right after Roy tried to shut the hood on Johnny's head.

~ There was some stock footage nostalgia in this one: we saw the fancy house with the white columns, a first- or second-season scene of them in the squad driving down the road, and we heard the usual stock audio file at the big fire at the end. Also, I heard "stat ident doctor in Room 3."

~ In that car accident with no victims... was it just me or did that yellow stuff *not* look like pieces of a car? And it wasn't just an ordinary accident; that yellow car was totally demolished. *That* didn't happen in a quiet dead-end city street. (Oh, and didn't you just love the "blood"? Red paint, or maybe ketchup, would be my guess.)

~ Anyone ever notice that Roy never tightens the chin-strap on his helmet? Johnny does, and Cap does, too. But Roy's strap is usually just hanging loosely—sometimes very loosely.

~ In the scene with the drunk in the building that didn't have a working elevator, all the stair scenes must have been filmed at the same time, then all the street scenes and scenes in the apartment were filmed together. Because when the guys are on the street or in the apartment, Roy has a watch on (left hand). But in all the scenes of them going up and down the stairs... and up and down again... no watch. But as soon as they get to the top floor where the guy lives—it appears. It's E! magic!

~ In the final rescue in the burning apartment house, the woman never told them which apartment she lived in. She also never told them her daughter is deaf. Isn't that the kind of information that might be considered, you know, important? Like the old guy who was blind, and the daughter didn't tell Johnny, and the old guy didn't tell him either?? Sheesh.

~ Also, I know it was fairly obvious, but I could *swear* there was a part of that scene with the girl where after she was reunited with her mother and points to Johnny and 'says' something, the mother says something like "you're right, he is cute." Does anyone remember ever seeing anything like that, or am I totally nuts? (And yeah, I did look up sign language signs for *cute, handsome,* and *good-looking,* and none of them match what she did. To me it looked like what she did indicated 'smooth,' but that's not right, either.)

~ Lastly, for some reason I think it's kind of cute when Roy occasionally uses the word 'ain't.' He did it in this episode, with the drunk, when he said "He ain't breathing." As a former English major, usually I totally frown on people using that word, and I might even make judgements about their intelligence and breeding. (Yeah, I can be a bit of a snob like that sometimes.) But for some reason when Roy says it, I don't have that reaction. Maybe because it's obvious that he's a thoughtful, intelligent guy, and he's the soul of polite (if sometimes unpolished) behavior. Plus, I just like him.

~ ~ ~

A pretty good episode, in my book. No silliness, no Johnny over-reacting to anything or being a buffoon. And yay,

May Fair

Roy's hair is back to its normal look!! (Warning: I think we'll see the horrible Roypadour / Pompadon't return soon enough, more's the pity.)

The theme of this one seems to be "Let's Tinker Under the Hood," as every time we see the guys at the station, that's pretty much what's going on. Including Roy trying to close the hood of the squad on Johnny's head. Scripted, or not? You decide.

(Fun fact: when Cap gives the response for that first call, watch the cord on his radio: it's not plugged in to anything. Also, there's a stock-footage snafu regarding the back bay doors: closed while they work under the hood and get in the squad, but open while they're driving out of the station.)

First call is for a whiny, entitled society woman who's pouting because her daughter-in-law has a backbone and won't cater to her or do things the "right way." Words are spoken, words are broken, and next thing you know, John and Roy find themselves in the middle of a family brouhaha. The mother, who ages from 53 to 55 in the space of two minutes, probably got off scot-free in the melee, as luck would have it. However, this mini-melee is the reason for a great scene at the station as the paramedics tell the story of their fun morning. Interestingly, Chet says "sorry I missed it"—not once, not twice, but *three times* over the course of that scene.

After the fascinating tracking-shot of Roy putting his shirt on, as he walks from the locker room to the apparatus bay, the tones go off and the guys are off again. (Roy has to finish buttoning his shirt as he gets in the squad. Love! That!) This call is a drunk guy on the 4th floor, in a building without an elevator. A pretty obvious goof: Roy's wearing a watch in the scenes on the street level and in the apartment, but *not* in the scenes on the stairs. Also, the second time they go up to the apartment, Johnny's in the lead on the narrow stairs, but when the scene changes, Roy's in front. I love Johnny's comment after the landlord tells them about the non-working elevator and the fact that there are tons of drunks there; he mutters "Looks like a real fun place." And I sure didn't envy Roy, having to give mouth-to-mouth to that disgusting, drunken lush.

At Rampart, Doctors Early and Brackett are trying to determine what's wrong with Donnie, other than having to put up with a horrendously awful mother, that is. Donnie's about eight or nine, I'd guess, and seems to have flu-like symptoms. I confess, I fast-forwarded through all her awful scenes with Brackett. Regarding Donnie, I'm no doctor (nor do I play one on TV), but in the treatment room I think Brackett was using the reflex hammer backwards on him. We don't see what he does with Donnie's shins, but when Kel moves to the boy's right elbow, he taps inside the elbow with the pointy end of the hammer, instead of the flat end, which I believe is more commonly used.

Now, about that mystery car accident... that isn't just a normal, run-of-the-mill collision on a city street. That is total annihilation of some sort of yellow sports car—the make of which didn't look familiar in the least. Whatever happened, that accident did *not* take place on that nice quiet street, because it would have been L-O-U-D. Even a disguised Valerie (remember her??) would have heard and noticed an accident like that as she watered her lawn. (And the less said about the "blood," the better.)

Back at the station, Mike's handing out plates of lunch, which looks pretty good. Roy's eating a stalk of celery and Johnny's about to get his plate when the tones go off. One thing I do wonder though... do men really drink coffee with lunch? I can see maybe having a cup *after* the meal, but every one of those guys had a coffee cup, and they hadn't even eaten yet. Seriously, they looked like a bunch of old hens enjoying some gossip during their coffee klatch. Maybe I'm so used to seeing people with to-go cups from coffee houses that I find it very odd seeing men with formal coffee cups—the small ones—with dainty handles and saucers and everything. (As opposed to the cardboard cups or mugs.)

The squad's next call gets cancelled, but since they're only a block or so away, Roy and Johnny decide to stop by the scene anyway, and it's a good thing they do, as the man (victim) is actually in worse shape than he or his daughter thought. The daughter, Betty, is recognizable by many as "Angelique," from the '60s TV show Dark Shadows. She used to scare the crap out of me when I was a little thing. Anyway, one thing I found odd about this scene: Johnny calls Rampart from the house phone (landline), and Brackett tells him to put on anti-shock trousers and start an IV with saline. Johnny says 10-4 and hangs up, telling Roy, "I'll go get the trousers." Now consider the conversation from Roy's perspective, or the victim's: all they hear is Johnny repeat the vitals, say 10-4, and tell Roy "I'll get the trousers." Is Roy supposed to use telepathy to figure out about the IV? And the victim and his daughter probably think Johnny's nuts for saying he's going to get some trousers. Which is all to say that, when calling in on a landline, people nearby do *not* hear the Rampart side of the conversation as they do when using the biophone.

Later, on the way back from Rampart, Station 51 gets called to a structure fire. The building looks like it was about to fall down on its own, but what I find really odd is the behavior of the woman who rushes up to the scene and can't find her daughter. The building is at least three or four stories, but at no time does Manic Mother tell Roy and Johnny which apartment, or even which floor, she lives on. Also, don't you think that the fact the daughter is deaf might be just a *little bit* important?? That's TWO major pieces of information that were easily available, since the mother was right there, and not only didn't she offer it (some mother *she* is!), but they didn't ask which apartment they should look in. (Some rescue men *they* are!)

In the background of one of these shots, there's a building with a sign for Barker's Home Furnishings. I take it that's no longer around? Also, when Chet is stuck in the roof, half in the building and half out, how funny is it to see the firefighters on the floor below spraying the hose between his dangling legs?

One thing I mentioned last time, and I'll repeat now. I might very well be going crazy, but I could swear that one time when I watched this episode, in the scene with the deaf girl, after Johnny reunites her with her mom and the girl signs something, I could swear that the mother said something like "yes, I think he's cute too," or "I agree, he's nice," or something like that. But when I watch it on Netflix, that scene isn't there, it just ends right after the girl signs and the mother laughs. Did I imagine that part about the mother's comment? Does anyone remember seeing it? If not, I guess maybe I did imagine it. (One of the hazards of having an active, creative imagination, I guess.)

Note: once again, no Morton.

* * *

[The deaf girl's] gesture definitely looked like a representation for "smooth," but in American Sign Language, that's not the sign for smooth. It's also not ASL for *handsome* or *good-looking* or *cute*.

I think there are other 'versions' of sign language.... maybe it was one of those?

5.9 The Lighter-Than-Air Man

I noticed quite a bit of stock footage early in this episode, starting with the very first scene when the squad was called out and Season 2 (or maybe season 3) Roy and Johnny got into the squad. Then we see the squad drive past the white pillared house... right before Roy callously mowed down some old man. (Seriously, why didn't either of them tell the cop, "we didn't notice because *he wasn't in front of our squad*"???)

The box of groceries Roy carries into the station looked pretty pitiful. Did you see the brown bananas? Who'd eat those?? And I can't believe he refers to the fridge as an "ice box." I thought that by the mid-'70s only people over the age of 60 called it that. (I know nobody *I* knew called it an ice box.)

I always have to shake my head at the bride-and-groom accident, in which the convertible has run into a fire hydrant and sheared it off, when Cap says to Chet "you open the door and the water comes out on your feet; is that how it works?" That's just too funny! One of those things that you wonder if it's scripted or just ad-libbed.

Speaking of bride and groom, I find it odd that they're driving together to the wedding. To the reception, yes, I can see, but the wedding?? Not usually, especially not for church weddings.

The little girl at the hospital who couldn't get in to see the Lighter-Than-Air Man and talked to Lieutenant Crockett... does anyone else remember wearing those yarn ribbons? I know I do. (And how did she get to the hospital all by herself? Rampart must be very kid-friendly, or right next to an imaginary elementary school, seeing how many kids apparently just walk right in off the street by themselves.)

I don't think Lt. Crockett ever mentions the 'victim's' name when he questions the paramedics, and yet Johnny and Roy mention going to see Mr. Medford.

I always liked the camper rescue that takes place right in front of the station. And Cap chiding the parents about the boy riding in said camper: "Now you know why it's illegal." (P.S., I had to laugh when Roy says "I'll ride with him in the ambulance," and Johnny responds "I'll follow in the squad." Well duh!!)

For last call, all the guys are in the kitchen looking at the layette Johnny bought, but when the alarm goes off we see them... coming out of the dorm?

At the scene of that last rescue, Cap knows the truck was carrying some unidentified pesticide, so he sends Chet out to see if he can find out what kind... but doesn't suggest putting on an air-mask! (I know, they'd already been exposed at that point, but still.... unknown substance means unknown effects.)

Lastly, Cap calls for other squads, but we never see them. I guess we just didn't have time.

~ ~ ~

The episode begins with the squad being called out for a "woman in labor," and we see the squad go through a couple of neighborhoods—in fact, they go past the fancy-shmancy white-pillared house, down another very nice tree-lined street with manicured lawns, and suddenly they're in some less-prestigious area where the kids apparently don't go to school until 10:45am.

May Fair

In any case, Johnny's in a good mood upon returning from that run, passing out cigars to anyone who wants one. (They've delivered babies before, so not sure what's so special about this one.) The mood is dampened, though, when he and Roy are called in to Cap's office and they learn of an old man who was the victim of a hit-and-run. "Gee, that's terrible," they say. What's worse, however, is that witnesses at the scene say that the vehicle in question was an LACoFD squad—number 51, to be exact. (Note: The kids were waiting on the opposite side of the street from where the guy supposedly was hit, so they didn't have a direct view of whatever happened to him; the squad was between the kids and the acrobatic guard.)

Roy and Johnny are understandably stunned by this news that they (supposedly) hit someone. (I mean, seriously, how do you hit someone who was never in front of your vehicle?) Roy is particularly shaken, since he was the one driving, and when the tones go off and the station is called to an accident, he tells Johnny to drive. (Yeah, he *must* be shaken up, if he suggests that.) Detective Crockett decides to go to the scene as well, for some strange reason.

A bride and groom driving to their wedding have hit a fire hydrant with their convertible, leaving a fountain of water spewing over the area. (Why are the bride and groom driving to the wedding together?? Isn't that kind of unusual—not to mention bad luck??) Anyway, the couple are bickering with each other and generally not being cooperative, until Crockett comes along and does his reverse psychology thing, getting man and soon-to-be-wife to stick up for each other. Johnny and Roy seem amused by this, which is very generous of them, considering; I don't think I'd have been so disposed to be pleasant to the detective. (I realize that Crockett's only the messenger on this matter and not necessarily the bad guy, but still. It's kind of hard to focus on the 'big picture' when you're more worried about being sent to the 'big house.')

In any case, one of the detective's 'threats' against the young groom is to cite him for driving without a license. Now, the guy *does* have a license, he just doesn't have it on him. Correct me if I'm wrong, but that isn't considered "driving without a license." As far as I'm aware, you might get a small fine for not having the license *on you,* but it's not the same as driving without *being* licensed.

By the way, watch for the fun interchange between Chet and Cap. Chet's bonehead move of opening the crashed car's door leads Cap to say, "You open the door and the water comes out on your feet; is that how it works?" That's just too funny! One of those things that you wonder if it's scripted or just 'popped out.'

After that call, the guys go to Rampart, where they ask Dixie if they can see Mr. Medford. (Funny, Crockett never told them the man's name, yet they know who to ask for.) I don't know how things were done back in the day, but in this day and age I'm pretty sure that whole scene would never happen in real life. They should never have said "I'm sorry" to the man, as that could possibly be considered an admission of guilt. I realize this was TV, it happened a long time ago, etc., but still, it seems obvious to me that it could be construed that way.

So, after Detective Crockett comes across the unattended girl in a big hospital who was there to visit some old man to whom she's not related, the action moves back to the station. Johnny and Roy are about to go back to Rampart (again) when a honking horn announces the arrival of a car pulling a trailer that's on fire with a boy inside. (Good thing the squad wasn't about to go on an actual call, right? I wonder what would have happened in that case?) Roy grabs an extinguisher and goes into the camper to find the boy, while Johnny alerts the Captain, who supposedly calls for the other guys to help out. I have to admit it seems to take a long time for Marco and Chet to show up. Cap drives the station wagon out of the way, Marco has the reel line in the trailer, and Chet opens a hole in the roof, and the flames are pretty quickly taken care of. What I find odd, though, is that those three (Cap, Chet, and Marco) seem to disappear after that. As the paramedics treat the injured boy, his mother is the one who works the O2 mask and holds up the IV bag, which I thought would be more *dis*couraged than *en*couraged.

Also, I found it funny: once Cap helps the parents into the ambulance, Johnny comes up and tells him, "I'm gonna follow in the squad." Well *duh,* doesn't the squad always follow to Rampart?? Also, Johnny must have backed out of the apparatus bay and gone around the station, since the trailer is still on the street out in front.

Must admit, I skipped past all the surgery on the boy. Not interesting to me, which I know is bad and shallow. So the next thing to note is back at the station, where—good news!—we see Marco seasoning some really yummy-looking steaks. Bad news: Johnny didn't use the trading stamps (ha!) for a grill; instead he picked up a Trundle Bunny Baby Layette. For the baby he delivered earlier. Yeah, that makes perfect sense, right?? But before the other guys can skewer Johnny and roast him on a spit, the station gets a call for a truck fire on a conveniently-empty onramp.

I have to say, I'm disappointed in Cap in this one. First a cop passes out, and then the truck driver also goes down. And even after they learn the truck is carrying some sort of insecticide, Cap *still* doesn't tell his guys to put their masks on?? Really, Hank, you're slipping badly. But I have to laugh at the generic-sounding company name that says absolutely nothing: Chemcorp, Incorporated. How funny is that? Sort of like CompuTech, or Amalgamated Global.

* * *

Excellent point about checking the squad for damage. That didn't occur to me since I had the impression that LTAM (Lighter-Than-Air Man) was supposedly knocked by the passenger side, although even if that was the case, the jutting mirror would have sustained some damage. (And Johnny would certainly have noticed some guy flying around right outside his window, y'know?) But yeah, now that you mention it, why *didn't* they even look curiously at the front of the squad???

> Their car is a dark blue 1968 Dodge convertible with the chrome trim on the driver's door broken off. Methinks we'll be seeing that car again in the next episode.

Hey, good call! That car probably came directly from the junkyard and will be used again for another car accident(s) until it's all but unrecognizable (like the yellow Lotus).

> [Johnny's behavior] Total disregard for his fellow FFs. They were all set to use the grill, with steaks ready and everything, and without their sayso he goes and uses their stamps for a layette for "his" baby. And if Roy was there and didn't like the idea either, why didn't he stop him? That whole thing left me very disappointed; epic fail for both paramedics!!

Yeah, it was too bad that they had Johnny do that. But I bet that Roy certainly would have tried to talk him out of buying the Trundle Bunny Baby Layette... unfortunately, you know how much luck Roy usually has trying to "reason" with Gage when he gets one of his hare-brained ideas. I think that's why Roy said something like "I don't think I want to see this" when it was time for the guys to unwrap the box.

May Fair

Poor Roy is put in a bad spot. Ya gotta wonder if he was sometimes secretly relieved when he pulled a shift with someone other than Johnny!

> At the trailer fire, I can only assume Cap called in a "still alarm" and requested an ambulance, and yelled orders to Chet and Marco; I was a bit disappointed that we didn't hear it. Also, apparently the father was named Charlie (what, again?) or Chuck, and the boy in the trailer was named Bobby. However, is it just me or did Roy call out "Chuck!" in the trailer?

Agree, I wish we'd seen a little more with the trailer fire. I didn't even catch that the father's name was Chuck, which as you say is the same as (yet another) Charlie. In the trailer, Roy called out "Son!" I thought that was odd, since he surely heard the mother call the boy Bobby, but whatevs.

* * *

I know, it was very odd that Cap, Chet, and Marco all disappear during the trailer rescue in front of the station. As I said, usually Cap keeps family members out of the way and the other guys are the ones who assist John and Roy, but this time the mother was helping them out (and getting in the way at times; Cap really fell down on the job).

At the truck crash with insecticide, after Brackett tells them to wear gloves, either John or Roy (can't remember which one was on the biophone) reaches into the drug box, presumably to get the gloves. And the next time we see them, they *are* wearing surgical-type gloves (although it was a little hard to tell, as the gloves are almost transparent). Nice bit of realism there, even if they really dropped the ball on the air-mask thing. After all, they had no way of knowing the stuff wasn't transmitted by air.

Earlier, at the station, who knows what happened to Johnny's cigar. Now you see it, now you don't!! Maybe he stuck it in one of those convenient ashtrays we keep seeing on the tables. Or maybe I should say *kept* seeing, as I don't know if they've been around much in season 5.

5.10 Simple Adjustment

~ Why does it look like Roy and John were taking notes from their calls on envelopes and scraps of paper? What happened to Johnny's little notebook, in his back pocket? (Or the one in the Biophone, depending on which reality we accept.) Writing on the back of envelopes and receipts is *my* thing, but I don't recommend it for paramedics.

~ In the scene when the guys leave Rampart in the squad to return to the station, and Johnny has his bright idea of recording the notes, did anyone notice that they seem to be driving out in the country? No commercial area, no industrial parks, just fields and trees visible outside Johnny's window, all throughout that conversation. Just what route does Roy *take* to get back to the barn, anyway?? (I'm assuming he didn't take the term 'back to the barn' literally.)

~ I love Roy's reaction to the idea. "I'm scared. You have an idea and I actually agree with you." Stick with that skepticism, Roy; you'll need it again in the future when Johnny has another 'bright idea.'

~ The scene in which John and Roy are installing the tape recorder in the squad (don't get me started on that; just a separate recorder would've been just as good and a *lot* more simple!), anyway, when Cap is asking what they're doing, listen closely, and I think you can hear Johnny talking over his own voice. This is when he's supposedly muttering--something about "out-of-focus," and "piece of junk." I wonder if it was just my version (non-Netflix) that was like that, or others? Also, when the thing blows up and he says "Oh, sheez," I wonder if they had to splice that comment over, um, something else he might have said.

~ The scene at the beauty shop was kind of funny when the woman called Johnny cute and Roy said "She's talking to you." Then she sees Roy and says he's cute too and one of them (Roy, I think?) says "he's cuter." Too funny!

~ Speaking of that lady, when we saw her in the hospital all I could think was "False eyelash war!!" And we thought *Dixie's* lashes were long... this woman's lashes just looked awful.

~ At the final rescue (ship on fire) I again saw that when the engine was backing up, the guys in engine jump-seats get out and (in some cases) hop on the back tailboard. Not sure if it's a matter of visibility, that they get in the way of the rear-view mirrors, or what.

~ The captain of one of the other engine companies was named Stone (according to his turnout coat), but it wasn't "our" Captain Stone. Another instance of the show getting maximum use out of the prop-coat.

~ Love the final scene, the freeze-frame, of Johnny looking directly at the camera. Too funny!

Because this episode *isn't* on Netflix, nor anywhere else, I've only seen it maybe two other times, back when I had MeTV. Even with bad quality, I'm glad to know I can watch it again if I like, because I do like some of the rescues in this one. Too bad it's not seen more often through usual channels like the NBC Classics site, Hulu, Netflix, etc. (And

I'm still curious as to *why* this episode isn't available more places?)

* * *

> I love listening to Captain Stanley take charge of the scene. At the ship fire he was telling all the engines that were coming in where to go and then telling all his men what to do. I just love it. He's so good at that and so in charge.

I love that too. Of course, I think it was standard procedure that the first captain on the scene takes charge, as he sizes up the situation and advises the other engines/companies how to proceed. (And since this show is about Station 51, they always seem to get there first—coincidentally, of course!) Then once the Battalion Chief arrives, Cap becomes just another captain on the scene, and the BC calls the shots.

As for the mic pack, sometimes it is placed more on the side, or even the back. In fact, many times I think it *is* on the back, but then when they bend over a victim, the pull on their shirt makes the pack visible there, so maybe that's why they did it in the front. I always think it's funny that these shows were filmed and edited with no inkling that they'd ever be A) still watched 40 years in the future, B) watched back-to-back, making some things more obvious than if seen once a week, and C) be able to be paused and re-wound, etc., to enable viewers to really *see* something rather than have it be on screen for only a second or two. If they only knew then what we know now...!!

Edit, because I forgot earlier...

> Even though Johnny is my ultimate favorite, I'm not sure he is "marriage material". I would probably kill him within a week or so. I also like Dr. Brackett but he might be a little too intense for me. Hank seems like

he's a nice balance. I'm sorry all you Roy fans out there, but he just seems a little too boring

I totally agree about Johnny, he'd need a "very special" kind of wife, one who won't throttle him on a regular basis. (*Is there such a woman??*) As for Roy... I think of him as more quiet and mild-mannered than 'boring' (wince). And you know what they say, "it's the quiet ones you have to watch out for."

~ ~ ~

I like this episode. I only wish it was on Netflix, because I have to watch it via an alternative method, and the film quality is just... subpar compared to Netflix.

I'd love to see the opening scene of this episode in better quality. The view is from the apparatus bay as the squad pulls up and backs in. There's a nice view of Johnny in the passenger side as the squad pulls up; he even turns to look toward the camera. I don't know that we ever see that view again in the series, do we? Usually we can't/don't see the occupants of the squad too well when they back into the station, and in some stock footage, there are obviously doubles in the squad, but it was clearly Randy this time. Hmmm, I wonder why that footage isn't used again—or at least more often.

I think I mentioned before that it seems odd that the guys' notes for each run are on little bits of paper and what looks like the backs of envelopes, etc. I know they keep the notes in their notebooks, so why aren't the notes all neatly kept that way? Also, I think someone mentioned last time that when they were in the office trying to write in the log, it seems odd that Cap 'orders' them to eat lunch with everyone else. Socializing with co-workers is fine, but paperwork has to come first, I'd think.

In any case, before that becomes an issue, the station gets called out for a car off the road. I have to wonder who called that in... there's no cop, and no passerby waiting to show the FD where the accident is. Anyway, a very familiar-looking blue convertible with a missing side piece of chrome is upside down with a woman trapped inside. And yes, someone really nailed that call—this is the same car that the newlyweds were driving in Lighter-Than-Air Man, and which was flooded with water from the hydrant. Good call!! As for the victim, all I can say is, it's a good thing she's wearing pants rather than a skirt, since she is pretty much hanging upside down. Also, I get a kick out of the guys putting the anti-shock trousers on her and leaving her fancy dressy shoes on. I guess if she'd been a man, they'd leave *his* shoes on, but hers look funny, sticking out as they do, and the sight of her looks awkward. Not to mention the shoes don't "go" with the brown anti-shock trousers.

Next we see the guys in the squad returning to Rampart. Maybe Johnny asked to take the "scenic route," as the view outside his window is certainly pastoral and rural. Definitely not their usual commute back to the station! Anyway, since Johnny hadn't contacted LA to say "Squad 51, available," Roy does it, and the sight of Roy with the mic causes Johnny's figurative light-bulb to go off and he gets his Big Idea. "We use the mic!!" he tells Roy, as if the rest is totally obvious. Roy's response: "Doctor, he was fine a few minutes ago but then all of a sudden he sort of left reality." Classic! Then Johnny explains his idea, and Roy's further reaction is funny too. "I'm scared. It sounds like a good idea, and I agree with you. That scares me." Yes, Roy, as well it should!!

From here things get a little less fun to watch. First of all, when they're both in the squad installing the recorder, at one point I hear Johnny more or less talk over himself, as if two bits of audio are dubbed at the same time. It's immediately after Cap says "don't immobilize he squad." But my problem with the whole tape recorder idea is that they really overcomplicate it. It would have been easier to just have an actual tape recorder in the squad, left under the seat or in the glove box; it doesn't have to be installed anywhere, much less wired. (In the final scene, they need a second device to play back the tape; if the recorder was free-standing, that wouldn't be an issue.) Anyway, the fact that they make it more complicated than it needs to be—and the resulting goof-ups—diminish my enjoyment of the storyline. Not to mention the fact that they apparently just give it up altogether. Whatever happened to persistence, and "If at first you don't succeed," etc.? Thomas Edison rarely got his inventions right the first or even second time.

Okay, enough ranting on that topic. In the middle of this muddle the tones go off for a call at a hair salon. I thought it amusing that when the call comes, the two guys are both in the squad: Roy in the passenger side, Johnny in the driver's seat. So what do they do? They switch sides! Johnny slides over to the passenger side and Roy gets out and hurries around to the driver's side. Wouldn't it have been easier to just stay where they were?? (Yeah, I know, they still had to get rid of some of their equipment and tools.)

Anyway, the hair salon call is funny. The woman says "Firemen, I love firemen!" to which Roy says to Johnny, "she's talking to you." And then she calls them both cute and sits on Johnny in the dryer chairs. This segment is a mini-PSA about the dangers of taking someone else's pills without a prescription. I do like the scene at Dixie's desk when Roy tells Dixie that "she called him cute, before she sat on him. Johnny always had a weakness for the subtle type." I think Johnny/Randy looked pretty genuinely embarrassed. And the way Dixie laughs, it made me wonder....

Back at the station, Johnny's about to demonstrate his tape recording machine for the guys. Just as he presses the button on the mic, the tones sound, causing Mike and Cap to jump, and Johnny just looks at the mic, sort of wondering how he did that.

The call takes them to a nice neighborhood where Helen Crump/Pete Malloy's unfortunate girlfriend Judy/wife of two other victims puts up a fuss because she doesn't want her father taken to *sniff* a public hospital. A bit taken aback, Johnny does his best to reason with her; meanwhile, Roy notices that dear old Dad is semi-coherent and asks if Rampart is OK with *him*, and they get the go-ahead that way, leaving Snooty Judy to deal with the humiliation of it. This leads to another mini-PSA at Rampart in which Roy vents to Dr. Early about victims who insist on wasting everyone's time by going to some other distant hospital rather than Rampart.

Final rescue is the big ship fire. (That's some bad ship, that is.) Cap takes charge until he decides to go in and help find the two missing men. I find it a little odd that he tells Johnny and Roy to let other paramedics take over their burn victim so they could go with Cap, since this show has always made it seem like treating a victim is sort of like being in a relationship (or starting an IV): once you start, you stick with it 'til the end. (Or, as the saying goes, you 'dance with the one who brung ya.') But I guess not. Anyway, they go into the ship and save the two missing guys and all is well there without too much drama. One question: When Cap yells to Marco and Chet, who are standing by the engine, what the heck is Mike doing in the background? Looks like he's using a mallet to tap one of the engine's nozzles. Also, note that there is a Captain Stone in this scene, to whom Cap passes the baton of authority for this fire. I guess they made good use out of "Stoney's" turnout coat, eh? The guy who plays this particular Captain Stone is in a number of episodes, so he's sort of a familiar face.

Okay, this is partly related to this episode, as it happens here, but I've noticed it before. Sometimes at a scene when the guys are evaluating a victim, Johnny will tell Roy the BP or whatever vitals he's taken, even though Roy's not the one who's going to call Rampart. It happens in this episode, with Helen Crump's father: Johnny tells Roy the pulse, pupillary reaction, and respiration, even though he (Johnny) is going to be the one to call Rampart. Roy's not the person who needs to know that info, so why does Johnny tell him? I don't think Roy ever does it (tell Johnny the numbers) when *he's* the one who calls Rampart. (Or maybe he does? I don't know.) And it's not as if these two can decide on their own how to treat the victim, either. Is that odd, or is it just me??

5.11 Tee Vee

First, I want to know whose bright idea it was to add that awful European-style "hi-lo" siren into the mix for LACoFD. I hate it.

Secondly, I think the director or whoever edits these things together needs to be retroactively (and metaphorically) shot. On that first call, barely two minutes into the show, they leave the station at 10:33 am.... bright sun. The next scene is from inside the engine (behind Mike) and it's late afternoon, almost sunset. Then the view switches to overhead and it's broad daylight again. They should at least have tried to keep their stock footage organized by time of day, to make scenes match. Maybe I'm just too picky, but I find that sort of thing pretty distracting.

Watching EMERGENCY! Seasons 4-6

I like the sewer rescue, but for one thing, I didn't see anyone bringing their air tanks back out to the surface. Also, I had to laugh because after they find the missing guy, roll him over, carry him back to the ladder, and have him pulled up via the rescue rope, *then* they call for the backboard. I hate to tell you, guys, but being careful of his back and neck *now* isn't going to help much.

So do we all remember those old console TVs, with the "rolling" pictures and that sort of thing? Luckily I don't think it happened to us very often... I don't think my dad ever opened up the set. (And after the "TV surgery" didn't work, how funny was it for the guys to be excited over a 26-inch screen??)

After the tape-recorder/radio fiasco of the last episode, whose bright idea was it to let Johnny get his hands on that TV, anyway?? You'd think these guys would learn! But then, I guess Roy knew what to expect, as he left the room and was probably just waiting outside the rec room for his cue. *Whoosh!* There it is, the set blows up, and Roy steps in with the fire extinguisher.

* * *

> And, I did love the final comment by Johnny, "when I am home, I'm certainly not watching TV". hahahahaha

Oh yeah, too funny! "But Johnny, without a TV, how can you invite a date to come in and watch a Polish art film??" *wink*

> Also, has anyone ever noticed that every time Johnny asks for "slack", he sounds very irritated about it. He does it every time. Roy simply and kindly yells for more slack and Johnny sounds so angry about it.

May Fair

I've noticed this once or twice, it's as if he'd asked for slack and nobody heard him or complied, so he has to ask again—forcefully. I probably assumed that's what happened, I don't think I realized it was a pattern with him. But I've definitely noticed it and wondered what had happened that he's so ticked off.

I know what you mean about the mudslide rescue. I imagine lots more stuff was filmed for this scene but just wasn't used, for whatever reason. Some of us have mentioned that we like those complicated rescues, the ones that can't be rehearsed, and this mudslide rescue falls in that category.

~ ~ ~

Once again we're back to the matter of the episode itself (rescues, etc.) being good, but the ongoing story indicated by the title is a little wearying. Yes, the story makes Johnny look bumbling and incompetent. *Again.* Big surprise, huh? Just the other day (previous episode) we see Johnny 'screw up' a supposedly minor electrical task. So what does he do again in this episode? You guessed it: screwed up a supposedly minor electrical task. Seriously, why do the guys on the shift ever even let him near any electrical appliances??

At the beginning of the episode, after their regular TV goes on the fritz, the call is to a fire in a manhole. I like this rescue, it's a good one, everyone gets involved in some way. I think I mentioned last time: Roy and Johnny pick up the victim, carry him through the tunnels, and he gets hauled up to the surface... and *then* they're concerned about putting him on a backboard?? Uh, don't bother with the barn door, guys, that horse is already gone.

Here's a theory I have, which I mention because this first rescue reminds me of it: sometimes at rescue scenes like this one, we see certain vehicles parked nearby (*cough*blue Chevy pickup*cough*). My theory is that many times these vehicles are used to carry production crew and/or equipment to the location shoot, and then parked in the area as convenient window dressing. When we see the squad at the second manhole, in the background there is a white truck (like a U-haul or moving van) parked down the street. I seriously doubt the owner of that house happened to have a large truck parked out front out of mere coincidence, so I believe it was part of the production crew. Same with the blue pick-up, which, YES, is present in this rescue, and can be seen behind the engine when Cap is on the radio and the squad leaves. Anyway, that's my theory about large trucks (and smaller pick-ups) near the scene of some rescues.

Back to the show... when they bring the victim to Rampart, as they come in the entrance, the gurney is accompanied by a nurse and some guy who looks like an intern (same kind of uniform that Morton wears), and I swear the intern looks like Gil, Johnny's old high-school chum-now-paramedic. It's *not* Gil, of course, and not even the actor who plays him, but it sure looks like him. With his LACoFD-approved haircut, he could have played a fireman. Anyway, they take the vic into Treatment Room #6, which is kind of unusual. I guess they have six treatment rooms when they want to, as I believe that particular room has been a number of things over the seasons, including a patient room.

But I like watching them bring a victim in to the treatment room. Once they get in there, everyone has a job to do: plug the air mask into the wall, hang the IV on a pole, take vitals, set up a particular test, etc. Most of those things are simple, but still, they (almost) always look quite efficient and professional. In fact, watching one particular scene in another episode makes me wonder if the show ever hired actual off-duty hospital staff for certain things. I'm thinking mainly of The Hard Hours, when the guy comes in to Joe

May Fair

Early's room to prep him for surgery by shaving him. We don't actually see any shaving, of course, but as he sets everything up, the guy looks like he really knows what he's doing. Yeah, I know, it could have been just some shmuck paid a few bucks to act like that, and in reality I don't know how they shave patients for heart surgery, but still, it looks authentic to me.

Back to the episode.... Once John and Roy leave Treatment 6, they pass by a janitor in white (who we've seen before at Rampart) mopping the floor. R and J are joined by Dixie and they turn into the main hallway for a walk-and-talk. The same "janitor" will soon turn the corner and pass them, walking toward the camera. A moment later he crosses in front of the camera and goes back up the hallway, this time stopping at a supply counter, which is less janitor-ly and more orderly. Then he turns back and comes toward the camera again, turning toward the emergency entrance alongside Roy. That's quite a versatile janitor, don'tcha think?

Elsewhere at Rampart, Dr. Brackett gets a fish-tank with some funky-looking fish, one of which bites him. This is a cute little mini-storyline, and some good continuity with him calling the Administrator, Mr. O'Brien.

Meanwhile, at the station, Tweedle-dee and Tweedle-dum are working on trying to fix the TV. Wouldn't you think the other shifts would prefer not to let the one-man wrecking crew to touch their stuff?? (To be fair, I should say two-man wrecking crew; Chet does manage, after all, to set fire to a pair of skis. Oops, that hasn't happened yet—never mind!) Anyway, as these two are performing their wacky wiring, in the background, Roy is at the counter with some sandwich fixin's (although I don't think he ever makes—much less eats—a sandwich). Cap, Marco, and Mike walk in, empty-handed, and walk to the counter, and less than 30 seconds

Watching EMERGENCY! Seasons 4-6

later (literally; I checked the time on Netflix) both Mike and Marco have complete sandwiches in their hands. More E! magic!! At that same time, Roy leaves the day-room. This ain't his first rodeo.... he knows exactly what's going to happen. And when it does, he returns with the fire extinguisher and does what needs to be done.

At Rampart, Morton deals with a man with "indigestion" and Brackett's fish bite is treated by Dr. Early with an "old wives' tale" remedy... that actually works. Take that, modern medicine!!

Squad 51 gets called out to see a man with an eye injury. (This is after Johnny calls some shady contact about getting a new TV for the station.) Anyway, I like the eye/glue rescue; it doesn't take long but it's interesting and different. I like how they have to break into the building (with the owner's permission), by Johnny breaking the glass with his helmet. It makes me wonder, though, what they do when they take him away in the ambulance. Do they leave the store broken into and unsecure? Call the police to let them know? It's not like they can just lock the door and close it behind them on their way out.

We next see the guys at the station when Johnny brings in "Uncle Ernie's" new TV... and the 26-centimeter screen. Needless to say, the guys aren't happy about *that*, leaving Johnny in the hot-seat once again. Then it's off to another call.

The "big" rescue of this episode is the mudslide, and the idiot husband who runs back into his house—the house with a friggin' gas leak in there, by the way—for a stupid clock. Once the house explodes around the guy, our intrepid paramedics run in to find him (should they have had their masks on?). That wouldn't be too bad if it weren't for the power pole that falls on the house. I know Cap had Chet switch off the gas and electricity, but I assumed that meant only for the house in question. Chet doesn't have authority to turn off power coming in from the pole, does he?? Anyway, when the pole hits the house, what do we see but men running over there with power tools, and hitting the house with streams of water. Water and sparks near live power lines... wouldn't that be problematic and a little, shall we say, dangerous? What am I missing here?? Also, as usual, loved the bubbling sound effects from the mudslide. Too funny!

* * *

Yes, it was odd that Johnny's "TV guy," Uncle Ernie, was talking in metric; I did wonder why on earth he'd speak in those terms. Besides, who discusses things like that without using the actual measurement word? You don't walk into Best Buy and say "I need a new TV and was thinking of going to 56." Or "Do you have any laptops that are 17? My 14 isn't big enough." No, you always use the measurement description, i.e., "inches."

Interestingly, at one time the US did make some strides toward officially switching to the metric system; I remember there being quite a to-do about it, heard about it in school, etc., and some places actually started converting and using the terminology. I don't recall exactly when that was, whether it was about the time of this show, but maybe it's possible. (Actually, I thought it was earlier.)

I wonder, though, maybe Uncle Ernie was really Ernesto? Do they use metric system in Mexico?

5.12 On Camera

First off, let me just say how pleasant it is to see Roy and Johnny have someone ride with them—a female, no less!—toward whom there wasn't any hostility. First it was the female photojournalist who thought everything was sexist. Then it was Karen, the trainee who was fine until she decided she shouldn't have to wait to act on her own, without instruction. So this young woman was a breath of fresh air. Even if she did have sports and athleticism on the brain. And I have to say, it was *very* refreshing not to have Johnny drooling after her or thinking up ways to ask her out.

Secondly, maybe it's just me—and if so, I'll stand still while you all virtually flog me—but.... I like all these guys at Station 51, think they're all cute and appealing (some a little more than others), but there's no way in the world that I consider them to be "macho men" or "he-men." Paula's comments and Roy's comments made it sound like people think these guys... *our* guys... are muscle-bound hunks of walking testosterone. Wha...?? I'm sorry, but when I think of the Station 51 guys, the word "macho" does *not* spring automatically to mind.

Okay, enough about that.

~ First rescue, with snake-boy. How funny to see a Gremlin in the driveway. Did all Gremlins have that stripe on the sides? I definitely remember seeing them, but don't remember if it was on all models.

~ At the scene with the boy over the cliff, they're trying to figure out how to get to the kid. Johnny turns and says something to the Captain, and Cap says "guess we'll have to." But I didn't hear what Johnny suggested. Doesn't matter, I guess, since we know what they did.

May Fair

~ I wonder how you train a friendly dog *not* to go to people who are calling to him? Most dogs are so friendly they automatically want to go to whoever is calling them.

~ This is one of the few times we see Roy writing something down while talking to Rampart. And he's not using the note paper in the biophone (which is clearly visible), or a little notebook like Johnny uses. He's got some sort of small clipboard. Not sure where that came from. Also, it looked like Johnny was writing something too, at about the same time.

Edited to add:

~ This is the second episode in which the "Mobile Intensive Care Unit" (or team) is mentioned. That's only *two* times in five seasons. (So far, anyway.)

~ I thought it was sweet/considerate/caring in the scene when John and Roy were down the cliff with the boy: I wondered where Roy's helmet was, then I noticed he was holding it over the face of the victim because as the Stokes was being lowered, debris and dust and stones were falling down, and he was shielding the boy's face. Yeah, I know that's his job, but it was such a nice considerate touch and excellent—albeit minor—detail. (Plus, if you were the kid/actor, I'm sure you'd be very glad he did that.)

~ ~ ~

I have to repeat some comments I made last time around, because they occurred to me again this time when I watched the episode today. So yes, here is a brief REPEAT:

First off, let me just say how pleasant it is to see Roy and Johnny have someone ride with them—a female, no less!—toward whom there wasn't any hostility. First it was the female photojournalist who thought everything was sexist.

Then it was Karen, the trainee who was fine until she decided she shouldn't have to wait to act on her own, without instruction. So this young woman was a breath of fresh air. Even if she did have a somewhat skewed opinion of FFs and consider them nothing more than daredevil jocks. And I have to say, it was very refreshing not to have Johnny drooling after her or talking about asking her out.

Secondly, maybe it's just me--and if so, I'll stand still while you all virtually flog me--but.... I like all these guys at Station 51, think they're all cute and appealing, but there's no way in the world that I consider them to be "mucho macho" or "he-men." Paula's comments and Roy's comments made it sound like most people think these guys—firefighters... our guys... are muscle-bound hunks of walking testosterone. Wha...?? I'm sorry, but when I think of the Station 51 guys, the word "macho" doesn't spring automatically to mind.

Okay, enough of the repeats, now I'll get to my current comments....

Did we all see Johnny trying to look casual in the background as Paula films that opening sequence? Then it's funny when she says something like "I hear you firemen get plenty of action off-duty too." Are we supposed to think she meant *action,* as in the boy-girl type? From the guys' reactions (or rather, their lack of reactions), I'd guess that suggestive statement wasn't really intended as suggestive.

One thing I noticed during The Indirect Method a while back was that Karen didn't wear a helmet while riding in the squad. I thought it was mandatory, and even guests have worn some sort of helmet almost all other times. (The other paramedic trainees, the screenwriter guy... even Leslie Charleson had her own helmet.) Anyway, I don't know if I mentioned it at the time we discussed The Indirect Method, but it occurred to me again today when we do see Paula put on a helmet. Anyhoo.....

Every time I see this episode, and the one with Gil, I have to wonder—and I'm sort of afraid to know the answer: when blasting a snake with a fire extinguisher, does it simply 'freeze' the snake temporarily, or does it kill it? Again, I don't want to know if the snake gets killed; I'm just going to pretend it temporarily freezes it, and I don't want to know any different. La-la-la, I can't hear you.....

Speaking of what the firemen do off-duty (sports-wise, that is), I wonder if any of the stuff the guys mention is something the actors do in real life? We all know that in real life Randy does enjoy outdoor stuff, so "Johnny's" answers were probably pretty real. And I smile every time I hear Marco mention soccer and say, "it's catching on, you know." Ha, yes Marco, soccer has certainly caught on in this country (although it took a few more decades).

I like the rescue of the wannabe stuntman at the factory. Even though that isn't really Roy and Johnny at that height, I think they do a pretty good job of making it look like it's them up there. (Not perfect, though, as it's obviously not Johnny doing the 'balance-beam' walk across the I-beam.) But the audio almost always matches quite well with what we see in the long-shots.

Next up (after an awkward scene when the guys were trying to be casual while eating lunch on camera) is a call for a fire in some park—Hillside Park*, I believe. The possible brush fire turns out to be nothing more than a smoking barbecue pit. Although how those people in the van don't hear the screaming sirens as Engine 51 approaches is beyond me. In any case, many fans will remember this scene from one of the bloopers in the blooper reel. One thing I've wondered, and might have mentioned before... why does Mike supposedly blast the air horn while driving down these unpaved dirt roads? It's not like they don't have both sirens going. And there's no traffic he needs to warn, or people/pedestrians they need to clear out of the road. They're in the middle of friggin' nowhere, and yet we hear the air horn! I think the audio editor gets a little horn-happy, as this happens in other episodes, too.

In any case, since the brush-fire call is a bust, the guys decide to check on a lonely bike and a barking dog, and soon discover a kid who has fallen off a cliff. I have to wonder, though, who are those people down in the bottom of the ravine? At one point I thought I saw a canoe or kayak down there too, so maybe there's a river that leads to the ocean? (Although I don't think we see any water down there, so that brings us back to, what are they doing down there?) Anyway, this rescue makes me wonder—again—why the Engine doesn't have a winch to help with pulling the guys up the cliff. (Fun note: that scene we see of Mike pulling the guys up by backing up the rig—we'll see it again in the episode with the sheriff's helicopter in the water.)

At Rampart, I like that they mention getting permission from the boy's mother to treat him. It's another nice touch of realism that Dr. Early has Dixie listen in on the call with the mother to verify the permission by phone. (But don't you think that was awfully quick?? No sooner does Early suggest this then the phone in the treatment room buzzes and the mother is being connected with him. Dixie barely has time to get on the other line; she was in such a hurry, she doesn't even press any buttons on her phone.)

* The only Hillside Park I can find now is a Memorial Park (cemetery) in Los Angeles (city, not county). Was there another Hillside Park back in the day? Or maybe they made up the name for that area and it wasn't a park at all?? (They don't normally do stuff like that, I don't think.)

5.13 Communications

This episode pretty much runs the gamut of different types of calls (or 'runs,' as they call them). Like the potential suicide, who they have to sit back and just watch until she loses consciousness.

~ In the first scene in the locker room, Chet is still in his civvies when the alarm goes off. Lucky the call is for the squad only... if it had been the engine, would he have jumped on Big Red in his jeans and pullover shirt?? Or would he have made Cap, Mike, and Marco wait while he threw his uniform on?

~ Re the first rescue, at the "record factory," every time I see this ep I always raise my eyebrows when Johnny calls an engine to assist them. I know they need all the extra hands they can get, but I'd think a construction person or engineer (mechanical, not firefighter) would be more helpful in this situation. But yeah, I get it, they don't have time to bring in any experts.

~ So now, in addition to St. Francis Hospital (it *is* St. Francis, isn't it?), we know that LACoFD also has paramedics working with "Pediatric Clinic." Also, this episode is another instance of "crossed transmissions" with the biophone.

~ After the discussion with Brackett, when Johnny and Roy are leaving Rampart they get the call about "a car on top of a house." We see the inside of the squad (from outside Roy's window) and Johnny picks up the radio and responds "Squad 51." Not only does his voice sound dubbed, but you can *see* that in the footage, Johnny is saying something else, something obviously more than just "squad 51."

Watching EMERGENCY! Seasons 4-6

~ Hate to say it, but I've seen that...*object*... in Johnny's pocket in almost every scene in the past couple of episodes, including this one. In fact, I thought he was going to offer one to the girl who'd taken the O.D. "A cigarette? Why, yes, I have a pack right here."

~ Speaking of... In the car-on-a-house rescue, Roy's reaction to the kid who offered him a cigarette is too funny. He tells the kid it's a "no-smoking" area, and then he mutters to Johnny, "Get a load of this kid trying to smoke." Too funny!

~ Another line that Roy says, I wonder if it was ad-libbed or not, is when he and John are visiting the kid from the record factory. The kid says, "I'd like to give you guys a million bucks apiece," and Roy says "you don't have to do that, right now." Johnny laughs at that, and so does the kid, and something about the way Randy laughs makes me wonder if maybe Roy's "right now" was ad-libbed. Or something. Watch Johnny's (Randy's) reaction, and even the kid in the bed, and see what you think.

~ Which brings me to the next thing... after they leave the kid's room, watch how they approach Dixie at the nurse's station. It looks for all the world as if they came from the emergency entrance.

~ Do people in LA really work on their cars so haphazardly that the cars fall on them? This run they have almost exactly mirrors a scene from Adam-12 in which a guy got crushed when the jack slipped and the car came down on him. In that one, though, the guy died. Luckily our favorite paramedics ensure that doesn't happen this time. (Although you'd think they'd have cleared the area of potential fire hazards before doing anything else, and allowing a fireball to erupt. Sheesh!)

May Fair

~ ~ ~

I like this episode; there's a little bit of everything in it, and one thing that is *not* in it is excessive, over-the-top silliness. (Yay!)

Chet's new-skis story is about as silly as this episode gets, and even that isn't too-awful bad. Other than Chet, as he attempts to perfect the skis, being careless where he aims his blowtorch—and the fact that the blowtorch was "on" the whole time prior to him using it—it's an honest mistake. (Also, I wonder if Marco skis, or skied, in real life. He doesn't strike me as the skiing sort.)

Bad news on this episode: Roy's hair. O Keepers of The Book, was this ep filmed at the same time as Pressure 165 and The Indirect Method, back during the dark days of the Awful Comb-Back (aka, the Pompadon't)? I hope so, and this was just a temporary aberration.

The first call comes when the guys are in the locker room. Chet's still in street clothes (blue penguin t-shirt and jeans) when the tones go off. Good thing it was just a call for the squad, as Chet was out of uniform! The call is to a record factory for a kid who got his arm stuck in some machinery. I was impressed that the factory looks quite real and seems to be in actual operation during the filming; maybe the show got permission to use one part of the facility while the regular operations were underway elsewhere. I confess I had to look up what a "worm screw" is... and I think it's funny that Brackett/Dixie don't blink an eye over hearing that the kid has "an arm caught by an 8-inch worm screw." (Wouldn't *you* ask??) Does everyone but me automatically know what a worm screw is? Anyhoo, when Roy gets up to where the kid is, he recites the whole spiel: "I'm Roy DeSoto. I'm a paramedic with LA County Fire Department." Seriously, Roy, all you need to say is "I'm

Roy, and I'm with the fire department." Better yet, "I'm Roy, and we're gonna get you out of here." Short and sweet.

That factory place is awful noisy, and I hope for the actors' sakes that they didn't have to do too many takes; I bet their throats hurt from all the shouting. And when Johnny's talking to Rampart on the biophone, "we" don't hear Brackett's responses, I don't think. Also, Brackett doesn't even ask where they are when he decides to take a road trip out to the scene. I guess he probably has Dixie call the dispatcher to find out where the squad was sent.

Luckily for the kid, by the time Brackett gets there, the guys have already worked out a reasonable solution to freeing him. Doc tells Roy that something has to be done *right now,* and Roy indicates that their plan is underway and asks Gage for a status update. This is where I have to raise my eyebrows again: I think it was awfully rash of Johnny to just "flip the switch" without any warning—to *anyone.* What if Roy had been reaching in to check the kid's arm at that moment? That was dangerous and would be inexcusable in the real world. But this is TV and we have E! magic, so things turn out okay for the kid. I still believe that there was some private joke or maybe an ad-libbed line when Roy and Johnny visit him in the hospital. The way Johnny (Randy) laughs when Roy says "you don't have to pay us a million bucks… right now" always makes me think there was more to it than a simple line. (Fun fact: in real life, the actor who plays the kid became a very well-known and successful musician. Good thing his hand wasn't really hurt!)

At Rampart we hear about a "communications" mix-up involving two squads and two separate hospitals, that luckily didn't have any serious repercussions, but which ended with the reminder that the paramedics should always respond on the biophone with their unit number, as in "10-4, 51." An instruction which I don't think we ever hear, by the way.

May Fair

They may say "10-4, Rampart," and while they usually do repeat any specific orders, especially for IVs and any other drug orders, I don't think I've ever heard them acknowledge with their squad number (either before or since).

Speaking of medications and musical kids, Dr. Morton is trying his bedside manner with a little boy who doesn't want his wound stitched up. Turns out the kid wants to be a violinist, and Dixie convinces him that he'll have trouble holding the bow if his arm doesn't get properly tended. (And props to the show for two cases in a row that actually have some blood and look at least a little bit like actual injuries.)

The next call for the paramedics is a "car on roof" call. Man, I hate when my car gets on top of my house; makes it so hard to back out. Anyway, Roy goes up onto the roof while Johnny checks the house, and it must have been a big-a$$ house, since it takes him soooo long. Roy finds two kids in the car, one of whom is of course a bratty wise-acre. The kids are both kind of idiotic and not really worth discussing. To me, the best part of this rescue is after the first kid carefully, slowly climbs out of the car... and promptly SLAMS the door behind him, causing the car to teeter. (Didn't I warn you, the kids were both stupid?) Anyway, Roy has a bit of panic in his voice as he yells, "Johnny? You wanna hurry with that rope?!?!" So what do we see next? Johnny comes sauntering up the slope, casual as you please, stopping to chat with the kid, and not hurrying *at all*. Yeah, wonder what he'd tell Cap if the car fell off the roof, taking Roy with it, I wonder? Anyway, I thought that was funny, and in general I wanted to smack those kids, especially the one in the front seat. I hope the cops showed up. (Side note: I wonder if LACoFD has to notify the sheriff's office if they respond to calls involving minors?)

Watching EMERGENCY! Seasons 4-6

Next we see Chet, who is again out of uniform as he's wearing a sweatshirt with his uniform pants while he pedals a stationary bike. Call me crazy, but that's as close as we ever come to seeing the Station 51 "gym," never mind a weight room.

Next is the call to the young woman (flight attendant) who took pills and doesn't want anyone to treat her. Other than being curious about the various books in her bookcase (and the Ringling Bros. poster on the wall) I tried not to get too caught up in the surroundings. Roy calls Rampart and tells Early that Diane has refused their assistance, so Joe just gives them some instructions on what to do as soon as she loses consciousness. Roy and Johnny talk to Diane until she passes out, although I have to say Johnny almost acts like it's amusing as he sort of taunts her, saying, "What? Did you say something about Indiana?" I know he was just asking questions to see if she could answer, but his demeanor doesn't seem to match the seriousness of the life-threatening situation. At least, that's how I saw it. But it's too bad the doctors couldn't keep her alive. Another case of the paramedics bringing someone into Rampart alive, only to have the docs lose the victim at the hospital.

I think this is the third episode in a row in which Roy wields a mean fire-extinguisher. First he used one to put out the fire in the exploding TV set (TeeVee), and then he used one to put the snake in a deep-freeze in On Camera. Maybe Kevin owned stock in the company that makes extinguishers??

We have a *very* nice shot of a sleepy-looking Cap getting up and responding to LA's wake-up call. I still wonder how the guys (real firefighters in the real stations, not the actors we see) keep from jumping out of bed and putting on their bunker gear out of habit, since (to me) the "wake-up tones" sound exactly like a regular call-out alarm. Oh well.

May Fair

Last call of the shift is an early one to a guy whose car fell on him while he was working under it. Due to some crazy calls and cancellations, the squad gets there first and Roy and Johnny work to get the guy out. They also, very uncharacteristically, leave an open container of flammable material very close to the site where a 3000-pound car is about to crash to the floor. Yeah, that sounds like them, right?? Especially since it seemed as if Roy was *looking right at it* at one point. Sure enough, as soon as Johnny's able to pull the guy free, the car slips off the jack and falls, sparking an explosion and a crazy-big fire. That's when the engine pulls up, and a cool-headed Cap calls for two inch-and-a-halves. (Or is it inch-and-a-halfs??)

This is where things get squishy. If you look very carefully as Cap, Chet, and Marco take their hoses into the garage, you may not realize you're witnessing a vast conspiracy. Well, maybe not a conspiracy, but certainly a sort of hoax. Sorry for being so melodramatic, but I was all agog today while I watched this. If you look really, *really* closely at the firefighters who attack the fire in that garage, it's obvious that it's not Mike Norell, Marco Lopez, and Tim Donnelly in those turnouts. I even have a crazy theory that Randy, thrillseeker that he is (or at least *was*, in his salad days), asked to take the role of Captain Stanley in this scene. Seen only from the back, the "Cap" in this scene has dark hair that's noticeably longer/shaggier than Mike Norell's hair. (Even if it's *not* Randy, I'm still pretty sure it's not Norell, either.) And the other firefighters are definitely not Tim and Marco. The scene was likely too dangerous to allow the actors to film it. Obviously, unless one pauses the scene and actually looks closely, these things really aren't noticeable.

~ Don't you just love hearing Chet say things like "dig it," and calling people "babe"? Not everyone can pull that off, but from him it seems totally natural.

~ Speaking of Chet, he was in civvies again in the final scene. Guess the guys were getting off shift and he was leaving the station.

5.14 To Buy or Not To Buy

Okay, I have problems with this episode, starting from the very first scene, and related to the title storyline: Roy buying a house. **First off,** if Roy was thinking about taking such a huge step, I'm sure Johnny would have been the first to know, rather than Cap. **Secondly,** most people generally don't decide on the spur of the moment to buy a house without doing any type of research on it (inspections, checking school systems, etc.). **Thirdly,** and most importantly, what kind of $#@%&! husband buys a house without discussing it with his wife?? (Unless you're Donald Trump or Warren Buffett and you say "Honey, I bought a house today; it's in Idaho, so now we've got the entire Lower 48 covered.") Anyway, I pity the average man who would even dream of buying a house without involving his wife and/or girlfriend. To me it's simply inconceivable, so I can't take any of the rest of it seriously. (Including the fact that "Ed Marlow," the paramedic trainee who'd served in Vietnam and was such a pain, changed his name and now sells real estate. Ha-ha, just kidding, Pratt does a great job as the slick agent.)

Okay rant over....

~ The first rescue, the house fire with the two girls: it looked like a 'real' house, i.e., not on the studio backlot. If that was the case, I wonder how nervous those other homeowners and business owners were to have that house set on fire?? Or maybe the whole block was being destroyed, who knows.

May Fair

~ I know we talked about this before, about why, into the house again to rescue the sister, Roy and Johnny didn't just go back up the ladder to the second floor rather than walking through the burning house and up the burned-out stairs. (Did anyone notice that the interior of the house was all burned, but the pictures were still on the walls? I'm pretty sure that defies some laws of physics.)

~ When they went up the ladder to get the first little girl, Roy's inside and Johnny's on the ladder. You can hear Johnny muttering "over my shoulder, put her over my shoulder," a couple of times—not really loud enough for anyone to hear, least of all Roy. And then Roy says (very distinctly), "I'll put her over your shoulder." I thought it odd that Johnny muttered that the way he did; wonder if he was talking to himself.

~ Did anyone notice that in the incident with the two driving schools, both pupil drivers were women?? And one didn't want to wear her glasses while she drove (i.e., she's too vain)? Another example of horrible (and outdated) attitude toward women. **Ugh.**

~ Johnny ate Roy's sandwich. And of course talked with food in his mouth. Big surprise!

~ What the heck was Chet doing with the coffee in a cooking pot?? He had to *ladle* it out, for crying out loud! That's not the kind of "coffee pot" people have in mind when they talk about coffee. Oh, and another multiple use of the word "sore" instead of *mad, angry,* or *p!ssed.* So I guess in Emergency!land, some people *foul up,* and others get *sore* at them. Is that how that works?

~ The rescue of the epileptic boy on the bridge: we've heard Randy say that he thinks of that film shoot every time he goes past that bridge or overpass. Didn't he say that it was actually a "small" adult? Maybe that was only in the scenes in which they were dangling and seen from a distance? Because in the close-up scenes, the person straddling that girder definitely looks like a kid to me. I do have a question about the ropes, though. Johnny was lowered down awfully smoothly considering that Roy was doing it manually and by himself; in real life it would have been a little more herky-jerky and rough.

~ Oh, back to the boy on the bridge... Cap said not to wait for the snorkel truck, but he did have Mike, Marco, and Chet get the other ladders out, which they did, and they leaned them against the bridge. My question: what good was that supposed to do??

~ ~ ~

I'm going to get this out of the way first, because it's the elephant in the room: I hate what the writer did here. What kind of husband does he want to make Roy out to be, anyway? What kind of husband thinks about buying a house... and actually goes out looking... and decides on one to buy...*without talking to his wife??* In other episodes, they go out of their way to suggest that Roy is a little bit henpecked and that Joanne "rules the roost," etc., but in this case they're having Roy suddenly and unilaterally make the single most important decision that will affect his entire family. Drives. Me. Nuts!!

Anyway... After a brief introduction to the logic chart—and Johnny wanting to show off how he can spell Chautauqua— the station gets called out to a house fire. A little girl is at the second floor window, so the guys throw up a ladder and go up there. (Listen as Johnny mutters "over my shoulder, over my shoulder," and then Roy says, quite loudly, "I'll put her over your shoulder." What's that all about??) Once they get the little cutie girl to the ground (and she really IS adorable) we find out that her sister Kathy is still up there and the girl couldn't wake her. So the guys go back into the house to get Kathy. Except they don't go up the ladder, which would make perfect sense and also be pretty easy; nooo, instead they wander through the house—the one that's *on fire!*—to get the girl. And Roy gets hurt in the process. By the way, anyone notice anything weird about the inside of that house??? (Hint: on the walls.) In any case, this is a good rescue and they get Kathy out in time and are able to successfully treat her. But wait! She's only 12 or 13... how can they administer an IV without parental consent?? That sort of seems to be one of those rules that conveniently get ignored when it can make for a more dramatic storyline.

Oh, and this rescue also gave us a chance to see Joe Early quick-waddle down the hall, which is apparently his way of running. Yeah, it's too funny to watch him.

After Roy gets his "injury" seen to, and a glimpse of really old stock footage of Roy and Johnny getting into the squad, there's another call for the paramedics. This time the car accident features a double dose of a horrible stereotype: women drivers who can't drive. (This writer ought to be flogged. Luckily he didn't write any other episodes of this show... although he did apparently write the movie Free Willy.) So the two women drivers were terrible stereotypes: the vain one who's more concerned with her clothing than with her safety, and also didn't want to be seen wearing her glasses... and the model who isn't really all that bad but is still a bad driver. What I do wonder, though, is: 1) why weren't there any cops at that accident scene? Isn't there a law that says they need to be called when there's monetary damages? And 2) were the instructors really going to just drive away and leave the wreckage of that bumper in the middle of the street??

Watching EMERGENCY! Seasons 4-6

The next scene features Robert Pratt as a real estate guy who's trying to sell Roy a house. We all remember him as Marlow, the disastrous trainee, and now he's getting his revenge on Roy by trying to sell him a house. I understand that in real life, Pratt and Randy are good friends (and were back in the day, as well), so I bet this was a fun scene for all of them to shoot. We also get the obligatory scene of Johnny eating (and talking while doing so), and I think we might have actually seen Roy take a bite of food too, believe it or not! And then after the guys leave the room, the real estate guy finishes the sandwich.

The next call is another car accident... with yet another woman driver who was at fault; what was this writer's problems with women drivers, anyway??? This call brings another heart-tugging scene from a kid, this time a little boy whose dog ran away when the accident happened. We don't know how long it took Roy and John to find the dog, or where they found him, or whatever, but it makes for a sweet, smile-inducing moment when Roy brings Feather into the hospital room. (Note to self: In addition to letting young unaccompanied children wander through the halls willy-nilly, Rampart also allows animals in its rooms, from monkeys to dogs to goats. Now that I think of it, a similar scene took place on Adam-12, in the E! crossover, as a matter of fact.) On the plus side, this scene does give us some nice views of our two adorable paramedics, so perhaps the lapse can be forgiven.

Cut to the start of next shift, when Chet is putting eggshells in the coffee to keep the grounds down at the bottom. But the real question is: why would you want to make coffee in a cooking pot so that you have to *ladle* it out?? To quote Hank Hill: "That boy ain't right." Anyway, Roy's in a bad mood because someone bought the house he was interested in, right out from under him. We soon realize who that "someone" is... of course! And after a minute or so, Roy knows too, and boy, is he "sore" at Johnny. Luckily for John Gage, the tones go off and the station gets called out to Johnson Canyon Bridge.

This is a tense rescue, as it involves a boy who's stuck way up on a bridge span and afraid to come down. Cap's willing to wait for the snorkel truck until he finds out the kid is an epileptic. Roy and John prepare to go up immediately and Cap tells Chet to call Rampart to ask if the stress of the situation can set off a grand mal seizure. Chet dutifully gets on the biophone and Morton answers. When Chet asks the question, what does Morton say? "Stand by, let me verify." Does that seem odd to anyone? Is it just me, or does it seem obvious that YES, stress is not a good thing for someone who's prone to suffer seizures?? Wouldn't that be the kind of thing that Morton—the *doctor*—should already KNOW, and not have to confirm?

In any case, Roy and Johnny go up on the bridge, and Johnny edges his way out to the kid. But the kid is starting to get agitated and no sooner does Johnny get to him than, yes, he has a seizure. Luckily John just has time to grab him and they both fall off the span, or whatever it's called. Poor Roy gets bashed into the support strut with the weight of Johnny falling, and he also has to somehow find the strength to lower John and Kid down to the ground before Johnny loses his grip. Once they get to the ground, the other guys take Johnny's burden from him and carry him away while Johnny follows so he can start treating him. Meanwhile, Roy's still up on Bridge-land, making his way back down by himself. This is one of those instances where it would make sense for one of the other (i.e., non-paramedic) guys to work on the actual rescue, so that the paramedics would be on the ground and ready to treat the boy *immediately*.

But all's well that ends well and later at the station Cap congratulates John and Roy for a good rescue. And then the bickering between Roy and Johnny begins, meaning all is once again as it should be.

* * *

> This storyline has always bothered me a little bit. Why would Johnny buy that house without first checking with Roy to make sure he didn't want it? Isn't that what a true friend would do? And what are we supposed to assume happened? Did Johnny sell it to him?

Yeah, I don't think we're ever supposed to know what happened with that house. Interestingly, I think it was only the *next day* that we find out Johnny bought it. He might have made an offer and/or verbal agreement, but there's *no way* he could have already closed on it so quickly, and yet it's presented as a "done deal." And for someone who didn't know a single, solitary, blessed thing about houses, or the market, or inspections, or points, he sure seems to have completed everything awfully quickly. (Either that or he has money to burn.)

The very next episode after this one is Right at Home, where Roy takes Evil Eddie home and we hear about the fireplace, the neighbor's goldfish, and a plate glass window. It's never specified whether he lives in an apartment or a house, but I always assumed he was describing a house.

In any case, no, we're not supposed to know, and no, Johnny wasn't a very good friend in this instance. (Not only for buying the house without checking with Roy, but also for not selling it to him without a profit.)

5.15 Right at Home

Okay, another one of my "not favorite" episodes. Mainly because of the Cousin Oliver kid. Yeah, yeah, I know that wasn't Cousin Oliver, but close enough, and he was annoying. I don't like conflict and people being put in bad situations, so this was just plain annoying. (Especially since Roy was being the good, decent guy that he is, and he didn't deserve the trouble he got for it.)

~ Brackett drives a Jag?? It didn't have the little jaguar ornament on the front of the hood; probably too obvious product placement. Someday when I'm super-rich, that will be my fancy car of choice. (Ah, who am I kidding?? Even if I had millions, I'd just buy a nice, two-year-old Toyota.)

~ I kind of like these episodes in which LACoFD shows off their toys: the choppers (brush stations), snorkels, boats, etc. Yeah, call me a geek, and it's nothing but a PR piece for the Department, but I find it interesting. And I thought it was cool watching the copters take off one after the other.

~ Boy, that Route 126 sure had some wicked S-curves, didn't it??

~ About that accident to which Brackett responds on the chopper.... a tanker truck and a camper... on a dirt road... and they couldn't avoid each other?? (Sort of like being in the desert and crashing into the only other vehicle within 30 miles.) Yes, there was a bend in the road, but assuming a truck or camper is travelling at normal speed, the odds of hitting someone else are pretty low. Except if you're writing for a TV show, however.

Edit: Oh, and I didn't like that storyline about the boy with meningitis. The one woman should have been up-front that she wasn't the mother, and the mother shouldn't have been quite so, um, crabby.

Watching EMERGENCY! Seasons 4-6

~ Also, funny to hear Stoker (supposedly) hit the air horn again on a lonely dirt road. Who did they expect would need to hear it??

~ Love how Brackett just opened the camper door with his bare hands, without waiting 20 seconds for Engine 51. There could have been a gas leak or some other bad thing he could have triggered by doing it himself.

~ Cap said "babe," again, when telling Marco they'd need safety lines.

~ Did the guys know that Brackett was riding with the chopper? I know they could see *someone* working on that man, but A) how did they know it was a doctor, and B) why didn't Johnny seem surprised to see Brackett at an accident scene?

~ There was some very obvious (and somewhat egregious) usage of stock scenes in this episode. The two that come to mind are the opening call, when we see Johnny heading toward the squad from the dorm (when he'd actually been in the rec-room), and the final call, when the guys were woken by the tones and got out of bed and into their bunker gear. Roy had red hair, and Johnny's hair was short. Oh, those action figures that have length-changing hair were at it again, except this time the color changes as well!

~ I did have to laugh too during that final alarm that woke them up. For one thing, the guys all grabbed their blue jackets to put on over their t-shirts, but at the scene they magically had their uniform shirts on. E-magic!! But the real kicker was that the alarm came at 11:12 pm! Sooo funny to think of these grown guys--all six of them--with lights out and already sound asleep just after 11pm, especially when most sixteen-year-olds stay up later than that. What, nobody even watches the late news over there??

~ ~ ~

Or, the one with Evil Eddie (the Cousin Oliver lookalike). I really don't get this one. At first, Eddie seems like a nice enough kid. He's concerned about his dad.... Roy goes out of his way to be kind and nice at the accident scene and on the way to Rampart... the kid is alone in a strange city... he even seems to appreciate Roy's efforts and responds to him... and yet he turns out to be a terror. To me it really doesn't track as a natural progression of events. Also, I don't like people being put in uncomfortable situations to begin with, and I *really* don't like that Roy was being kind and compassionate—and look what he got in return. That really steams my onions.

Oh well... on to the rest of the episode. So Doc Brackett rode with the LACoFD air support people. Sounds like fun and he certainly looked like "Cool Kel" in his jumpsuit and dark shades. Although I confess to being a bit confused—the copters carry some medical supplies, including a defibrillator. And yet there's not a paramedic on board most of the time, so I guess the crewmen are medically trained to some degree? They'd have to be, I would think, in order to use the equipment. And if so, couldn't the engine crews get some of that same training since every station doesn't have paramedics?

Anyway, we get some nice aerial shots of the LACoFD "camps," shots which, ironically, are filmed by other helicopters. Then Copter 10 gets a run to an accident, and speaking of ironic, I find it hard to believe that in the middle of nowhere like that, on roads that must have a very low speed limit, these two vehicles couldn't manage to avoid each other. But then we wouldn't have the drama we so love and enjoy, right??

I do like this rescue, but I still find it strange that Johnny doesn't register even mild surprise at seeing Dr. Brackett so far from Rampart. Not even "Oh, hi, Doc." Also, Copter 10 doesn't look all that big, and yet in addition to the pilot and crewman, it manages to transport a doctor, a paramedic, and two victims to the hospital. Maybe inside it's like the TARDIS.

Okay, so, after Copter 10 takes off, the pilot says "Copter 10, 10-8 to Rampart with two victims." At least, that's what it *sounds* like he says; according to the CCing, he says "Copter 10 *heading* to Rampart." *Heading* makes much more sense than 10-8, but it really does sound like 10-8.

Once at Rampart, we discover that Roy and Eddie both apparently like grape soda, and the PMs and Dixie discuss what's going to happen to Eddie until his mom comes for him or his dad is released from the hospital. Roy doesn't exactly jump at the chance to open his home to Eddie, but is talked into it, and begins to believe it won't be a problem. (Hahahahaha! Fat chance, Roy.) Anyway, here's another mystery for all the E!nuts out there... another one of those "what did he say?" questions. At Rampart, after Johnny teases Roy about his "dehydration" and Roy wipes off part of his grape mustache, Dixie returns and says to Johnny, "You told!" Johnny shrugs and says... what?? What is his reply to Dixie? I know what the closed-captioning tells me he says ("Mothergate"), but that word makes absolutely *no* sense at all. So I'm taking suggestions on what he actually did say. Anyone? ... Beuller??

Next we have a woman bringing a young boy in to Rampart who has meningitis. Dr. Early goes to get an authorization signed so they can do a lumbar puncture, and yet the woman seems oddly reluctant to fill it out. Finally, however, after asking a bunch of questions, she signs it and Early goes and does his thing. Later on, another woman comes in and says

May Fair

"How's Benny?" The first woman, Martha, who I hate to say looked a little old to be the mother of an eight-year-old, turns out not to be Benny's mother at all. That 'honor' belongs to the Johnny-come-lately who had been out of town. Martha the babysitter is the one who brought the kid in to Rampart when he fell ill. Now, I'm not excusing Martha at all—there's absolutely no excuse for her not telling Early that she wasn't Benny's mother. And no, it wasn't just a misunderstanding; it was actual deception or withholding information on her part. On the other hand, the mother isn't exactly blameless, either. What kind of parent goes off for multiple days (or at least overnight) and doesn't leave the sitter with a name or phone number or *any* idea how she can be reached? So there's plenty of guilt to go around, but I have to give the prize to the mother, whose behavior is incomprehensible and inexcusable. (Also, did Martha sign the mother's name, or her own? Must have been the mother's name—forgery!—otherwise Early would've, or should've, noticed the different name.)

Now fast-forward to the next day (next shift) when Roy is listing all the ills of Evil Eddie, the Spawn of Satan. Eddie demands to see the engine and Chet says, "how bad can he be? I'll take him," and Roy predicts that Eddie will insist on blowing the air horn. On his way out, Eddie tells Chet that "Mr. DeSoto is really mean." Wha—?? Roy, *mean??* That's gotta be the most absurd statement ever. In any case, within minutes the air horn sounds, and soon Cap comes in and tells Roy that something has to be done with Eddie. Hmm, now that I think of it, why did Roy bring Eddie to the station to begin with? Did Joanne refuse to deal with the kid while Roy went to work? Was Roy planning to take Eddie on runs with him and Johnny? On a related note, did they leave Eddie at the station when Roy and Johnny went to Rampart to talk to Dixie? And what if the engine had gotten called out, too?

In any case, it's a good thing Dixie picked up Eddie that afternoon because that night the guys get a run that apparently wakes them all up from a deep sleep... and it's just after 11pm, for heaven's sake. We get some old stock footage and bad continuity here, but eventually the engine and squad end up on a very unattractive back lot where a house is fully involved. And of course the man of the house is still inside. But all in all it's a pretty good rescue and fire scene, even with the bad special effects of the fire on a neighboring roof. We hear more of the stock audio, but also, I was impressed to see a Captain manning a hose here. (Not Captain Stanley in this case.) All in all, it's a good one, and our guys are the heroes once again.

Finally, the next day they go to Rampart where Roy's reluctant to see Dixie, and afraid he lost her friendship, poor guy. But no, Dixie had Evil Eddie firmly in line and even got the bra—er, I mean *imp*, to thank the guys for their help. Quite a miracle, indeed! Her explanation is cute, though, even if it isn't exactly on a par with dealing with Eddie.

5.16 The Girl on the Balance Beam

As has been noted on the Least Favorite Episode thread, there's a lot to dislike about this one. It *is* heavy-handed, and shmaltzy, and way too much time is spent with this girl that we never really care about. (At least, *I* don't.) Also, another reason not to like it: *not a single scene* takes place at the station. Not. One. All the time was sacrificed for this girl and her awful father. (And by the way, what is the point of that discussion Johnny had with Dr. Morton? It came from out of the blue and disappeared right back there again, never to be referenced again.)

May Fair

~ As Johnny was hurrying into the gymnasium, right after the opening credits, we see him bend down to pick something up and put it in his pocket. Wonder what that was??

~ He used the biophone notebook.

~ On the rescue to the movie studio, how old was that angel-girl on the wire supposed to be? From her whimpering and whining I thought she was about 12, but she seemed too full-grown to be a tween. Also, she was a horrible actress; was she supposed to be passed out or just scared as they brought her down? Her hands were more or less limp, but then she'd whimper some more. Then her arms were around Roy but she was quiet. I couldn't figure out *what* was going on with her.

~ Okay, I'm just gonna say it: the drunk guy played by Ronnie Schell was *hilarious*. Can't remember the last time I actually laughed out loud while watching TV, but today I did. Wonder how much he was ad-libbing. "That water's cold! I don't know how to swim, officer." "Boy, if I was my friend, I'd trade this in." (It was his friend's car.) A couple times I saw Roy/Kevin trying not to laugh.

~ But where was Vince during this scene? A truck and car in an accident on a large street, the guy was drunk, and not a single cop in sight? Not likely! (P.S., we get a good view of Stoker's turnout coat from the back; it's so *clean*! Unlike Cap's or some of the others, which you can barely read because they're so worn and dirty.)

~ Had to laugh at the gymnastics stuff. First of all, I feel like NBC/Universal was trying to cash in on Olympic fever since this ep aired in early 1976. And that was the summer of Nadia Comaneci, who, incidentally, was FIFTEEN when she won Olympic gold. So this chick Nancy on Emergency!

would have had to already be world-class in January if she wanted to be in the summer Olympics in '76. Plus, I thought it was funny to see the lame scoring they had, and the announcer declared she was performing "superior moves." Sounded like they didn't even bother using real gymnastics terminology.

~ When we see the ambulance (and squad) taking Nancy to Rampart after her second fall, did something fall in front of the camera? At first I thought it was my mouse pointer, but I replayed the scene and maybe it was a piece of paper fluttering in camera range? Took me by surprise.

~ I do like the final scene at the railway fire. Cap had to get tough with some of the railway workers and Chet stepped in to help get the job done. Roy got blasted and was awfully cute stumbling around like a drunken sailor.

~ ~ ~

I'm afraid some might be a little more forgiving with this episode than I am... I think it's right up there (or down there??) on the Least Favorite list. There is one bright spot, though, which I'll get to shortly.

Perhaps it's foreshadowing for season 6, but this episode shows us the "set up" of the first rescue. I bet the powers that be were trying to cash in on the fact that 1976 was an Olympic year; in any case we have this weak storyline of a bratty girl who insists on trying something she hasn't worked on with her coach, and she gets hurt in the process. Come to find out her dad is one of "those" sports parents. Or, as some have said, a moron. As unlikable as they come, and I really find no redeeming quality in him. And I gotta say, when he picks his daughter up at the hospital after her first visit, their whole conversation is kinda creepy. Maybe it's actually *my* family that's dysfunctional, but I can't imagine a father and daughter talking like that to each other. Well, maybe creepy isn't the right word, but at the very least, their conversation is so cheesy. "Can I convince you to come home with me, because I'm lonely. The hospital release forms say that you belong to me." Umm, no, I'm gonna stick with *creepy*.

And yes, the Tinkerbell rescue... I can't tell if she was supposed to be 12 years old or 22. She's whining and crying like a little girl, but her body looks, shall we say, full-grown. It's just a stupid scene. Poor Roy, who has to bear her full weight all of a sudden. And that director lady.... I hate it when people give our guys a hard time by saying things like, "About time you got here," or whatever it is she says. I wanted to smack her.

Had to laugh, though, when the next call comes in. We see Station 51 from across the street (not the inside), and I half expect to hear Sam say "Exercise caution when departing, as there is a gray car rolling slowly past the station." Seriously, I thought that car was going to stop, and maybe be another still alarm for the station to deal with (like the camper fire).

But the call is actually for a "vehicle fire with possible injuries," and THIS SCENE is the best one of the episode. It, and it alone, truly does save it from the bottom of the pile. Ronnie Schell (who's been in three other episodes) is a drunk who hits a truck while driving his friend's car. And he is *hi-lar-i-ous*. I bet it was a hoot to film that scene; I wonder how much ad-libbing he did. Toward the end, I think Kevin had a hard time keeping a straight face.

In that scene, as Stoker wielded those Jaws of Life, I noticed that his turnout coat was almost spotlessly clean and very new-looking. I think I mentioned it last time, and it was just as obvious this time around. Also by the way, the stealth truck (blue pick-up) went past the scene not once, but twice. Same with a blue beetle (lighter blue than the victim's car).

John and Roy are just talking about getting a bite to eat for lunch when they get another call, this time to a train fire at a dockside rail yard. It's a good dramatic rescue, as of course there's some sort of dangerous stuff (this time ammonium nitrate) that's endangering the whole area. I also like Chet doing the "heavy machinery" thing. Who knew that knowing how to operate a crane also gives you the know-how on what to do with a *train*. (Yeah, somehow I don't think it would have been quite that easy in real life; doing the one really isn't the same as doing the other.) But as all the FFs are hosing down the train, Roy uses bolt cutters to open one of the cars, and as soon as it opens, there's a big explosion. Which was impressive, I must say. I did think, however, that Marco should have picked his hose back up instead of running willy-nilly toward everyone else. But I have to say, Roy is *soooo* adorable when he's a little dazed and confused.

I'll also add that I love watching Cap gesture where he wants vehicles to go when he's in charge. He does it in this rescue, with one of the approaching engines, and he also gestures to Chet when it's time to move the train car out of the way. He's so authoritative! Rawr!

Lastly, just voicing displeasure--again—that not only does this episode open somewhere other than the station, it also closes somewhere other than the station. In fact, there's not One. Single. Scene. at Station 51 in this episode. And we are not amused.

* * *

Well she certainly changed her tune after they took Tinkerbell down- in fact, she started coming on to Roy as an envious Johnny looked on, totally oblivious to Dixie saying "go ahead 51" repeatedly over the biophone. Score another one for Roy and his charisma!

True. But I guess I didn't read that scene quite the same way. I know she was crowding Roy's personal space (can't blame her there!), but the way she talked ("go ahead, take your time with her, we're on lunch break"), I just figured she thought she was being generous, as in, "you have plenty of time to deal with this chick, we don't need her back for another hour." Either way, no matter what the scene meant, she was clueless.

Yeah, that mention of Texas City is/was a good reminder of what they try to do to avoid disaster. These days, they would have Cap reference West, Texas, where a similar deadly explosion happened a few years ago. Not nearly as deadly as Texas City, but a tragedy nonetheless.

5.17 Involvement

Yay, an episode back on Netflix!! Thank. God.

However, it was an inauspicious beginning, as the very first shot of the episode was an old stock scene of short-haired firefighters and paramedics getting into their respective vehicles. In fact, once again, there were a lot of stock scenes in this one... and, based on hair length and facial hair, they were all old. Shame on those editors!

I liked the first rescue (the nurse who took pills and then her apartment caught fire) because it shows a little bit of what firefighters do at the scene once the fire is out. They often reference things about clean-up (like when Cap calls in that "fire is out, Engine 51 out 30 minutes"), but we usually don't see it. (Probably because it's boring, but still... it's nice to flesh out the whole firefighting process a little, at least once in a while.)

When the nurse was brought into the treatment room, they mentioned the Bird respirator. This is the one I screen-capped a while back that was so amusing: the Bird Animal Anesthesia Ventilator.

And did anyone recognize the paramedic who brought in the young paraplegic girl? He's better known for another show he was on quite often, whose character earned the nickname "Boom Boom." (Hint: Adam-12)

During the retired nurse's speech to Dixie, I found the timing ironic that she was talking about why she tried to commit suicide. Luckily for her this was a friendly, family show and things ended well for her... better than they do for others in real life.

The lady wrapped in cellophane... why didn't they just call it cellophane? I don't think it's a trade name in the US. Or instead of "plastic" they could have said "plastic wrap." Saying someone is wrapped in plastic could mean any one of a dozen things, none of which would be very good for that person, I don't think. Anyway, Roy turned her over and listened to her breathing from her back. They almost never do that, that I recall. Also, I really wanted to be her when they "felt her up" trying to determine how far up the plastic wrap went.

I like the CO rescue. Although it was funny, after Roy said the front door was locked, Johnny said, "windows are locked too." Actually, he'd been running his fingers over the *screens* in the windows, not the actual windows themselves. And Randy himself had a serious situation with CO in real life... I wonder if this episode was filmed before or after that happened?

The final accident, with the liquid hydrogen and the "invisible fire," for one thing it would have been kind of cool to see an example of the invisible fire. (And yes, I realize how contradictory that sounds, "seeing" an example of something described as invisible.) Not that I don't believe them, but still, it'd be cool to get an idea what they were talking about.

Oh, and at that scene, am I the only one who saw just the one driver? What about the gas truck driver? Or the driver of the other vehicle, the one that exploded? Did I miss something?

Lastly, this is the *second* episode in a row in which *not a single scene* took place at Station 51. Not a new scene, at any rate (see paragraph #1 above in reference to stock footage). I wonder what gives with that? Guess they wanted to beef up the Rampart scenes, maybe.

~ ~ ~

I like this episode, with one major caveat: no scenes at Station 51. We see stock footage of the guys getting into the engine and/or squad when the tones go off, but that's all it is: stock footage. No original scenes filmed at the station. Same with Girl on the Balance Beam, I believe, so that makes two in a row. I'm beginning to get Stoker withdrawal (heh), because even at rescues we don't 'see' Mike very much, much less hear him.

But the call to the apartment building is good. Upon arrival, Cap notes that there's no real smoke, much less flames, so they go in to check it out. Roy finds some smoke coming from under a door and in the apartment there are drapes on fire. I really like watching what they do: Johnny goes to the couch and picks up the unconscious woman there, and Roy and Cap start pulling down the drapes and stamping out the fire. Cap calls the engine for X, Y, and Z equipment and everyone gets to work. And I like seeing that work. I like watching what they do after the fire is out, and the fact that Cap calls for a carpet runner or whatever it was, etc. This shows that firefighters don't just bust in, spray water all over the place, and then leave; they clean up afterward, to some degree. It's nice to show us that from time to time.

So anyway, Millie was the head nurse at Rampart, although obviously Roy and John didn't know her. Was she head nurse in the Emergency Department, or head nurse of the whole hospital, I wonder? In any case, did we all notice that we never actually *see* either the electrodes being applied to her chest, or see the chest thump, or her getting defibbed, or even see her receiving chest compressions? Roy was "pushing" on her (ha!) pretty darn hard in the treatment room doing the CPR, and yet, we never actually see *Millie* during any of this activity; we only see the people who are doing it to her. More proof that the network was pretty loath to show a female body being subjected to that. (Except for the infamous naked-from-the-waist-up woman incident.)

Anyway, I don't know how Dixie knows that Station 51 brought Millie in after there was a fire in her apartment, as nobody asks Roy or Johnny how they found her, and they didn't offer the info. In addition to E!-magic, maybe there's also an E!-grapevine. (Way back when, didn't one episode make a point of showing us that there was an LACoFD scanner at the base station? I'm sure that was the case, but that has *never* been seen or heard or referenced since.)

Anyone notice the "hotphone" in Millie's ICU room? Maybe those phones are in ICU only because I don't recall seeing one anywhere else.

Also at Rampart there's the story of Jean, a paraplegic (I hate when people add an extra syllable and pronounce it "para-pa-legic," which seems to be every time the word was spoken in this one). In any case she's a little brat who's indulging in the world's biggest pity-party. Don't know about anyone else, but I'd like to shake her and say, "look, chickie, nobody *likes* hospitals or *wants* to be stuck in one, so quit being a prima donna. Put on your big-girl pants and deal with it."

In any case, Dr. Morton seems to have the most cogent question of the episode, one which, unfortunately, goes unanswered: what was the girl doing in a swimming pool? I would assume it was some sort of physical therapy, but if that was the case I'd think they would have stated that right away. (Side note: fans of Adam-12 may recognize the paramedic who brought Jean into Rampart. The actor, Claude Johnson, played Officer Brinkman on that show. It's good to see him here on the sister show.)

Next up for our intrepid paramedics is the "woman down at a grocery store." This is the woman who's all wrapped up in plastic wrap, sort of a do-it-yourself "fat-wrap." I admit I was jealous of the woman, mainly because both John and Roy run their hands up and down her body. (*sigh*)

Back at Rampart, Dixie gets the bright idea to pair Millie with problem child Jean. One needs to feel useful and needed, and the other needs to be taught a lesson, so why not? Dixie brings Roy and John up to meet Millie (while she's conscious, this time), which is nice, especially when they do their "aw, shucks, 'tweren't nothin'" thing. They're too cute!! (And Johnny seems to have lost the HT... he had it when he left the base station with Dixie, but when he got off the elevator, his hands were empty.)

I really like the CO rescue. Did we ever determine the timeline in regard to Randy's CO incident? Anyway, even though it's a sly mini-PSA, it's still a good scene. Although, when they first go into the house, I thought they could have picked up the poor dog a little sooner. Especially since it's, you know, right in front of the vent. But at least they do get the dog out and treat him, too, which is really adorable.

Finally is last call for the car that crashed into the tanker. Over the past couple of episodes, how many times have the guys gotten called out while they're in the squad??? In this episode alone we saw three of those in-cab shots that I love (see screen shots). Anyway, the car crash…. I might have mentioned this before, but I have to wonder: we see three vehicles (two cars, one truck), and yet the only "victim" at the scene is the guy trapped in the car. What about the other two?? And if this accident has too few victims, it somehow also has too many engines. The original call came only for Station 51 (which was odd enough, given that it was a 3-vehicle thing), but anyway, after the explosion, we see another engine rolling up to the scene. Maybe Cap calls for back-up?? If so, I didn't hear it.

In any case, this scene features another instance of "what'd he say???" I can't tell what was said, and Netflix's closed-captioning only says "indistinct chatter." It's right after we see the cars backing away from the scene, and as Stoker runs up with the Ajax tool. I think it's Roy's/Kevin's voice, but not sure what he says. Maybe something like "Ah, not springing enough with this." Yeah, I know, that doesn't make any sense, but it's sort of what the words sounded like. It might not have been a scripted line, maybe just something that the mics picked up during filming. Anyway, I just wondered.

(Last note: I loved the houses in the background of those scenes. They were some of those "stilts" houses, on an ugly slope that doesn't even provide a nice view.)

5.18 Above and Beyond, Nearly

~ Spaghetti and chili? Did I hear that right? This is what happens when Stoker and Marco fight for cooking privileges.

~ So Houts was Chief Engineer. As opposed to some other kind of Chief, I'm guessing.

~ The Chief gives Roy and Johnny an award for going "above and beyond" the call of duty, but the guys unfortunately don't recall the incident that earned them the award.

~ "It's not my hat." Classic line. Along with, "Get your hair cut, Gage."

~ The old dancing coot... was he wearing a puka shell necklace? I had one once, I thought it was a "big deal" when a boy gave it to me.

~ Too funny when Brackett's rushing to the elevator for the dental-office emergency, and he practically flings one woman out of his way. I would hope that Fuller spoke with that extra beforehand to let her know he might do something like that, or even suggest she stand so that he'd *have* to do it.

~ Do most hospitals have dental clinics? I can maybe see a dental school having a free (or inexpensive) clinic as a sort of training ground, but I've never heard of a hospital having one before. (But what do I know??)

Watching EMERGENCY! Seasons 4-6

~ Speaking of the dental clinic, the check-in desk of the clinic looked suspiciously like the check-in desk in the Emergency area, complete with the door behind and to the left of the desk.

~ Final rescue, of the climber on the cliff-face: I like that rescue, has plenty of complications, including the fact that it got dark pretty quickly, but a few things about it I just don't understand and I wonder about them every time I see it. 1) If the chopper was called, why not just have the chopper either hover so that they could be lowered down directly to the victim, or at least have the chopper take them to the top of the ridge and climb down (which, as we saw, was MUCH easier than climbing from bottom up), and once that was done, 2) was there a reason they didn't have themselves pulled back up to the top? Not enough manpower for pulling them, maybe? I can't imagine the chopper doesn't have a winch or something. It just seemed to make more work to lower them down and have the chopper go back down and then back up again.

~ Still on the final rescue, I notice they put in an esophageal airway. At one time, didn't they need Rampart's permission before doing that? I'm thinking of Marlowe, the Vietnam-vet trainee, who was about to insert one without clearing it with the hospital. Maybe the policies changed over time as far as what needed authorization and what didn't. Also, aside from the esophageal airway, nothing that Roy and Johnny did on the side of that mountain needed to be done by a paramedic, and yet again we have the most highly-trained guys risking life and limb to get to what could easily have been a dead body. Either or both could have been seriously hurt trying to get to this guy, and another squad would have had to be called, and another 20 minutes waiting, etc.

May Fair

~ Maybe the point of this rescue in this episode was to show that even if that fancy-shmancy award was a mistake, Squad 51 does deserve accolades, even if they come only in the form of a handshake from a grateful friend.

ETA: During the cliff rescue, the scene was dark and the footage not very good (again, not Netflix) but it kinda looked like Johnny had a pretty good wedgie going on. Not sure why, since his belt was above the waist, but that's what it looked like to me. (Not that I was looking, you know, in that particular direction or anything, mind you....) *whistles and walks away*

* * *

Yes, that rescue did take as long as two rescues in a normal episode. In fact, I glanced at the time remaining when they started and thought, "ooh, there might be another one after they get this guy down."

You're right, maybe they (TPTB) wanted to show that the guys occasionally have to "free climb." (Which they did do again, in daytime, in "Santa Rosa County.") But it really didn't make any sense not to wait for the chopper, especially with the danger involved, which Johnny so *helpfully* pointed out to Roy as they climbed. *insert eyeroll here* And did I see they were not wearing gloves? I realize you have to have precise finger work but you also have to have a clean, dry grip, and be able to handle a rope as well.

I know Kevin's thing was a dislike of heights, but I wonder what he felt about climbing like that. They didn't go very high, but it *was* a pretty tricky climb, and as far as I could tell, that really was both of them.

Yeah, all the stock footage we're seeing these days is starting to get annoying.

I really liked it when they showed the long shot of the squad coming back to the station and backing in, with lights on. Definitely more interesting than the standard shot of them just backing up the driveway.

I noticed that too. Neat to see such a different angle. Why don't we see something like that more often, rather than four-year-old footage of the guys getting into their respective rigs?

By the way, in that scene, were those the little raised reflective markers on the floor, maybe used to help guide the squad and engine to correct parking spaces??? I'd never seen reflectors like that in the station before, but it totally makes sense to use them. Also, many of us already know that on streets and highways, white reflectors are for lane markings, yellow is used to show the yellow line separating direction of traffic, and red means "do not enter," but DID YOU KNOW there are other colors used as well? A blue reflector in the roadway indicates the location of a fire hydrant on the shoulder or curb, and green means that emergency vehicles can open gates to a gated community. (Thanks to Wikipedia for that. I don't know if I've ever seen/noticed green reflectors... which says more about where I live than anything else, I guess.)

~ ~ ~

The title of this episode refers to a commendation that our favorite paramedics receive, lauding them for going "above and beyond" the call of duty on a particular rescue. After one of Marco's chili-with-spaghetti lunches, Cap is astonished when Chet says that Chief Engineer Houts has pulled into the station. After a moment of panic, the Station 51 guys hurriedly line up in the apparatus bay, where Johnny's insistent that what he's wearing is "not my hat." Two items of note on that deal: 1) for the mad scramble to line up at attention, we have that horrible "circus" type of music. I hate that music, it means that something very silly is going on and I probably won't like it. And 2) are they really called hats? In the military they're called *covers*, and a lot of police departments refer to head coverings as *covers* too. In any case, regardless of what they're called, Johnny got the wrong one. And he told the Chief about it too, for some reason. (Makes you wonder who got *his*?)

So the Chief gives them their commendations for a really brave and dangerous rescue, and while all the other guys are happy and proud, Roy and John are a little perplexed. (Keep an eye out: when the Chief is reading the commendation, check out how Cap looks at Mike questioningly. Stoker sort of shrugs, and it's just TOO. FUNNY.) In any case, the guys can't remember exactly which rescue they're being honored for, so the rest of the episode is spent with them wracking their brains to figure it out. And don't anyone tell me they didn't discuss it on the way to the first rescue, because *you just know* that they would.

And that call is to a place which is apparently a senior center. First off, when the alarm sounds at the station, it looks like Johnny turns as if to give 'his' hat to Roy—as if Roy can do something with it, right? As it is, they apparently take their hats in the squad with them. (???) And at the facility, Roy pulls in and blocks in a number of cars with the squad. But the victim here is a 94-year-old man who hurt himself while dancing (and wearing a totally hip-looking leisure suit too, I might add). It's kind of a cute rescue, but very fluff-ish and not much to it. About the only thing of note is that apparently Roy's idea of a "splint" is to tape a chair cushion around the guy's ankle. (Uh, yeah, pretty sure that's not gonna cut it, Roy.)

At Rampart, Johnny is confused when people stop him in the hallway to congratulate him. Seems Roy told "the gang" about their commendation, hoping one of them would say they remember the event for which they received the award. After a silly conversation in the enclosed base station (while pretending to smile the whole time, as if that's necessary), the guys find out that neither Early nor Dixie can help them remember.

Upon returning to the station, R and J head immediately for Cap's office, and it looks like Johnny waves at someone before entering. (Well, maybe not waves, but certainly raises a hand in greeting.) I suppose it could have been at Cap, who was sitting in the office, but that seems a little unlikely. Anyway, Johnny thanks Cap for submitting them for the commendation (hoping to learn from him which rescue it was) but Cap insists he had nothing to do with it... except he wants to hear all about this amazing and memorable rescue. So the guys are stuck between the proverbial rock and hard place, since they have no idea, and nobody left to ask.

Meanwhile, back at the ranch—er, I mean Rampart, there's an emergency in the 3rd floor dental clinic. Robert Fuller gets to expend as much energy as we ever see him exhibit on this show as he runs from his office, down the crowded hallway, and to the elevator, where he grabs a woman by the arm and literally flings her aside. Then it's a tense five second wait until they arrive on a floor that looks suspiciously like the Emergency department, and go into the dental office. This is a good scene, they take all sorts of precautions but when they get the victim back downstairs and run more tests, seems his only medical problem is that he faints like a goat. Ya gotta wonder, though, what those other patients waiting in the dental clinic thought when they saw "one of them" being taken away on a gurney, unconscious, and with an IV in his arm.

May Fair

At the station, John and Roy eventually confess to the other guys that they don't remember the supposedly outstanding rescue they performed to earn the commendation. Turns out, none of them remember it, either (which would have made *me* feel better), although they do try to hash it out. Their trip down memory lane is interrupted by Sam, who calls both the engine and squad out to a climbing accident out in the middle of hell's half-acre. (Speaking of, that location reminded me of the place where they found the "hermit" in the cave.)

There are some things about this rescue to like, but watching it this time around, I found those things fewer and farther between. In fact, I got downright impatient and skipped around. First of all, I can't figure out why they thought it would be faster to free-climb (and possibly risk their lives) rather than wait for the chopper which was already on its way. Even if they *hadn't* slipped back down the cliff-face, they wouldn't have reached the victim any sooner than they did with the chopper's help. So why risk life and limb with no actual benefit?? Second, it seems odd that, at the top of the cliff, Marco and the chopper guy have to man three lines by themselves. What about the pilot, couldn't he help? And what is it with LACoFD anyway, that none of their big equipment have winches?? At least getting back down to ground level with the vic was a lot easier than getting *to* him. And thank heavens for Light Unit 103. (I guess they have to remember to say Light *Unit* 103, so people don't think they're a radio station. Yeah, I know, that's pretty bad.)

I think the purpose of this rescue (in addition to just being dangerous, and proving that 'our' guys really do deserve commendations) was to show off the night-vision thing that the choppers can do. Although I did notice that, oddly, after they make a big point of show them using the goggles on the flight to the top of the mountain/cliff, they do *not* wear the goggles on the way back down to pick up the victim and paramedic.

But one of the reasons I don't really care for this rescue is that, it t..a..k..e..s s..o..o..o..o l..o..o..o..o..o..n..g. It is easily 1/3 of the entire episode. And maybe that wouldn't be so bad if we could, you know, actually see something. Not only is this rescue at night in the dark, but since the episode isn't on Netflix, the quality of the scene I watched was awful. (I imagine it's the same on TV, although I hope the DVDs are better.) I honestly couldn't tell what was happening in some parts.

I do wonder, though, about Lite 103. Er, rather Light *Unit* 103. You think they only have one shift that works overnight, say 6pm-7am? And maybe they have a lot of downtime if most of LA County's big accidents happen in the daytime and not at night?? (Ha, just kidding.)

5.19 Grateful

As has been mentioned on the "Least Favorite Episode" thread, Grateful is on the short list for a number of fans. I can't really say that I disagree, but possibly not for the same reasons as others have. (Even the fact that it was written by Mike Norell can't really save it.)

Actually, I like the first rescue the best, with a car that has crashed into a restaurant. John and Roy each working with a victim, not really being able to help each other very much, at least not until they're able to get the woman, Amy, out from under the car. But it was a hectic scene, everyone had to be drafted to help in some way, and that's the kind of thing I like.

May Fair

I found it interesting that the couple's names were Amy and Carter. I'm sure there are no political subtexts in this fact, since the episode aired in early 1975 and Jimmy Carter didn't get elected President until November, '76. Still... interesting.

The two old coots at Rampart: The show got a bit meta and did a sly PSA to tell people not to try, in real life, any 'emergency' life-saving measures they might see on TV. Like chest-thumps. Which have been shown on a show called Emergency! They should do a disclaimer like the one on Mythbusters: "Please don't try anything you're about to see at home. We're trained experts."

Also, I know we've discussed in the past the occasional unfortunate cultural stereotypes on this show (and on Adam-12 as well). In this case, it's the old coots (who I'll call Zeke and Otis). They obviously live in LA county, or they wouldn't be going to Rampart, and I realize that LA County at that time had some rural, undeveloped areas. But where, exactly, in LA County were these codgers from?? Does the county have an annexed area in, say, Arkansas or Tennessee? Did the Clampetts fly Zeke and Otis in from Hooterville on their private jet? Otherwise why did they talk like they were from Deliverance??

We saw Johnny flip out his trusty notebook. (Yay!) He keeps it in his right-cheek—er, I mean, right-side back pocket. Too bad we didn't see an extreme close-up in slo-mo as he whipped it out. (The notebook, I mean... when he whipped out the *notebook*. Keep it clean, people!)

So the Merkles had just moved to LA less than a week ago, and yet they know their way around pretty well. They were able to meet the squad at the scene of the kid with the eye injury, even though Roy and Johnny responded to the call from Rampart.

The boat rescue. Not the most riveting rescue they've been on, which is too bad since it was the 'big finale.' I know we've discussed this one previously as well. But this time, did anyone hear some strange echoing of voices around the time when the second boat got to them? Sounded weird, but that might have been due to technical issues in my particular viewing experience. The echoing effect didn't last long.

Speaking of the boat, Johnny and Roy sure dried off pretty quick, as two minutes after they got in, they were nice and dry.

And no, I didn't see anyone say "thanks" to the boat guy. Hopefully someone (the Cap?) did and we just didn't see it.

Bad news: Johnny's "object" was back in his pocket in this one.

* * *

I do feel the ending of this ep was kind of a cheat, though. Instead of actually *solving* the problem, the guys at 51s were just happy that the problem got 'shifted' elsewhere, since the other station would now have to put up with the Merkles. That's kind of a crappy attitude. (And yes, I can be a Goody Two-Shoes when it comes to stuff like that. I'm all about fairness and not wanting people to be uncomfortable.)

~ ~ ~

The title of this episode refers to the annoying PITA couple Amy and Carter Merkle. (Yes, their names are Amy and Carter.) Station 51 rescues them after a drunk driver apparently takes the phrase "drive-through window" literally and smashes into a pizza place, hitting the table at which the Merkles are sitting. It takes the Jaws of Life to get Amy out from under the vehicle.

May Fair

At first Carter seems to be fine, except he's anxious about his wife—hysterically so. I can understand being concerned about a loved one, but to me, this guy seems inordinately panicked and downright whiny. Obviously I'm not in his shoes, but I hope I wouldn't react that way if I ever had a loved one in a dire situation. He's even worse than the "Debbie! Debbie!" mother. Anyway, he soon keels over and Johnny fears it's his heart, but turns out he's only hyperventilating. Dr. Brackett prescribes the old "breathe into a paper bag" remedy for him. (Don't they have to attach the electrode thingies to transmit data to Rampart? We see Brackett reading the EKG strip, but the guy's not hooked up. I thought the paddles only show the *paramedics* what the heart was doing, and didn't send to Rampart.)

There's some funky editing going on in this scene. We hear Cap tell Rampart the vitals on "victim 2," which is Amy, and *after* that we hear Roy relay those vitals to Cap. Also, while still under the car Roy asks Vince to get him a stethoscope and BP cuff, but it's not until after they extricate Amy that Roy takes the stethoscope from around Johnny's neck; no word on what Vince did with the stethoscope. I think the scene was probably filmed okay, but just put together clumsily and out-of-sequence in the editing room. And one more nitpick about this rescue: the opening credits are so LARGE and they kind of obscure the action behind it. Normally it's not much of a problem, but in this rescue it's difficult enough to see what was going on under that car, and it seems that every time a name comes up on the screen it's on top of Roy trying to work on the woman.

Another funny thing I noticed.... in the ambulance, why did Carter have his arm up in the air? He'd had it up on the back of the ambulance seat, but while Roy was talking to Rampart, we see Carter with his arm raised and his hand balled into a fist.

Up to this point, other than the man's annoying demeanor, I like the Amy-and-Carter rescue. After this, however, their storyline takes a big downhill plunge. I'm sure their actual rescue was based on a 'real' rescue from some logbook somewhere, as they all apparently were, but I sincerely hope that the rest of the Merkle foolishness didn't really happen—in fact, I doubt it did. For one thing I can't imagine anyone being idiotic enough to do what they do: follow the squad and engine around on their rescues. And for another, I can't imagine any fire department captain worth his bugles allowing them to do so without putting a definite stop to it. Roy and Johnny should have been more firm with the Merkles, and if they couldn't, then Cap should have stepped in—and I don't mean by talking around the issue in generalities and using phrases like "I really wish" or "I don't think," as he does here, but in using the actual, forceful words: "Stop. Doing. It." If he mentioned legal ramifications to both the Merkles and the Department, I'm sure that would have done the trick. But he pussyfoots around it and doesn't get the point across. And the end of the episode still bothers me, since the Merkles never do learn the lesson; the problem doesn't get "solved," it gets "transferred," and that's no solution at all.

Okay, now, back to the show.... Fast-forward about a week or so, and we see the guys at the station where Roy and Johnny are peeling carrots and Chet presents Johnny with a riddle. Roy and Marco quickly let on that they know the answer, but *you just know* that's not what John Gage wants to hear. He insists he'll be able to solve it on his own but before he can, the Merkles invade the station and the rest (of the episode) is history. In any case, the guys are very soon looking forward to the prospect of a home-cooked meal. Anticipation which they will soon come to regret.

At Rampart, the "old coots" arrive, and I'm a little disappointed they weren't driving the trusty blue Chevy pick-up. In any case, one runs into Rampart, and it's funny to see Dr. Early grab him by the shoulders and shake him in an effort to find out "what's your problem?" and when the man says "I've got a massive coronary," Early shouts "Get a gurney for this man!" We all know this scene from the infamous blooper reel, but eventually they get the correct person into the treatment room. This storyline was a sly meta PSA against trying what you see on this show at home, especially when Dixie tells Joe, "I hope I don't have any friends who think they can learn that sort of thing [CPR, precordial thumps, etc.] on TV." In other words, "you may see it every week on this very show, but don't do it in real life!"

The next rescue we see is Squad 51 responding to a "child with eye injury." A boy, about seven or eight, was practicing with a BB gun—at his mother's insistence—and there was some sort of strange accident which caused a BB to graze his eye. This rescue reminds us that the writers not only don't know how to write a reasonable woman character, but they also rarely write a reasonable husband-and-wife couple. It's either a boorish bully of a husband with a weak jellyfish of a wife, or a boorish bully of a wife with a weak, henpecked husband. The parents in this case fall into the latter category. On the plus side, sometimes the writers have the weaker spouse finally grow a pair at the very end and stand up for him/herself, as well as the child. That's what happens here, when the husband states firmly, "The doctor is right." I do wish that Dr. Early, too, had been a little more forceful with the mother, and when she asks "is that your medical opinion"—that the kid is just doing what they want only to please them—I wish Early would say, "no, those are your son's words." Not sure why he doesn't, but I'd think that would be the best way to get the mom's attention.

In that scene in the treatment room, did anyone think the eye doctor ("Jean") who examines the little boy looks familiar?

She also plays the psychiatrist who helps the paramedics in Isolation, when they're stuck at that remote station for a day or two.

(Note: I'm purposely not mentioning the Merkles' intrusion into little boy's rescue scene.)

The final rescue gets our guys in Copter 10 to respond to some sort of accident. Halfway there the call is cancelled and the chopper turns around, but while flying over Lake Castaic the pilot spots a boat on fire. He brings the chopper low enough and close enough that Roy and Johnny can drop into the water, and they find a guy swimming away. Another boat happens to come by and they get the driver to help them get the guy on board and then get closer to the burning boat when they find out that (of course!) there's someone else on it. The boat's tank explodes as they get close and Roy uses a small fire extinguisher on the fire while Johnny gets the other victim, and they speed away to safety where Copter 10 is waiting to take them to Rampart. (Roy left the boater's fire extinguisher on the burning boat; oops! Also, the guys are already bone dry as they get the second victim.)

The paramedics arrive back at the station, and even though Roy says the rescue was "wet and wild," they are, again, totally dry. In any case, they're thrilled to find out that the Merkles will no longer be a problem, and they learn why not—which is kind of a cheat, in my opinion. Finally, Chet reminds Johnny that he never gave an answer to the riddle (Chet called it a puzzle) from earlier, even though I'm pretty sure it was probably the previous day when they first talked about it. So Johnny admits he doesn't think there's an answer to the riddle, Chet tells him the answer, blah blah blah. Freeze frame and end of episode.

Notes:

May Fair

~ Hal Frizzell plays an ambulance attendant in this ep, and he actually gets to speak a line or two. On the other hand, Angelo DeMeo plays an orderly or something, and apparently draws some blood for testing.

~ Did Copter 10 have a co-pilot? Usually the choppers do have at least a 2-person crew, but I didn't see anyone but the pilot.

~ I find it hard to believe that Amy could be *that* bad of a cook.

~ Yet another episode in which I didn't hear or understand a particular line. In the very last scene, after they tell the story of what happened with the Merkles, Johnny pats Cap on the back and says... something,... to which Cap replies "For which we can all be grateful." (Hmmm, *grateful*. I just noticed that he used that word.) Anyway, I'm not sure what Johnny says. It sounds like "Credit future runs thin these days." But that's obviously not right. Since this ep isn't on Netflix, I couldn't check the closed-captioning, so in addition to your ears, perhaps those of you with DVR or DVD can check to see what *your* closed-captioning says. *** Subsequent study by eagle-eared fans reveals the line as "My, my, gratitude sure runs thin these days." ***

5.20 The Great Crash Diet

~ I wonder, when the guys first call in to Rampart, they always say "This is Squad 51" when usually nobody is in the little room to hear them. Then they have to repeat who they are.

~ I too liked the first rescue, at Oceanside Park. I like that the show depicted the FD as doing things outside the station:

checking hydrants, fire inspections, etc. This gets them (and us) out of their usual ruts.

~ At the station, it's funny when Chet patted Cap's gut, and Cap said "quit that!" So cute!

~ The boy who ate the cinnamon dough—was his moaning annoying enough? I know people moan when they're uncomfortable, but he was going way overboard. Also, this show isn't known for its special effects, but his gut really did look distended. If it was a flesh-colored prop, it looked real enough.

~ Had to laugh when Johnny, of all people, was telling Morton that "Chet has a tendency to overreact sometimes." Wha—?? Pot, meet kettle! Hahaha!

~ The older woman having the heart problem… notice we didn't see the patches being put on her. Johnny very strategically blocked the camera's view as he slid the patches under her blouse. And I'm a little surprised he didn't send Chet and Marco outside while he checked on Pregnant Patty's dilation.

~ Did anyone notice that after Dixie talked to Obstetrics about the baby, she runs into Roy and Johnny leaving, and the mother is wheeled out of Room 2, then Dixie goes into Room 2. Not sure why she went in there, as Brackett and Preggo Patty are in Room 1.

~ Speaking of Dixie, she told the guys that Morton was "in Kelly's office." Since when does she call Brackett "Kelly"? To the doctors she calls him Kel, and to the paramedics she usually refers to him as "Dr. Brackett." (Or maybe even Kel, I don't know.) But I don't recall her ever calling him Kelly.

~ The show made a point of showing us that Cap took his gloves off to disengage the car horn. That didn't facilitate his injury, did it? I don't think those gloves would have shielded him from the electricity. Would they? But anyway, it was kind of freaky to see the spasms he had. I have to say, though, that I think ALL the Station 51 guys would have been at Rampart to check on Cap. They all went to the hospital when John got hit by the car, didn't they?

* * *

> Stoker "gurgle gurgle", lmao!! Not to mention he was the only one completely dressed during Chet's demonstration, lol.

I noticed that too!! While he pretended to button his shirt a little, he was sort of turned away from the camera, probably to hide the fact that he was fully dressed, and not gonna stoop to taking his uniform off or untucking or even unbuttoning it. (More's the pity, right?) But seriously, I think maybe Stoker thought too highly of the uniform (which he earned the right to wear) to mess with it that way.

> Good auto accident rescue! Everybody clicked together, and Mike had a bunch of lines on the radio reporting the fire.

Yeah, this was Stoker's moment to shine!! With the captain incapacitated (in-Cap-acitated??), the engineer takes command of the scene, and he did it like a real pro. We love ya, Mike!

* * *

> Agree, no idea why the biophone wasn't used for both patients.

I kind of assumed Johnny used that landline so that A) he wouldn't have to schlep over across the room to the biophone, even if it wasn't that far away, and/or B) he didn't have to relay the info through Roy if things got hairy. After all, Roy was using the biophone for a possible heart case and needed to send an EKG to Rampart. Also, he might need the phone at the same time as Johnny if things went south. (After all, John had no way of knowing that both were going to end up talking to Brackett. Too bad we didn't see the good doctor with one phone to each ear. Oh wait, when they call in on the biophone the doctor's at the base station and doesn't use a handset. Never mind!)

I liked that phone Johnny used. I hadn't seen one of those in ages either, but I always liked them. I've heard them referred to as French phones, but I don't know if that's really what they were called back in the day.

Note: in the episode they didn't call it Marineland, it was called Oceanside Park or something like that.

~ ~ ~

Let me just take a moment to thank the Netflix gods that this episode is back on the 'flix. No more horrible quality video and the return of too many screen-pics.

Between all the dried figs and alfalfa sprouts, this is sort of an Issues episode—not just because of the importance of a healthy diet in general, but because of the facts that came out about the lives of firefighters. Stress, irregular sleep habits, inhalation of smoke, chancy diet…. all contribute to health issues and burnout in firefighters and other emergency responders. In the first scene we hear that someone from Rampart is going to visit the station to talk to them about a study that's taking place. This leads to some ribbing of Chet and others, and is mainly notable for the final few seconds of

May Fair

the scene, when Cap pats Chet's gut and Chet returns the favor, prompting the great Cap-ism: "Quit that!" I think that's so cute!!

Roy and Johnny go to Oceanland Park to do some sort of inspection, and of course while they're there, there happens to be an emergency in one of the huge habitats (morays, and maybe something else). Roy and Johnny borrow some scuba gear and go in to assist one of the workers who's trapped in one of the tank's features; it's not a huge rescue, but it does have the benefit of getting our guys soaking wet, which is always a plus, amIright?? I'm not sure why Johnny requests that the engine respond to the scene, not sure what they could do, but it's interesting to see Engine 51 take off from where they were supposedly checking hydrants. (The footage of them driving off is from another episode, where they were waiting for word on the girl threatening suicide.)

Back at the station Dr. Morton addresses the group about the health issues mentioned above. This is the scene that someone clued me in that Roy is wearing slippers. (Actually I think they look more like sandals, but it could really be either one.) I suppose it could be argued that he was letting his shoes dry out after being soaked at Oceanland Park, but that doesn't quite explain it. In any case, just after Stoker serves an ironically rich and artery-clogging lunch, the tones go off and the paramedics are on the run again. (Good to know that in addition to his wonderful spaghetti, Mike makes great chicken, too.)

This call is to treat a boy who ate two loaves of raw cinnamon bread dough. Personally I don't get why he would've been tempted to do it, but that's beside the point. I do have two things to note about this call: at the house, the boy was being annoyingly annoying with all that melodramatic groaning. Did the director really coach him to do that?? And secondly, I'm hoping his "stomach" was some sort of prosthetic. Man, that was freaky looking. In any case, the guys transport the kid to Rampart and later they run into Dr. Morton, who mentions that there seems to be some "dissension" among the guys at the station about the diet, and that Chet is the only one taking it seriously. Johnny and Roy trade "oh, brother" looks, and when Morton questions them about it Johnny says, "You don't know Chet, he has a tendency to overreact sometimes." HAHAHAHAHAHAHAHA!! Does Johnny really say that with a straight face? Oh man.... "Pot, meet Kettle." Don't get me wrong, I'm glad it wasn't Johnny who was taking an idea to the extremest extreme, but ya gotta admit, it's ironically funny to hear John Gage say that someone overreacts.

In any case, back at the station, Johnny wants just one of Stoker's chicken drumsticks before they put the new diet into action, but unfortunately they find that Chet has thrown out all the leftovers. There's nothing to eat but some crackers, which Johnny chomps in Chet's direction... and shows us more masticated cracker than any of us ever want to see. Needless to say the guys go to bed hungry.

The next afternoon (after Roy's calves' liver lunch, which Cap said was delicious) the whole station gets called out to a possible heart attack. Not sure why the engine was there, although it always handy to have Marco and Chet around to do this and that. And Cap contributes by handing Johnny the French phone. ("What kind of a phone is this??") In any case, Roy treats heart-attack mom while Johnny deals with the pregnant daughter and checks her lady parts—with Cap, Marco, and Chet all within uncomfortably close proximity. Anyone else find it odd that Johnny asks the woman "what's the month?" I half-expect her to say "October." (He means "how many months are you," or "how far along?") In any case, both patients are transported safely to Rampart, where the pregnant daughter is wrapped up tighter than a burrito.

Literally, from her neck to her feet; all that's visible is her head. Brackett even checks her out from the side, sort of like lifting the bedspread to see where all the dustbunnies are. I just thought that was strange.

Next we see the station where the guys are apparently doing some sort of calisthenics or other exercises in the apparatus bay. (What happened to this weight room we've heard so much about??) Note that while the other five are in various stages of undress (but, sadly, nothing too eye-opening), Stoker is still 100% in uniform. Yes, he is supposedly buttoning his uniform shirt back up, but I bet it was never unbuttoned to begin with. Mike Stoker was a *professional,* someone who worked hard to earn the right to wear that uniform, and my guess is he wasn't about to be seen out of uniform, no matter what. (Well, that's *my* sense of it, anyway, that he's far too squared-away to be seen at less than his professional best.)

Next we see Chet about to serve some god-awful meal that nobody wants to look at, much less eat; did he go to the Amy Merkle School of Cooking?? Roy takes him aside to chat with him, but I'm disappointed that Roy doesn't take the conversation to the next step. He says "We know you mean well, and we appreciate your concern." And then he stops. He should have followed that up with, "You're taking it too far; instead of going so far overboard, let's stick to making small changes." Bad, Roy; you blew your chance! Luckily, he and Johnny are able to escape the lunch by going to Rampart (probably with a swing past a burger joint on the way) to tell Morton about the monster he's created. Dixie tells them that Morton is "in Kelly's office." This always throws me when she says that. She *never* calls him Kelly; it's always Kel. (Or Dr. Brackett when talking to patients.) But John and Roy tell Morton about his monster and then leave the hospital.

They get a call about a car accident and meet up with the Engine at the scene. Some guy in a fancy car (with a carphone, no less!) has called in the accident and he also actually helps a bit later on. I do like this rescue, it's got a little of everything, and it's definitely an "all hands on deck" kind of situation. Roy and Johnny are dealing with the injured driver when suddenly one of the loose power lines falls and does two things: sparks a fire in the nearby brush, and it hits the car, on which Cap is leaning with his bare hands. (And he yelled at Johnny that one time about not wearing his gloves! Cap took his gloves off to disconnect the car's horn and never put them back on.) Anyway, Roy works on Cap while Johnny stays with the driver. Meanwhile Mike takes charge and directs Marco and Chet in dealing with the brush fire. ** Love, love, *love* seeing Mike take command of the situation. Squee!!** Anyway, Cap has spasms as Roy treats him and checks his heart, but luckily things seem to be pretty okay. I did wonder why we didn't see Chet, Marco, and Mike at Rampart... in real life you know they'd hang out a while to see how Cap is.

Quick bits:

~ I find it funny that Roy says of the crash victim: "age about 42." That seems odd; I'd stick with "round" numbers: 40, 45, 50, etc.

~ Another instance (two, actually) of "who said it." When the power line falls and sparks a fire, I thought it was John who said "we got a fire." But CC says it was Roy. (Also, when they get the call about this accident, it sounds like Roy acknowledging "Squad 51" instead of Johnny. Oddly, the CC on Netflix attributes it to "dispatcher." Hmmm....)

~ Also think it's odd that when the power line hits the car Johnny has to tell Marco to stay in the car. You'd think Marco would know better than to get out right then.

May Fair

* * *

> The calves liver lunch really threw me for a loop. That doesn't seem like an average type meal a firefighter would prepare or eat. And Roy has never come across as any kind of "seasoned" cook.

I just assumed that Roy made this dish as part of the new trial diet. I bet it was basically a "liver and onions" meal, which is probably not that difficult. I just looked up calves liver and apparently it's just veal.

As for Marco, maybe his first instinct was to get out to help Cap. Also, now that I'm thinking about it, when exactly *was* it safe for them to get out of the car? The power line was still "hot," and it was still touching the fence, which was still touching the car. So I don't understand how that worked in this scene.

> I wonder if those kinds of things irritated in real life Marco Lopez, Mike Stoker, Tim Donnelly, and Michael Norell. Being out-shined by Randy and Kevin?

Interesting question. On one hand, Roy and Johnny have been the "star" firefighters from Day One and the other actors knew that going in, so I guess they knew that without the stars, they (Mike S, Marco, Tim, Mike N) wouldn't have a job.

Speaking of that last car-crash rescue, a couple of things struck me about it. Check the scene when the guys first arrive, and how the shadows fall. Then check the shadows later on in the scene. Totally different. Probably took hours to shoot a scene that supposedly played out in 30-45 minutes. (I'll post some comparison pics.) Also, on first arrival at the crashed car, Roy tries the near-side passenger door, only to find it jammed, so he announces that it's stuck and runs to the squad for tools. Meanwhile, Johnny comes around to the passenger side and says "maybe this door is open." Thirdly, Cap knows there's a loose power line. Why doesn't he have it cut down so that it won't fall on the fence, exactly as it did?? They've cut lines before. And he didn't notify the power company as he usually does. Ah well, as he lies at Rampart hospital, he'll wish he did!

Edit: Another thought. We've all seen (and I personally love) when one or the other of the paramedics "borrows" the stethoscope from around the other one's neck. But in this rescue, we see that they definitely *do* have a second stethoscope and BP cuff. Roy gets one out of one of the other boxes (Trauma box, maybe?) so that both victims have BP cuffs on their arms and both paramedics have stethoscopes.

5.21 Tycoons

Does nobody in LA County know how to make a pot of coffee?? Every time someone says "I just poured the last cup," they never bother to make more. That's just plain inconsiderate. And as someone said on a thread long ago, why do they bother with little puny coffee pots? They need a friggin' urn.

The fire-safety inspection of Davey's Dogs was funny. Disgusting and slightly nauseating, but funny. And John and Roy said, "Who'd buy a place like that?" "A total idiot." Then later on Roy says "I think I just figured out what idiot we were talking about.".... too funny!!!

I've always liked the lawnmower rescue, not sure why, exactly. I wonder what they would have done if the guy's heart had stopped? Can't do chest thump... can't do compressions. Guess they just had to hope that didn't happen.

We saw the Bird Animal ventilator again. Probably same footage as last time.

About the status board in the Rampart base station... I'd think that Brackett, Early, Morton, and "even" Dixie have better things to do than stand around moving those magnetic "fire" and "rescue" pieces on the board, even when they're standing right there. That could be a full-time job in itself on some days. I bet it's not usually accurate after the first half-hour of their shift. I suppose the theory is that as they stand at the base station answering a call, they can update the board, but you know how those things go in real life. Or *don't go*, is more like it.

In the previous episode Chet was on a healthy-eating kick, which was extreme even by California standards. But this week, he's all about the chili-dogs. Go figure!

So according to Johnny, whoever bought Davey's Dogs went from being a total idiot to having a gold mine. Funny what a single bite of hot dog will do for you!

Roy and Johnny ate *twice* in this episode: the hot dog at Davey's, and then sandwiches at the station. (You can even hear the crunching of the lettuce as they bite in.) In the latter scene, it was sooo funny when Johnny said "Come on, Roy, do you want to be a fireman all your life?" And, predictably, Roy looks straight at Johnny and says "Yes." *smile* He sounds so cute, like a little boy who wanted to be a fireman since he was a kid.

That evening/night, when the squad was pulling into the house on the call with the baby, you catch a glimpse of an RV/camper parked across the street. It made me think of the

Watching EMERGENCY! Seasons 4-6

RV that Kevin and Randy used as a dressing room. (I think it was Jim Page's camper, maybe?)

And about that baby rescue: anyone else think it funny that Johnny and Roy just took off with the woman's baby?? Yes, they're paramedics and they did talk to a hospital, but it looked odd that they just carried the kid off. And later at the hospital, Roy should know better than to tell the woman "Dr. Early took care of your baby." Don't use past tense, Roy!! I would've thought the same thing that mother thought.

One thing I don't understand. Well, two things... first, after having seen the conditions in the kitchen at Davey's Dogs, I can't believe Roy and Johnny actually agreed to eat there, regardless of what Chet said. In fact, I would've had doubts about it *because* of what Chet said. But the second thing is, what made anyone at Station 51 think the hot dogs they cooked would taste anything like the ones that Hobson cooked? It's not the *building* that makes the hot dogs, it's the person who makes them. Just because a bunch of firemen buy Davey's Dogs doesn't mean that the dogs will taste the same as they did before, when the other guy made them. In fact, who knows, it's probably all the piled-up grease and unclean preparation surfaces that gives the dogs their unique flavor. Clean that up and you'll change the taste of the product.

* * *

> Ok, first off, what is "51's women's auxiliary"? Did they do firefighter stuff or what?

As far as I know, there isn't a 51s women's auxiliary. Never mentioned before or since this ep. I assume Johnny (I think it was him) was just ribbing Cap that the young woman with the fire extinguisher would be handy to have around.

May Fair

At the lawnmower rescue, I too wondered about defibbing the guy. Sending electricity into someone who has a piece of metal in his chest sounds a little dicey to me. (But then, what do *I* know??) Just like the chest compressions… if the guy is dying, you have to do *something*, right?? And the whole point of defibbing is to jolt the heart into some sort of rhythm.

> Johnny was gathering up the equipment, he picked up the trash they littered around the lawn and stashed it in the defib case.

They actually do this pretty often, at least, I've noticed it a number of times. Maybe the camera is focused on the victim being loaded into the ambulance and we just see it in the background, but they've definitely shown it before. Maybe LACoFD has that policy that campgrounds have: You bring it in, you take it out; leave the place like you found it. One major exception to this is the episode Smoke Eater, when the guys worked on the heart victim in his home, things went south, defibbing didn't work, they had to do CPR all the way to the hospital, etc. The scene ended with the cranky captain standing in the man's living room, surrounded by all the trash and debris of the rescue efforts, which ultimately were in vain. (That was done for effect.)

The Bird Animal ventilator, I think we concluded/verified that "Bird" is the brand name. Still not sure what the word "animal" is doing there. Unless they also make ventilators for carrots and potatoes.

And I too noticed that, on the night-time ride to the hospital with the baby, the squad's passenger (Johnny) didn't have a baby in his arms, much less giving one mouth-to-mouth, when we saw Squad 51 arrive at Rampart. In fact, I wonder how far back they had to reach in the stock-footage vault to find the scene of the squad backing in at the hospital with *both* Johnny and Roy inside? Especially at night?

~ ~ ~

Another money-making venture features in this episode. A while back was the floor-cleaning business, which Roy wanted to start slowly and maybe—*maybe*—later they might bring in others. Now it's a hot-dog stand, which, upon first seeing it, Johnny says "What a dump." Later, when Roy wonders who'd buy a place like that, Johnny says "A total idiot." Then, in a nice touch of continuity, when they finally marvel at Davey's "fantastic" chili-dogs, Roy says "I think I just figured out who the idiot is."

Getting back to the first scene, the guys run into Cap in the day-room, and once again, there's no coffee. Cap took the last cup and guess what? He didn't make any more. "That figures," Johnny says, but guess what? He doesn't bother to make any more, either. What is wrong with these people!!! And what about that fancy double-cooker type of coffee maker they have? What's the point of having something like that if they never actually make more than three cups of coffee at a time??

Okay, I'm done ranting now. Anyway, first call is to a fire in an alley, and when Station 51 gets there they find a small trash fire that has effectively been put out by a gung-ho woman with an extinguisher. There are some cute scenes of Roy and Johnny teasing Cap, but otherwise this is truly a non-event (although Cap does have Marco give the dumpster a good washing, just so they can say they did something). As the paramedics walk back to the squad Johnny says "Good thing Cap cancelled the truck company," and Roy responds "Yeah, we'd have heard about that for years." Really, I'm not sure why they would feel embarrassed... it's not like *they* put in the call and made it sound bigger than it was. Also, if I was Stoker I'd be mad: Johnny said something about *five* guys standing around in full turnout gear. Is he excluding Mike? Or the captain??

May Fair

After this call is when they go to Davey's Dogs. I wonder what was the deal with the place, if what we see is really the inside of that building, or if they just made it look like it? If we see the real inside of that building, I hope it was condemned or actually for sale or something.

Leaving Davey's, they get the call for Lawnmower Guy. I like this rescue, as it's not simple and straightforward. I could say something about the very little blood we see in that wound, but I'll let it pass this time. Although I did think that based on the wound, the object embedded in his chest would have been larger than that tiny piece of nail we see later. In any case, I'm surprised they actually used the defibrillator on him, since who knew what that would do to the object in his chest. But I guess he would definitely have died if they *hadn't* defibbed, so it was a chance they had to take. If that was the case, though, I'd have liked to see a little more drama about that.

Check it out: when they take Lawnmower Guy to Rampart and into the treatment room, Roy takes the tubes that I think were attached to the O2 tank... and it sort of looks like he just sets the tubes on the floor or something. I know there are supposedly air hook-ups in the wall or maybe some machine for respiration (the Bird?) or something that the victim can be plugged in to, but I don't think Kevin did anything with the tube(s). I think he just sets them down and makes his exit.

On the plus side, we finally have proof that yes, there actually *are* other doctors who work at Rampart, as all the operating rooms are tied up, so of course Brackett and Early need to do surgery themselves, in the treatment room.

Next up is the guy with a mysterious wound to his leg which he doesn't want looked at. He's being held by the cops on suspicion of burglary and so far the only evidence of the crime is in his leg... and it's a bullet. He doesn't want the 'evidence' to get in the cops' hands so he tells Brackett to back off. But of course Kel is able to reason with him, or, more truthfully, scare him straight.

Later, John and Roy are having a late evening snack (Roy actually eats! You can hear him crunch the lettuce!) as Johnny works up his Station 51 Enterprises idea. But even though Davey's hot dogs/chili dogs are good, Roy's not having any of it. Can't say I blame him... buying the building doesn't mean *their* hot dogs will taste the same as Davey's do. For all they know, the five years' accumulation of grease and crud (and dead flies??) could be what gives the chili and dogs their unique taste. (Charming thought, isn't it?)

Anyway, this conversation is interrupted by a call for a baby with breathing problems, and in a very unique situation, Dr. Early tells the guys to bring the baby right in, in the squad, without waiting for an ambulance. They mention a "peds airway" which Johnny apparently inserts in her mouth or throat. (??) Not sure how that affects (assists or impedes) Johnny doing the rescue breathing on the tot, but he's able to sustain it all the way in to the treatment room. (Luckily the victim is so small that he can carry her and run at the same time. And a careful viewing shows that the baby was actually alert and happy during the rush down Rampart's hallway—a real cutie.) I did wonder though: Roy carries the baby out of the woman's house; why doesn't he just keep her and let Johnny drive the squad??

When the mother arrives at the hospital, it's somewhat realistic when she addresses Roy and he says "This is Dr. Early, he took care of your daughter." His use of the past tense is kind of a bonehead move, though, as she thinks her baby has died—which I would have thought, too—but happily, no, that's not the case. Turns out this is probably a

May Fair

case of what will later become known as crib death, or SIDS, which as far as I know is still pretty much a mystery to doctors. (And a potentially horrible threat for new parents.)

At the station, Roy seems to be the last holdout standing in the way of Station 51 Enterprises, but as the others try to convince him the tones go off and they're called out to a structure fire at a chemical plant. Luckily there isn't an instance of "someone left inside," but there are other things here that make it busy. By the way, have we ever figured out why the FFs in the jumpseats run back and get on the tailboard when the trucks/engines back up? We see it twice at this fire, and we've seen it in other eps as well. Anyway, at this fire they're dealing with 'normal pentane,' which apparently is different from outstanding pentane and lackluster pentane. (Ha-ha, yeah, I guess that's not funny.) So the guys carry their hoses up to the roof of the building, and Roy and Cap actually fight the fire while the other guys turn off some valves. And of course what does John Gage do but break one of the valves, and just see what kind of trouble he gets in: it causes an explosion which becomes another fire that leads to yet another explosion and fire that needs to be dealt with. Bad, bad Johnny! In any case, this all seems to be much ado about nothing, as no sooner does the ladder truck get into place than ¡voila! the fire is out. Seriously, once that happens the whole fire is out within a minute and a half. Amazing, huh??

Last scene is at the station. Roy finally decides he's going to buy into the hot dog stand thing... when Cap comes in and says the place burned down last shift. Final glimpse is the sight of Chet, Roy, and Johnny as See No Evil, Speak No Evil, Hear No Evil. (Marco's sitting at the table, but he's just window dressing.)

~ No Dr. Morton in this episode.

~ Fun fact: If you look closely, a crew member is visible on the roof of that building.

~ Speaking of Mikes, we don't see Stoker at all, except at fire scenes; I think his only line was over the radio to Cap.

~ The answer to Roy's question is: Alexander Hamilton is on the $10 bill.

5.22 The Nuisance

Okay, we all know the importance of this episode: 1) Johnny gets hurt (it's #3 in the "Johnny in Jeopardy" trifecta), 2) the introduction of the bane of every paramedic's existence, Brice, and 3) Randy directed it.

~ Middle-of-the-night call... I wonder why the engine got called out on a run for a spaced-out woman at a bar? Because they needed everyone there for Johnny's injury, that's why!! Of course, Stoker never made it out of the engine. I hope he had a book stashed in the cab. Or maybe he just listens to the radio.

~ Spacey-lady's sister came in and ordered a beer... she neither paid for it nor took a sip. As soon as her sister "came to," she was outta there.

~ Love the look on Roy's face as he leans over Johnny in the middle of the street. I bet that no matter how professional he is normally, in that situation, his mind probably went blank and for a brief second or two he was *not* thinking like a paramedic. (Even though he had the presence of mind to shout for the Trauma Box.) Would've liked to see a scene in the ambulance, but that would've required Randy to be on-screen, and the whole point of the accident was to free him up so he could direct.

~ Weird seeing him lying there in the treatment-room-turned-OR with his *eyes taped shut*. Freaky-weird. Have we ever seen that done with any other patient at Rampart, under *any* circumstances? I don't think so, not that I recall.

~ Randy must've liked the hand-held camera shots, as we got plenty of shaky, moving cameras in the treatment room.

~ Had to laugh when Johnny was telling the woman "It's hard to think of you as a physical therapist." I kept expecting him to finish the sentence with "You look more like a stewardess to me." And later on, when he was trying to shush her, he called her hon. "Not now, hon." (I don't think I'd like that, if I were her.)

~ Anyone notice how short Johnny's hospital gown was in that first scene when the girl and Dixie walked in? Good thing he was wearing boxers underneath. (I hope....)

~ The drill-sergeant nurse... her lashes were worse than Dixie's.

~ Roy and Brice— er, I mean DeSoto and Brice: so glad our boy finally told him off. You go, Roy!! Also, usually Johnny keeps his helmet on the back window-wall of the cab, but neither Roy nor Brice kept theirs there.

~ Arriving at the scene of a rescue, Roy said on the radio "Squad 51 at scene." I don't think we've heard that since the first season, have we? Maybe Brice insisted on it?

~ When Brice was getting respiration on that guy, I thought he placed his hand rather high up, more on the chest, whereas when Roy takes respirations, he does it on the belly.

~ At the "big fire" that Johnny was watching, as the guys were being put in the ambulance I saw a guy whose turnout indicated his name was Stone... again. Yep, definitely re-using those prop turnout coats!

~ Lastly, I don't recall soap operas back in the day spending so much time in a therapist's office. ??? Most of them had hospital settings (which would've been fun for some meta-meta references from John Gage), or law offices or just the local millionaire's mansion. You'd think they could've done a better job with that, right??

~ ~ ~

Every now and then I watch an episode and notice or realize something that I hadn't before, and that's what happened when I watched The Nuisance today. It's nothing major or earthshaking, but sometimes we just accept a storyline or plot point without question, and it's nice when the light bulb goes off and we can connect the dots.

In any case, we all know what happens in this episode, and the setup at the bar with the spaced-out woman at 2:00 in the morning isn't all that important. What *is* important is what happens when the guys of Station 51 leave the scene. Johnny walks around the squad to put some of the equipment away and *bam!* he gets hit by a hit-and-run driver. Obviously the other five members of Station 51 (and Vince) rush to give assistance, but of course Roy reaches him first. I always like how he leans over his partner and asks questions about how he feels, where he hurts, etc. (This is the first scene where I began my oft-repeated mantra, "I wish this was on Netflix!!")

We don't see much of what happens immediately after Johnny is hit, but we do see him get loaded into the ambulance. I wondered today why another squad wasn't called out on this accident? Yes, it's true, Roy is arguably the best paramedic in LA County and he is *right there*, but there are two—no, three—reasons why another squad should have been called out. 1) The drug box got splattered all over the road, so a good portion of its contents is unusable, and Roy might need it; 2) Roy is just one guy, and paramedics work in pairs. I realize this isn't a very important reason, and one paramedic could, in normal circumstances, easily give perfectly excellent care, but then there's 3) the emotional connection. Not only did this happen to Roy's partner and friend, but he witnessed the violent accident, which could put him in some degree of shock as well. After all, there's a reason why doctors don't treat family members. I do realize, though, that time might have been a factor in this case, as Johnny was suspected of having internal injuries. But still… from a purely procedural perspective, another squad *should* have been called out.

In any case, it would have been interesting to see the actual treatment Roy administers at the scene, not to mention the ambulance ride to Rampart. However, that would defeat the purpose of the accident: Randy minimizing his time onscreen so he could direct. Also, it's kind of a nice realistic touch when, as he's being loaded into the ambulance, Roy asks John how he feels and Gage replies, "I'm trying to think of something funny, but I hurt too much." Yeah, I can totally see him saying that.

I also like watching Roy help out in the treatment room. Seeing him in his t-shirt, suspenders, and bunker pants wasn't unpleasant either, don'tcha know. Johnny's looking bad, but Roy is looking gooood. Also, I think it's interesting that Dr. Early says that if John had a ruptured liver or spleen, he'd have pain in his left collarbone/shoulder area. Is that still an (unscientific) indicator of that sort of injury? Good to know.

Watching EMERGENCY! Seasons 4-6

After the creepy scene of Johnny with his eyes taped shut during surgery (we've never seen that with any of the other surgery patients), fast-forward a couple days when the rest of the guys are at the station for next shift (it's shift-change) and Dwyer #2 tells Roy that Brice is going to be his partner for the duration. First of all, not sure why everyone else seems to know about Brice, and yet Roy—a fellow paramedic, no less—doesn't even seem to recognize the name. On the plus side, though, I think it's at least a nice touch (realistic) to see not just one, not two, but *three* members of the other shift in that scene. A very minor detail, but again, it adds realism that bolsters the claim that 'our' guys are not the *only* guys who work there.

So we meet Brice. He's blunt, brash, and a pain in the ash. He's the Sheldon Cooper of LACoFD paramedics, and poor Roy is Leonard. Brice even sprays Johnny's helmet with disinfectant before he uses it. Bottom line: it's obvious that Roy's gonna have his hands full.

Back at Rampart, Johnny's wearing a skimpy hospital gown while watching some horrible-even-for-1976 soap opera. He meets a very attractive physical therapist, and I thought his first words to her were going to be "you remind me of this stewardess I once knew...." Yeah, I probably made that joke last time. But it's interesting that Gretchen Corbett appears in both the first and last episodes of season 5. Also, did you get a load of that TV remote? It's the size of a small brick. We didn't have a remote at our house at that time— we still only had four channels, I think—but my parents always said that that's why they had *us:* to get up and change the channel. It's also about this time that we meet the real nuisance: the mean nurse. I don't even think she has a name, does she? Of course, we've never seen her before and never see her again, but I like to think that this woman was specifically assigned to patient John Gage by one Dixie McCall. I do wonder, though, if the nurse really had authority to "kick out" the physical therapist. I wouldn't think so.

At the station, Cap asks Roy how he's getting along with Brice. Roy says "Fine, no problem," and then says "We get along fine, but I might have to bust his nose." And finally, after a run in which Brice terrifies the victim, Roy lays it on the line, the way we've been hoping for him to do all along. "I can give you twelve reasons why your way is wrong, but I'm gonna give you just one: I'm the senior paramedic," he says, "and as long as I am, we're gonna do things *my* way." Go, Roy! And might I add, "rawr!"

The scene of Johnny seeing the news item about the big fire is interesting. For one thing, when they show a bunch of different trucks/engines arriving, that sort of reminds me of the Steel Inferno movie. Which hadn't been filmed yet, so I don't know why it would remind me of it. But it's also funny/interesting/ironic that the physical therapist chooses that moment to want to talk to Johnny about... well, them. Unfortunately for her, for once in his life, Johnny doesn't really want to talk to the attractive woman who is expressing interest in him. He calls her "Hon," and then pretty much tells her that his buds are in trouble and he can't pay any attention to her at the moment.

Meanwhile, back at the fire.... The firemen have to ventilate by opening doors and stuff inside the building, and that's what Station 51 guys are doing. Chet's with Cap, doing something or other, but Roy, Marco, and Brice are together lugging a hose through the building. Roy says something about "be careful of this floor," and later, while we're seeing Chet and Cap, there's a big explosion-type noise. When Cap goes to check on it, he and Chet see a caved-in floor and that's supposedly where our guys are—they fell through. (This is the penny-drop scene for me; I never really realized how or why the guys got injured.) Anyway, Cap calls for assistance, and once he gets the blueprints and finds where the guys are, he requests the K-12 and tells Chet to go meet the guys bringing it because, "They ain't gonna find us up here." (Another instance of 'ain't'... I thought that was cute.) Also, when the news guy is showing the injured FFs being brought down, he misidentifies the ambulance drivers as paramedics. In any case, the injured guys are Roy and Marco. Not surprisingly, Brice somehow comes out without a scratch.

Final scene is at the hospital, where Roy and Marco are probably in for overnight observation and Johnny comes to visit. Nurse Nuisance comes in and runs him off for his bath, and when Roy protests, she says "you wait, Steve Stunning, you're next." That puts the fear of God into Roy and Marco, which is no surprise. But to me, the big question is... who gave Marco a dozen roses?? Roy only has an ugly plant.

Other:

~ Nurse Wretched has lashes that rival the beautician who went crazy and pulled her boss's wig off.

~ Funny page over the PA for Dr. Roberto Almonzo. The funny part was, it didn't tell him anything. It just says "Dr. Roberto Almonzo, Dr. Roberto Almonzo."

~ The Public Information Officer on the TV broadcast is listed on imdb as being played by "J.B. Friend." I know we debated this matter before, but thought it was worth repeating.

~ Another sighting of a firefighter named Stone at the fire scene; someone wearing the "Stone" turnout coat. As I've said, they sure got their money's worth out of props

Season Six

Yes, it's the last of the regular seasons of Emergency! Chin up, ladies and gents, we still have a number of episodes yet to enjoy. Note: The order of episodes in this season varies; imdb not listing them in the same order as the Netflix or the DVDs, etc. So the order you see them in may vary.

This last season brings three major changes that I can think of off the top of my head:

1) We see the 'set-up' of some of the rescues (which sort of began toward the end of Season 5).

2) Dixie no longer wears her nurse's cap, although the other nurses do. (Maybe it's Head Nurse privilege?)

3) The paramedics have the paramedic sticker on their helmets, making it easy to find/identify them at a hectic and smoky disaster scene.

Have I missed any other changes for the season?? (A certain four-legged change will appear soon.)

6.1 The Game

Okay, so this episode starts the final season, but it's not one of my favorites. In fact, this one may be in my "bottom five."

~ When Roy and Johnny are up in the tree with the Jersey roof-man, it was funny to see Roy kind of "feel up" the man's thigh in order to find any possible breaks. Lucky man!! Also, I have to say, I love when one of the FFs gets behind and holds the ladder while Johnny or Roy climb up. They sort of plant their feet and pull back, and it looks cool. (Yeah, I said that: holding the ladder looks cool. Whaddaya gonna do about it??)

Edit: When the mom drove away in the van and the rope was still tied... what are the chances that she'd pull down a whole full-grown tree? More likely her bumper would fall off.

~ The status board at Rampart's base station: Station 51 wasn't at the top, as it had been previously. Did they get 'demoted'?

~ When Johnny was in the shower at the station and Roy dumped the bucket of water on him... I assume that was in the script, but I like to think (i.e., wish) it was just a prank Kevin pulled during filming. Loved his sly smile as he walked away (toward the camera). Of course he had the t-shirt on and towel around his neck.... rawr!!!!

~ At the stadium, did Johnny do the Heimlich on that guy in the tunnel? It's possible, since the Heimlich was 'invented' (is that the right word?) in 1973, so by the time this episode was on, it would have been known in the emergency medicine community (if not the general public).

~ The fan who sat nearby asked Johnny to bring him a hot dog next time they went on a run. Don't vendors come around selling hot dogs and other food or snacks? He doesn't even need to leave his seat.

~ I guess our guys on "Team 8" would still call Rampart while at the stadium, since that's where the biophone is wired to transmit, but would Rampart really be the nearest hospital to the stadium? I have no idea where the *fictional* Rampart is supposed to be in relation to the Coliseum. (But obviously UCLA Harbor General shouldn't be that far away.)

~ We had a page for Stat Ident Doctor.

May Fair

~ We also have Treatment Room 7 now? Is that new this season too??

~ Scenes of the game: was it my imagination or were the teams facing in opposite directions half the time, even in the same "half" of the game?? Red team facing left, then right, all before half-time. Not sure about college rules back then, but I thought they switched sides at half-time, not each quarter.

~ The heart attack in the press-box. With that announcer doing the play-by-play while the guys were working on the heart victim, I thought their vitals might be mixed up with the announcer saying "That was number 34, he ran 42 yards, and now the team is at the 27." Can you imagine hearing all that when you're trying to remember BP and pulse and respiration numbers??

~ The final scene at the Coliseum always bugs me. You can't tell me that during the 15-20 minute drive from Rampart to the stadium, they didn't know the game was nearly over, or had just finished, or whatever. And to have absolutely NOBODY left in the whole stadium... it strains my credibility beyond reason. Not to mention they'd have noticed heavy traffic, and there being no cars around when they got out of the ambulance. Speaking of... where did the ambulance go? Weren't they supposed to hang around? And how did Roy and Johnny get to the stadium before the game in the first place? *That's* how they get home.

Sorry to nitpick, but that scene really bugs me and pushes the whole episode from *meh* to *bleah*. Add to that the generic comments that Early and Dixie were making during the game... I'm just glad to get to the other episodes and forget this one altogether. Very few highlights in this one for me.

* * *

What is a Stat Ident Doctor by the way?

I don't think we've ever figured that out for sure. The usual page is something like "Stat ident doctor, Room Three." One guess might be that a doctor is needed in Room Three, stat, and he should identify himself immediately upon arrival—and by 'identify himself,' that may mean to let the switchboard or 'someone' know that Dr. Estrada is taking care of the patient in Room Three. . (Maybe...?) I know that sounds odd (and unlikely) but sometimes there are similar calls on Adam-12, when the dispatcher doesn't call a particular unit, but announces a problem somewhere and says "unit responding, please identify," or something like that.

You mention how Roy pushes Johnny from the staff room at Rampart before Johnny can tell the doctors that they really haven't seen much of the game. Usually it's Johnny who tries to do stuff like that, and Roy who wants to be honest about things.

~ ~ ~

I think I'm on record as saying this isn't one of my fave episodes. It starts out simply enough, with Roy and Johnny bringing some groceries (ingredients) for Marco's lunch. Meantime, Cap comes in and tells the paramedics that they've been chosen to work the "big game." (I hate that phrase; I don't think I've ever heard anyone in real life say they're going to "the big game," or getting ready for "the big game." I've only ever heard it on TV.) Anyway, the rest of the station guys are envious that Johnny and Roy are going to be there in person. Roy's quick to remind them that they'll be "on duty" while they're there and it won't be all fun and games, but hey, they'll *be there,* at the stadium, seeing the game *live,* and that's gonna be exciting in itself, right?

Meanwhile, with the new format of the show, the scene cuts to somewhere in suburbia where we have to listen to some gosh-awful music while Joe Homeowner stupidly tells his Bart

May Fair

Simpson kid to "tie me off somewhere strong" and then doesn't watch or even look where he does it. Turns out, the kid ties the rope to the family van and when mom takes off to spend dad's hard-earned money, dad gets pulled into a tree. (He should thank his lucky stars: he landed in a *tree*.) By the way, I noticed that the ignition in the van is to the *left* of the steering wheel, rather than on the right. Was that a thing, back in the day? I don't recall ever using my left hand to start a car. Maybe it was a van/truck thing??

Anyway, Station 51 arrives and saves the day, with Johnny climbing up the neighbor's ladder and tying off the victim (for real, this time) and they lower him down. He's got a broken something-or-other in his leg, but at least he and his family have broken the ice with their local fire department in anticipation of a long and hopefully-not-painful relationship. By the way, when the scene ends, with the mom driving off with the rope still attached—probably now tangled in the tree—we see Johnny cringe... and then a freeze-frame. They don't normally end scenes with a freeze-frame, so I wonder if there was a reason for it. Probably not, and we'll never, ever know anyway, so I guess it's pointless to even ponder it. Forget I asked.

Next we have a nice scene at the station in the locker room (or, as they call it, the wash-room) as John and Roy are getting ready to go to the "big game" and Marco and Chet are gonna get together with the other guys and have burgers while they watch on TV. Is this the only time we ever see the shower being used? I can't think of another time, offhand. But it's nice to see Roy shaving. And when he dumps the cold water on Johnny in the shower... priceless! Love that little grin he gives. I assume that was scripted, since Johnny (Randy) wasn't *really* in the shower, but it was a nice, funny touch.

I'm sure this episode played well in the SoCal area, but since I'm not a big college football fan, I really don't much care about the game, nor was I interested in seeing the Trojan on the horse. (Heh.) Anyway, all the scenes of the actual game do little for me. I also don't like the fact that the game was sort of an excuse for butt-shots and awkwardness as the guys get to their seats, leave their seats, come back to their seats, etc. Also, I don't think too many football games have instances of people saying "down in front." It's a stadium, you fool, if someone in front of you is standing, you can stand too.

It's funny when the woman in charge is briefing all the personnel; you can tell that Johnny's getting antsy and wants to get to his assigned area. 'Johnny, antsy?' you say? Naw, that never happens! I do like the choking guy in the tunnel... they don't mention the word Heimlich, do they? I don't think so. It was a relatively new procedure, but I'm sure the paramedics would have been among the first to be trained on how to do it.

Next, after more awkward climbing around to get to their seats, comes a guy with trouble breathing. After just about preparing to put electrodes on the guy to check his heart, they find out that he has a habit of "breathing too fast." This is a big tip-off to the guys, so they grab a paper bag that they happen to have (or find) and have him breathe into it. Yep, that's it—he's just hyperventilating. I do wonder though... shouldn't he have held the bag over his nose as well as his mouth? The point of the bag is to re-breathe your own CO_2, and it's kind of difficult to breathe in what's in the bag, if the bag isn't over your nose. Duh.

Anyway, back to the game. I do wonder if the football players who were mentioned by name (by the broadcasters, etc.) were actual players on USC or Stanford. I heard one named Lopez, another named McKay. I assume they were made-up names, but maybe not. After the hyperventilating guy, Roy and Johnny get moved down to the 50-yard line. Yay, finally they'll get to see some of the game, right? Wrong. Seems that

May Fair

no sooner do they get to their new spot when a player runs out of bounds right toward them, and as bodies start to fall, Roy and Johnny fall with them, and so does a nearby photographer, who doesn't get back up again. So the guys have their next victim to deal with—with the assistance of the coordinator woman, who is also some sort of medical professional. By the way, the scenes we see of the guys standing behind the team bench and then treating the victim there on the sidelines are obviously fake, and not filmed during a real game. Yeah, I know I'm not telling anything you don't already know. Also, I did think it was strange, in the ambulance when we see the victim he doesn't have shoes or socks on. I suppose Rampart might have ordered the guys to check his Babinski reflex, but I don't think we heard that, did we?

Once the paramedics get back to the stadium, they're hoping their run of calls has ended, and Roy is having trouble with the sorriest-looking hot dog you've ever seen. However, no sooner do they try to relax and enjoy the surroundings than they get called up to the press box for a possible heart attack. I like this rescue, too. It's busy, it's crowded, it's hectic. It's also proof that no matter the urgent situation, life (and college football) goes on.

But this is where the wheels fall off the wagon for me: the final scene at the stadium. It's totally unrealistic and I can't seem to suspend my disbelief enough to let it slide. Skipping past it, we see the final scene—next shift at the station. It might as well be the very next day, based on the way everyone is talking about the game as if it just happened, and John and Roy are trying to not admit that they didn't really see any of the game, and wish they'd watched it on TV.

* * *

>And just what is an "emergency hospital" anyway? Is that a New Jersey thing?

Watching EMERGENCY! Seasons 4-6

I took his words as meaning a hospital emergency room. Actually, *way* back in the day, I'm pretty sure not all public hospitals had emergency departments—there were also private hospitals, and many of them didn't handle emergency cases, either. So just because there was a hospital a mile away didn't mean a person could go there if he had a household accident. Maybe that's what Jersey Joe meant, that he found a hospital that treats emergency cases. Or, again, it could be that he meant emergency room.

Speaking of that phrasing, it sometimes still throws me when the guys tell someone they're being taken to Rampart Emergency. As if that's the name of the hospital. If someone I know got hurt, I wouldn't say they're being taken to Presbyterian emergency.... I'd just say Presbyterian, and the "emergency" part would be implied. Other times, they'll say Rampart General, which obviously makes more sense, and the "general" implies that the hospital handles all types of patients, including emergency cases.

> Perhaps that coordinator kept calling Team 8 just because she had it in for Johnny and Roy. Later she'll make them go through excessive paperwork for their supplies, but that's another episode.

Wow, that was her?? I didn't know that. Of course, we only saw her very briefly in The Game, and I didn't pay much attention, I was watching Johnny be all gaga about being at the Coliseum. Good catch.

> And last but not least, where was Mike Stoker, not only at the end but in the whole episode?

Yeah, this does happen sometimes. There are other episodes (there was one recently, can't recall which one offhand) in which we see Mike doing his thing at the scene of a fire or accident, but he's not in any of the 'filler' scenes at the station.

I guess that's what happens when a guy is juggling two careers.

6.2 Not Available

Yay, an "issues" episode, about the coverage of paramedic squads and the process of responding to those calls. Turned into a bit of a PSA when Roy started quoting numbers (first to Chet and then to Cap and the others). 60,000 calls per year, handled by 31 squads. That's just over 1,935 calls per squad. That's per *squad*, total. Divide the 1,935 of squad 51's calls by three—for A, B, and C shifts—and that's over 645 runs per year for John and Roy. If they work every third day, that's about 121 days per year, so handling 645 calls in 121 days is over five calls per day/shift. That might not sound like a lot, but I don't know if that includes "Station 51" calls, when the engine goes out as well... the five calls per day/shift might be strictly paramedic calls. And Roy also said that their paramedic runs increased by 40% each year... (probably due to a television show that made everyone aware that LA County had a paramedic program; I bet even county residents didn't know about it before the show came on.)

Okay, enough with the math, my head is starting to hurt.

~ William Boyett was in this episode, as Captain of 39s. I don't think we ever saw his face clearly, but boy, you can't mistake the voice. From a sergeant at LAPD to a captain at LACoFD, and later a chief...not a bad career progression.

~ A while back we discussed using landlines rather than biophone, and it turns out that the paramedics can use something called "phone patches" to put over the landline receiver and somehow hook it up to the biophone to patch the patient in and send EKG. At least, that's how it looked to me like it worked.

~ Another scene of Johnny talking with food in his mouth. This time it looked like Randy was eating his actual lunch, as he seemed to be pretty thorough with that sandwich, and apparently enjoyed it as well. "Tuna? Really?"

~ We also saw Johnny use the mapbook while driving to a couple of their calls. It kind of looked like he was using his pen to trace the route, although maybe the pen was closed and he wasn't actually writing in the book.

~ Usually I don't care much for a lot of Rampart scenes, especially ones which don't begin with Squad 51 bringing in a victim, but the old lady and her daughter was kind of interesting. Love how Brackett shook his head when the old lady said "who's gonna drive me home? It's almost time for supper." Note: behind her, the clock said 11:00, so by supper I assume she meant lunch...?? Anyway, it would have been interesting to see a little bit of follow-up. Why is it the cases that are boring always get the full treatment, when things that are halfway interesting don't??

~ Once again Roy makes an Executive Decision and calls Rampart to suggest something outside the box. Thankfully it worked out fine. I wonder if the fainting woman finished her potato chips before she got to Rampart?

~ I like the outside-the-jailhouse rescue. I wonder if there's a reason Roy did it instead of Johnny? As far as I could tell, that really was Kevin, or if it wasn't, the camera angle was vague enough so that it could have been. (I choose to believe it was.) Anyway, this whole episode did seem to have a Roy-edge to it. I wonder if that was deliberate or just how it naturally turned out.

~ On the roof of the jail building, they didn't even look twice at the ladder the convict used to get over the side. I suppose it's policy to use their own equipment unless absolutely necessary; after all, the last time they used a 'civilian' ladder, Roy got electrocuted. But man, that ladder they used was *narrow*. I think I mentioned before how narrow their ladder was, but I also know they have more than one ladder on the engine, so the 'skinny' one happened to be the one they used here.

~ So, in addition to spaghetti, Stoker makes good tuna salad. In fact, Johnny used his favorite word and said it was 'incredible.' Good to know!

* * *

> Wasn't this the first time we've heard the guys listening to other calls over the station radio/intercomm?

Do you mean the calls the other stations/squads get? We sometimes hear them in the background, but usually not very distinctly. I think we can only hear them when it's convenient to the plot. (Like the time when Johnny was mopping and there was the call about the Samoan fire dancer.) Also, the same goes for calls heard over the radio in the squad. Usually "we" (and they) can only hear LA's portion of the calls, and not all the other stations' responses. But when it's important to the plot, *voila!*, the old E!-magic kicks in and we can hear everything.

Speaking of Johnny's hair, it was pretty unkempt, fly-away in this episode.

* * *

> they look like "Lucky Strikes" ... it fits, lettering across the top and a circle on the middle of the package. Soooo,

> not only are those in fact cigarettes, but I think we know the brand now too.

So Lucky Strikes is the likely brand, eh? At one point, I thought it might be Vantage, since those also had a large circle on the pack, with lettering above. Not sure it really matters, I think Randy has been effectively 'busted' already for having his cigs on him all the time, but you and your hubby sure have a keen eye. I did manage to notice the 'object' in Johnny's pocket in that final scene, but to be honest my eyes kept drifting back to the CoV. You know, the one on Roy's naked chest. Naked and furry.....

> Did Mantooth really bang his head on the oven or was it scripted? I thought it was not part of the script, but was left in.

It's very possible the knock on the head wasn't part of the script, but was left in. I've noticed other things which I'm not sure were scripted but left in because either A) it seemed natural or was funny, or B) wasn't worth doing a whole new take, or C) both of the above. Those are the fun things, the things that (true or not) make this show seem all the more real.

Edit: I just rewatched the scene of Johnny cleaning the oven. Right after he bumps his head Johnny asks "who was that call for" (or words to that effect), and Roy answers "39." Roy (Kevin) has kind of a bit of a smile as if maybe that *wasn't* part of the script and he's watching Randy play it off. Again, that could be very incorrect, but sometimes that's how I choose to think of things. 'Cuz I'm weird like that.

~ ~ ~

Here's a nice Issues episode, with some angst and concern over sufficiently covering the LA County area with adequate paramedic coverage. It's good to see the occasional reminder of the paramedic program's growing pains... and the realization that no system is ever going to be perfect.

Had to laugh at the opening scene with Johnny working on the oven and Roy cleaning the stove hood. I can't remember the last time I did either of those things in *my* house, I can't imagine doing them somewhere else. And while these manly firemen routinely perform these chores at the station, what ya wanna bet they balk at even a little dusting or washing dishes at home? Ah, well, that's human nature, I suppose.

I know this is the second episode of season 6, but it's the first one in which we see the helmets with the new paramedic stickers. They make it much easier to identify the paramedics in a crowd of firefighters. (The green numbers really didn't do the trick, imho—*if* that's why the numbers were a different color.) By the way, when Sam gives the address of the first call, I have to laugh at his pronunciation. "Conkwistador" instead of "Conkeestador."

Anyway, I like the first rescue. Since our guys are filling in for another squad, it takes a while for them to arrive, and the woman (victim's sister-in-law) is not happy about it. Engine 39 has done what they can (hi, Sergeant MacDonald/Chief McConnike!) and they all work together in what is an incredibly small, crowded room (house? bedroom?) to assist the patient. When Johnny gets on the biophone, they hear another squad talking to Rampart... have we ever heard that before? I know other squads use the same frequency, etc., but I don't think we've ever actually *heard* them. Just this time, for storyline purposes, I'm sure. Anyway, Johnny gets on the landline to Rampart, where Brackett is apparently talking to Squad 14... although a minute later he responds to Squad 39, on the same line?

There's some good medical mumbo-jumbo in this call. For example, Roy notes that "the pulmonic component of the second heart sounds unusually loud." (Man, I really hate when that happens. My second heart is always being louder than my first, and sometimes they just can't keep their components to themselves.) Also, the guys use a "phone patch" to somehow hook up the landline through the biophone to Rampart. Or something. I wonder if that's something relatively new in their toolbox, as I don't think we've seen it before. Have we??

At the hospital, Johnny runs into the guys from 39s and they trade call-stories. Did anyone notice their handshakes? With one guy, it's a regular handshake. With the other, it's a more hip, bent-elbow hand clasp. (Can ya dig?) In any case, their conversation spurs John and Roy to talk to Brackett about the paramedic coverage issue. Brackett agrees there *is* an issue, but for the time being doesn't have any answers or suggestions. Note: there are two instances of the phrase "bad scene" in that, er, scene.

Also, I had to laugh... in preparation for the guy's arrival at Rampart, Dixie commandeers a passing orderly to assist her in prepping a room. Funny thing is, his name is Mike. This show already has two Mikes (Stoker and Morton), and even though we don't see Morton in this ep, we get this new, additional Mike. Maybe *Mike* is the Rampart version of *Charlie*...?

Speaking of Rampart, then we have the situation with Florence and her daughter May. Mother Florence insists she's always had a "weak chest"... meanwhile she probably outlived a couple of husbands. Daughter May is cowed by mom and taken for granted by her, and before long it's the daughter who suffers a heart attack. And good ol' mom's reaction? "Who's gonna drive me home? It's almost time for dinner." (Dinner, at 11am?? Ah, well, 'supper' is probably at 4pm, so I guess that works out.)

May Fair

Next up for John and Roy is having to act in place of Squad 39; on their way to their station they get a call for "woman unconscious." She's on the sidewalk in front of a store, doesn't seem to be in bad condition, but she gets a preventive IV and transport to the hospital—along with her groceries, of course. I was impressed that the guys actually thought to ask if she's pregnant; I think that's a first for them. (Note: I always laugh now when they mention a "syncopal" episode. For the longest time I thought they were saying "sinkable" episode... which sort of means the same thing, as they both mean loss of consciousness, fainting = *sinking*. Hence *sinkable*. But no, the real word is *syncopal*.)

But while transporting this minor call to Rampart, the guys learn about a serious accident that their engine has responded to, and to which Squad 64 would be delayed. Once again Roy takes the initiative to act outside of prescribed guidelines as he and Johnny send Potato-Chip Patty to Rampart on her own and they respond to Engine 51's accident. (Roy does run the idea past Brackett first, of course.) By the way, how hot does Cap look when he's disheveled after talking to the crash victim? In any case, the guys are able to reach this accident victim and treat him quickly, and at Rampart, Brackett agrees that sometimes breaking the rules is what it takes to do the job well and possibly save a life.

At the station, the guys are still debating the hows and whys of the problem of available coverage by paramedics, repeating the rule that once an IV is set up, someone has to accompany the vic to Rampart. Now they know that there are times when that rule can be bent, and that might make things better from time to time.

Last rescue is at the local jail, where an inmate attempted an escape and is now stuck on a ledge. Up on the roof of the building, Cap tells Mike to put the engine's ladder next to the other ladder, the one the prisoner used. (Haven't we mentioned how *narrow* that ladder is??) I thought it natural that they used their own equipment rather than what's found at the scene, but then what do they do but use the rope they just happen to find there. "Yeah, it's safe," Chet says. Really? You want to risk your life on equipment chosen by a dirtbag prisoner and that Chet declares safe after a 5-second assessment? I'd go with the FD rope, thankyouverymuch. Anyway, both Roy and Johnny are wearing safety belts, but Roy's the one who goes over the wall on this one. Which I find interesting, as in instances when a rescue is a "one-man job," that one man is usually Johnny. But I think Roy does a good job. When he reaches the prisoner, he's hot and sweating and anxious, because the guy's obviously terrified beyond reason, but Roy stays cool until the poor victim literally jumps on him and hangs on for dear life. (Who can blame him?) Luckily the two of them are brought safely back into the jail building. And we—the viewers who can appreciate such things—are richly rewarded with the sight of shirtless Roy exhibiting his CoV at Rampart as Dr. Early assesses him for damage. I know the rescue was hairy (like his chest; yeah, that's corny) but in this case, Roy's risk was definitely worth it... at least for *us*.

* * *

CoV is "carpet of virility"... in other words, a hairy chest. I believe the term comes from the TV Tropes website (which is hilarious, by the way, although definitely a time-suck, and therefore not to be risked unless one has time to spend wallowing in it; you have been warned!).

6.3 Unlikely Heirs

So the guys finally get some serious coin, eh? $20,000 left to them by the mysterious "bum," and headquarters says they can keep it as long as they "don't spend it on themselves." Okay, I can see that. Maybe the first thing they can do is run down to Service Merchandise and buy a nice big COFFEE URN for the station. That way someone isn't always saying "I just poured the last cup." (With "and I was too lazy to make a new pot" being implied, apparently.) But it's nice they can give some money to charity, and buying something for the station doesn't qualify as being "for themselves," since 12 other guys are going to be able to take advantage of it.

~ Anyway, the first rescue, the refinery or whatever it was where this mattress-man was, sure looked familiar. I'm willing to bet the filming location is a place we've seen before, more than once.

~ I've often thought that Cap must have good eyes. He can tell which engine or truck is arriving at the scene from a half-mile or a mile away, regardless of visibility conditions (angle, sun, etc.); he's able to address them on the handy-talkie them and tell them to cover the south exposure, etc. (Yeah, I know, he's aware which trucks and/or engines have been called out, and can recognize a truck from an engine a mile off. But still.)

~ Brackett got a haircut.

~ "Season Six: Time for a Wedding" ... this is the episode I always have to laugh at, with the Case of the Swooning Bride and the elephant in the room that nobody addresses. We have a young woman, who apparently has fainted a number of times in recent weeks, and nobody—not mother, or paramedic, or even the doctors, I don't think—anyway, it never seems to occur to anyone to ask if she might be pregnant?? Come on, I know this was a family show, but you know that would have would have been one of their first thoughts. But this is a family show, and of course no young woman could ever have a baby before she's married. It's inconceivable!! (See what I did there??) In any event, that's not the issue here, so it's a moot point. I will say that, if I was that bride, and my honeymoon plans were already ruined, I wouldn't settle for a rinky-dink wedding ceremony in the hospital. I bought my gown and veil, doggone it, and I'd darn well want to wear them in a church. Especially since I don't want my 'wedding night' to be in a hospital bed.

~ Speaking of the church... looks like the studio had a small budget as far as extras were concerned. That wasn't a big church and it wasn't even close to half-way filled.

~ Yikes, it was the return of Evil Eddie, the one-boy hellion. Except now he calls himself Andy and he steps on rusty nails. I did think it was funny, though, that he pinches Dixie to show her how much the shot hurt.

~ Also, this episode had Simba, the ventriloquist cat. We see the cat, we hear the meow, but Simba's feline mouth never moved. Who knew that E!-magic extends to our four-legged friends??

~ When the station got called out on that last call, anyone else think it was strange that Cap said to put the money in the squad? Yes, the squad will be where the firefighters are, but it's also likely to be unattended for an extended amount of time; not exactly the best place for safekeeping. I'd have re-wrapped it and put it in the freezer. Or, if it had to be taken on the call, at least it could've been locked in the drug-box.

~ And when Johnny got in the squad on that call, I assume he was supposedly 'doing something' with that money, because it looked like they made a point of showing him sit in the squad. If I didn't know better, I'd think he was putting on his seat belt, but most likely he was supposed to be rewrapping the money or something.

~ ~ ~

May Fair

First of all, THANK YOU to all of you for your kind words about my rambling, dissertation-like posts. I love watching this show and delving into the "hows and whys" of what happens in each episode. (Although it reminds me that I may need more of a life.) Anyway, we still have most of the sixth season to go, so.... on with the show!

So we start at the station, where these hard-working guys are earning our equally-hard-earned taxpayer dollars by sitting around watching Chet and Marco arm-wrestle. "Kid" Kelly handily beats his opponent, and when he starts to brag a bit, Johnny takes him on. Luckily for John, the tones sound before Chet can officially beat him.

The call is to an "abandoned plant," which looks oddly familiar, no? It wasn't quite so abandoned the two or three other times the station responded there for various fires, explosions and other sundry disasters. Anyway, Cap starts his guys after the fire, but I'm a bit surprised at not seeing any air masks being used here; just because there's no apparent toxic stuff doesn't mean they can't suffer from smoke inhalation. Also, Cap must have great eyesight... he can recognize trucks/engines from 200 yards away as he communicates to them on the HT.

Roy and Johnny find an old guy passed out in one of the building's rooms and carry him out to safety. Marco and Chet put out the fire in the room and toss the mattress out the window for safety's sake, later discovering it's full of money. Luckily for us, Cap's an honest man and has Marco call the cop over to keep watch over the money before handfuls of it mysteriously disappear into those capacious turnout coats.

The old guy (I'd call him a bum, but it's tough to consider anyone with that much money a bum) anyway, at Rampart, his conversation with Dr. Brackett is kind of funny. Best line is when Brackett rattles off various tests to be performed and mentions possibility of pulmonary edema.

Max: More medical mumbo-jumbo designed to confuse the layman.

Brackett: Yes, sir, but please allow me to say it. I spent most of my youth learning the proper pronunciation. [Too funny!!]

Next we see a sort-of-typical 1976 wedding. Anyone remember that kind of dress, with the Empire waist? I do, I wore one in my sister's wedding. And the hats.... oh, lordy, the floppy hats! (Thankfully ,we did NOT wear those in my sister's wedding.) Also, in the wedding scene, did it seem odd to anyone else that there were so few people in the church? I went to a wedding last fall and there were four times that many people, easy. Anyway, I'm not going to rehash the point I'm sure I made last time, about everyone ignoring the possibility that the bride could be *gasp!* pregnant. Instead I'll just ask this: would *you* want to be married while you're in the hospital? It's not like the young woman was terminal and wouldn't be released in the near future. I mean, what kind of wedding night can they possibly have? And since the groom's trip was likely going to be cancelled, why not wait the three weeks and have an actual wedding in an actual church?

Next we see Max the anti-bank fanatic visit the station. He expresses his gratitude to the guys who saved him and tries to give them some of his money, but Cap and the others tell him it's against the rules to accept money (gratuity). The conversation is stopped when a call comes in for a woman with breathing trouble (really? the engine gets called out on that??) and turns out that a little old lady gets upset and breathless when her cat gets away from her. But this cat, Simba, is special: he's a ventriloquist! When Chet finds him behind a shrub, we hear a distinct "meow"... but Simba's mouth doesn't move! What a trick!!

May Fair

But the engine *has* to be called with the squad, because the station has to be empty so that Max can leave a bundle of 'lettuce' in the fridge's crisper. Generous gesture? Yeah, sure, but Cap can't just accept it, so he decides to call headquarters about it. Before he can do that, though, the tones sound and they're off again. (They put the money—twenty-thousand smackers—in the squad. Which will be left unlocked and unattended at a busy, hectic scene. Yeah, good choice!)

At the site of the last rescue, a plane crashed into some sort of warehouse with (of course) flammable material. There's a very familiar blue Chevy pickup parked nearby, along with a VW van which also looks vaguely familiar.... Anyway, a man and woman are stuck in the plane which has flames licking around it. The woman is annoyingly vocal, screaming "get me out" repeatedly, even when she can plainly see that a number of capable men are working to do just that. (I will give her props, though, for telling them to get her hubby out first, since he's unconscious.) When they do get to work on getting the husband out, I wonder why they don't use the firefighter carry. Instead of having *two* men work to awkwardly carry him out, *one* of the guys could have had him put over his shoulders and taken him out that way, easy-peasy.

Finally, Cap hears back from 'headquarters' that, since the situation has no precedent, the guys of Station 51 can keep Max's grateful donation. Caveat: they can't spend it on themselves. So a "nice" argument ensues, as they discuss which causes should receive their donation. Question: doesn't it occur to them that they could still divide the money six ways and each FF could donate "his" portion to the cause of his choice? It doesn't *all* have to go to one place.

Quick bits:

~ So far this season, the ambulances no longer say Mayfair on them. I wonder what prompted the change, and whether it will stay this way going forward.

~ When we see Johnny drive into the driveway at start of shift, we get a glimpse of the gas pump next to the station. I guess they normally try to hide it, which is why it's sort of hidden among some trees.

6.4 That Time of Year

The title refers to vacation time, when every employee looks forward to getting away from it all. For all our sakes I'm going to skim over the fact that Roy seemed to be "deciding" the vacation destination on his own, even though he did "run it past" his wife... once he'd already decided. **(Very generous, I'm sure.)** Also, what were Johnny and Cap thinking, suggesting Hawaii and the Swiss Alps?? They know how much money Roy makes; did they really believe he could afford to take four people to either place?? Also, once Roy heard about the farm, he got all excited. "The kids have always wanted to see a farm." Really, Roy? Where are you raising them, some blighted, inner-city part of LA?? You live in LA County, for god's sake, and it's very obvious that parts of the county are (were, at the time) quite rural. You've never driven the kids past a farm before? And by the way, when he says "farm" in this context, I wonder if what he really meant was more like a ranch. I've heard of people taking vacations at ranches of various types, but I don't think I've ever heard them referred to as farms.

Anyway, back to our regularly-scheduled review....

May Fair

~ So the "swinging singles" club is already swinging at 1:00 in the afternoon? This was obviously before SueEllen became Miss Texas and met J.R. Ewing.

~ Did they ever explain what happened to Roy in the club? I think I remember something about his air tank malfunctioning or something... or did I just make that up??

~ Speaking of that fire, I thought it was funny to see the place full of firefighters, shouting, lugging hose, etc., and Johnny's looking under dang tables for the missing man. Also, he opened a door, yelled "anyone in here?" and closed the door again. I'm sorry, but if that's how LACoFD searches a building, I'd think they'd have a higher death toll.

~ Who saw the ill-fated AMC Pacer, when the girl drove to the Emergency entrance at Rampart? It was our friend Ronnie Schell again. He went from being a weed-smoking computer nerd to a hilarious drunk guy who shouldn't drive and is now a gourmet who doesn't know when to quit eating pie.

~ At the scene of the martial arts incident, did anyone notice when Johnny had to get Roy's attention he said "Roy? Get out of the way." Not sure if his being in the way was scripted or not, but it was funny. Speaking of cute/funny, when Johnny and Roy were in the locker room and Roy said he'd been getting vacation suggestions for three days, he said "I don't want any more suggestions!" And he did a little shakey/dancey thing for emphasis. Too funny!!

~ Speaking of that martial arts thing, the old woman was referred to pretty consistently as Mrs. Pastone, except for one time when the instructor called her Mrs. Preston.

~ We see Johnny buckling his imaginary seatbelt again. Either that or he's doing something that really shouldn't be seen on primetime TV.

Watching EMERGENCY! Seasons 4-6

~ I like the final rescue with the hang-gliders. It's a complicated one, and Roy and Johnny each have their own victim to treat. We hear Roy keep up a continuous chat with his victim, asking questions, asking him to move this or do that, and also instructing Marco on how to help as well. Poor Johnny gets a victim who's unconscious, but Chet helps him out. At one point we see the "unconscious" victim move his legs and 'help' Johnny and Chet position him for the portable stretcher... so considerate of him! (And they really had him bundled into that thing like a cocoon, didn't they?)

~ Once they got him up to the top, at first I assumed it was Johnny who knelt next to the vic and set up the oxygen, but when someone else with dark hair knelt beside the guy, I realized the first guy was Stoker. He just went right to work with the O2... almost like it's his job or something. Go figure!

~ I'm guessing that Kevin's issues with heights didn't apply to situations like this. I get the impression he didn't have a problem with rappelling, maybe having a mountain or a cliff literally under his feet was enough for him not to feel so exposed and vulnerable, like one might when sitting at the top of a 250-foot crane. But I don't know, that's just conjecture on my part.

* * *

What I didn't like about the "vacation nonsense" was that Roy was making this decision. By himself. Oh, sure, he "ran it past" Joanne, but we all know that any good wife would be just as interested and involved in deciding where to go on vacation as her husband. Do these writers not think that women can make decisions or have useful input on issues like this, that once they say 'I do' they relinquish all rights to be involved in big decisions??

~ ~ ~

May Fair

This time I'm not going to harp on the issue of Roy deciding—unilaterally—where his family is going to spend their vacation. I still think it's stupid and unrealistic and six kinds of wrong, but I'm accepting that it's just a plot device and not worth getting worked up about. [Deep breath in... deep breath out....]

Anyway, in the first scene, the gang's hanging out at the table after lunch, looking at vacation brochures (or, as Johnny calls them once or twice, folders) and Johnny's going around pouring everyone a cup of coffee. Thought that was odd, especially since nobody seems interested in drinking it. Anyway, by the time he realizes he hasn't poured a cup for himself, the pot is empty. That's when the tones go off, so it doesn't really matter anyway.

The call is for a fire at a singles club, which Johnny says would probably be crowded. (And he knows this, ...how??) It's just after 1:00 pm, so just like the wild parties these guys have been to in the middle of the day, singles clubs apparently flourish at that time of day. Boy, you LA people really know how to live.

At the scene of this fire, we see a vehicle in the parking lot that's familiar to a lot of Adam-12 fans—always nice to see. But tensions mount when Sue Ellen Ewing (Linda Gray) worriedly tells the paramedics that a cute guy she just met is still in the building; he'd just left for the restroom when the fire started. John and Roy go in to search, and everyone is wearing their air masks, thank heavens. I have to chuckle when one of them (Johnny, I think) looks under tables in the main dining room, as if an adult would actually be hiding underneath one. Especially when firefighters with hoses are standing just a couple feet away while booths and chairs are burning around them. Upstairs we see the guys do a thorough search of the restrooms, but downstairs, Johnny just pushes a door open and yells "Anybody in here??" Seriously, he doesn't actually go inside, he just stands there and yells and then closes the door again. Also, we see footage reused from other fires, including Cap and Chet doing Cap's little trick of opening a door, running the hose full-blast for XX number of seconds, and closing the door again. (The theory is that the resulting mist or fog will help tamp down the fire.)

I think I missed hearing it this time, but I swear that when Roy gets lightheaded and has his episode, that there is a reference to some sort of glitch with his air tank. Or maybe I'm confusing it with the time that Johnny's air tank has an issue? In any case, you'd think Cap would make it a priority to find out why one of his guys is uncharacteristically overcome with the heat for no apparent reason.

Next shift, Roy tells Johnny that he's been getting so much advice about vacations from everyone and his brother; it's funny to see him do his little dance when he emphasizes, "I don't want any more suggestions!" Can't think what it reminds me of when he does that, but whatever it is, it's darn cute.

Next comes the healthy, robust former Marine teaching a bit of self-defense to a bunch of little blue-haired grandmothers. Of course, we know something's going to happen to require the services of the paramedics, and since little Mrs. Pastone keeps telling us how her heart's palpitating and her knees are quaking, etc., we're supposed to think that that something is going to happen to *her*. Well...*psych!* It's the gung-ho martial arts instructor who goes down. Although why he was sprawled out on the grass instead of the large mat on which he'd been standing, I don't know. In addition to cracked ribs, he apparently also suffers a little brain lapse, as he refers to Mrs. Pastone as Mrs. Preston. And then Pastone again.

Back at the station, Roy's overwhelmed with the vacation decision, and surrounded by brochures (not folders). Johnny's been pressing a trip to Hawaii, although how he thinks a

May Fair

humble civil servant with a family can afford a vacation in Hawaii... I'll never know. Then Johnny starts talking about the travel articles in the newspaper and derisively mentions that one person recommended going to a farm for vacation. A *farm!* Johnny's tone says it all—for him—but Roy's face says the opposite—for *him*. As for me, I have to wonder: by farm, don't they really mean ranch? Working ranches, dude ranches, whatever you want to call them, I think that's how they're referred to, isn't it? Much like a farm, but less tilling. Plus, ranch just sounds better. (Confession: I wouldn't mind taking one of those ranch vacations. Preferably one where you can do some nice, gentle horseback-riding.) Anyway back to the show, where we finally have a winner in the Vacation Roy-stakes.

Last call is for some downed hang-gliders. I have to say, I think (theorize) that the filming location for this one was right next to the place where they responded to a call off a cliff with the trainee, Marlowe; a comparison of the location and the white buildings will tell the tale. Anyway, the glider rescue is another one of those complicated, busy, all-hands-on-deck rescues that I love so much.

~ John and Roy each have their own victim to deal with.

~ I find it odd that the more severely injured guy was put in the collapsible stretcher.

~ Chet and Marco know how to rappel, too. All the more reason that they can be the "action guys" sometimes, rather than *always* having Roy and Johnny be the ones.

~ Is it just me or does it seem that when they put a cervical collar on a victim—who might possibly have a spinal injury—they really can't do it without moving/jostling the head. I think I've mentioned it before that if the victim's neck wasn't hurt *before,* it certainly would be by the time the collar's put on.

Finally, at the station, Johnny's smugly sitting back, taking credit for Roy's vacation when the man himself walks in. Roy acts like things are hunky-dory and his time away was "just fine," but finally he admits it was less than ideal and recounts the litany of ways the vacation went south, and Johnny gets a look that says 'Hey, don't look at me!'

Oh, and once again, there is no coffee.

* * *

> At the hang glider rescue: When Chet says "You were rough on him." and Johnny says "It was either that or he falls.", what was it that Johnny did? It looked liked he was just trying to keep the hang glider from falling.

Yeah, that comment might have been referring to getting the guy unhooked from the glider; it was probably not pleasant for the guy. I thought Chet said it as they were cocooning the victim into the stretcher thing.

Fun fact: after the glider falls to the bottom of the cliff, the camera pans back up to where we see both groups of people from far off (a long shot), we can see that Johnny is trying to maneuver his victim a little, and we can see the "unconscious" victim moving his legs to assist in getting him in position.

* * *

> Regarding the fire at the singles club, that guy that Sue Ellen just met saw the smoke as he was heading to the bathroom, but decided to leave without telling/warning her. She thinks he is a nice guy! She should have kicked him in the a$$.

I know, right? I thought the same thing—he knew the place was on fire and didn't bother looking for her. What a catch *he* is! (Although I'm not sure J.R. Ewing ends up being much better, y'know?)

6.5 Fair Fight

Directed by Kevin, which is always interesting. There were some things to like about this ep, and some not as interesting to me. Basically, it was sort of a meh-sandwich: I liked the opening action, and the final rescue. The in-between stuff.... not so much. (I was going to call it a crap-sandwich, but I guess it wasn't all *that* bad to deserve that description.)

~ Loved the opening scene, of the overhead view of the squad and engine backing into the station. Have we seen that before? If not, I wonder if it was Kevin's doing. Probably not, but what the heck. And if they're just now getting back, who went down the driveway?

~ Nice shot of Johnny getting out of the squad, framed by the 'window' of the engine, with Chet in foreground. And I had to laugh: they come in and talk about "cleaning up oil slicks".... and they're not in the least bit dirty. No dripping turnout coats, no messy shoes or pant cuffs. LA County must have the neatest oil slicks in the country.

~ First view of Henry, (un)official Station 51 dog. Actually, he's the Station 51 *Couch's* dog. As many hijinks as this group gets into with Henry, it seems odd that he's only just now making his first appearance.

~ At the first alarm, with the fire in the industrial park, Johnny uses the heavy equipment to open the "secret room" door, and as he goes in he slips and falls. Not sure if he was supposed to do that, I'm betting that was an accident, and they just went with it. Roy says "Johnny, you all right," but with the air mask on and the muffled sound, you can almost imagine he said "Randy." (But I'm pretty sure it was 'Johnny.')

~ More stock footage being used, kind of noticeable as the squad zips down the road, but that's nothing new. Funny to see the 'old' white numbers on their helmets though.

~ The part of this episode I don't like is the "fair fight" couple. I don't like confrontation to begin with, and also, I think it's rude and just plain bad manners to argue and fight in front of strangers. (I know, that's a prissy and simplistic attitude, but it's all I got.)

~ Funny that Captain Hookrader was mentioned. Now that he did not retire, they still have to deal with him. When we first met him, I thought he worked out of another station, but in this ep he was referred to as Captain of B or C shift, I believe.

~ That last call at the cave-in, was off Little Seco Road (sp?). I know we've heard that road before, but have no idea what episode.

~ Also funny... Johnny tells Roy that the victim has 'possible broken ribs' and difficulty breathing on the right side.' Roy translates that to Rampart as "large discoloration on the chest." I realize it's possible that broken ribs can lead to discoloration of the chest area, but that wasn't what Johnny described.

~ Have to say I loved hearing the "on-air" transmissions from Johnny on the HT, and Roy on the bio-phone. I don't know why I think that's so cool, but I do. It does lend a good authenticity to scenes, imho.

~ And I have to wonder.... I hope Stoker had a copy War and Peace stashed under his seat in the engine. On this last rescue he had time to get through the "war" part. (Seriously, what does he do in situations like that when he's not needed and simply stays with the engine??)

* * *

> I was a little disappointed, as we all have been before, that they didn't show the actual rescue of the victims and Johnny from the cave-in. That was kind of a letdown after all that. At least show us one of them being pulled up and how they went about it

I know. I guess the assumption is that once the digging crew got through, the victims were just transported out. Would have been nice to see, but I guess the 'important' part was handling the cave-in. Gotta inject those bits of drama to keep us on our toes. (Hey, I wonder if this should be included as a minor instance of JiJ... not enough to make it a quartet, but definitely related to the others via the 'danger' to Johnny.)

~ ~ ~

'Fair Fight.' Or, Hello Henry!

On one hand, I don't really care for this episode, because I don't like personal conflict, so the couple's constant arguing makes me uncomfortable. Not to mention the fact that I don't believe in conducting private conversations/disputes/arguments in front of other people. However, I do like both the first and last rescues, so those calls do pretty much cancel out the rest of the unpleasantness.

I do have to chuckle, however, at the continuity error in the very opening scene. Start with an overhead shot of the squad backing into the station, and the engine right behind. It's really a nice shot, taken by chopper, I wonder why we don't see it more often. Have we ever even seen it before this episode?? Anyway, on the back of the engine, we clearly see the guy who sits behind the driver (in other words, the Marco) standing on the tailboard as Big Red backs in. Then cut to inside the apparatus bay and both Chet and Marco getting out of their jump seats. Wha—?? I guess Marco jumped off the back of the rig and back into his seat. By the way, I still don't know why they get on the tailboard when backing up to begin with. The only explanation I can think of is maybe for visibility purposes, but I wouldn't think that would really be an issue.

Anyway, we find out that Station 51's been out cleaning up an oil slick since their shift started, which has only been a little more than an hour. Must not have been too big a slick if they're already done. Not to mention they're all nice and fresh and clean—didn't even have to wash off their boots! So upon entering the dayroom, they all stop short when they see... a big ol' basset hound on the couch. Nobody knows where he came from or how he got into the station. And later on, after Chet leaves a plate of food on the floor, nobody can explain where the plate and/or food went. In a nice (albeit rare) bit of continuity, Cap even mentions Captain Hochrader, a.k.a. Captain Hook. In the end, they decide to call the dog Henry... with Cap throwing in a warning that he doesn't want to hear anyone refer to the mutt as Hank.

In any case, before they can discuss the dog's origins in depth, the alarm sounds and they're off again, this time to a structure fire. I don't think they ever specified what type of building or business this is, but did you see the names over some of the doors in that building? "Comp Parameter Analysis" (I assume Comp means Computer) ... "Electronic Miniaturization." Sounds pretty technical. Not surprising, then, that there's a room in the building which only three people have ever entered, and there's some question as to whether someone might be stuck inside. First of all, when Johnny finds a guy who was trying to bus down the door to the secret room, why is the guy just cowering in the corner? He was right next to a window, for heaven's sake, and apparently has an axe in hand.

May Fair

Why cower and hide when he could actually get out and maybe find some help? Ah well, it was good for the story, so....

By the way, did we all enjoy seeing Johnny slip and fall after breaking down that door? I bet that wasn't supposed to happen. Also, I'm guessing the FF who goes with them through the window when they're breaking into the secret room is there to man the hose and protect the guys. Yes? No?

After the locked-room mystery, once John and Roy get the clearance from Cap, they respond to a "man with head injury," which is the first of the Hubbard calls. But I think what's good is that the guys are still dirty and dusty from the fire when they get to the Hubbards'—some actual continuity! I bet they smelled like the proverbial smokestack, but them still being messy and sooty is a nice, authentic touch. On their second visit to the Hubbard House of Hell, I think it's funny when Johnny says he'll call for an ambulance. He gets on the landline, dials, and says, "Is this LA Dispatch?" LOL, am I the only one who finds that odd and/or funny? If he dialed LA Dispatch, that's who he should have reached. And I'm betting that however LA Dispatch answers their phones, it's pretty obvious that you've reached LA Dispatch. (Now I'm going to quit saying LA Dispatch.)

Last call is to an "unknown-type rescue," and the address is a few miles off Little Seco Road. Now, I don't remember which ones, but I know for a *fact* that they've responded to other calls on or near Little Seco Road—it's an odd name and sticks in my memory. Anyway, this one is a cave-in; some sort of mining or construction site, and two guys are stuck, luckily right under some sort of ventilation pipe. Johnny figures he's slim enough and can go down the pipe so he volunteers to help the two guys out. Now maybe one of you learned people can educate me a little: the foreman guy drops a rope and tells his guy to "grab the downhaul." Then 'downhaul' is mentioned again a minute later. I looked up the word, but only came up with the meaning of some sort of rope for sailing. So, not sure how it was used in this context. Anyone know??

In any case, Johnny's got the drug box, blankets, and the HT lowered down to him, and Roy has started relaying info to Rampart. We hear him giving vitals of the more-seriously injured guy, and we hear Rampart mention O2, and apparently Rampart also prescribes an IV with D5W as well, although we don't hear it. In any case, imagine my surprise when Johnny tells the less-injured man, the one who's *not* unconscious and with probable internal injuries, that *he's* going to get an IV. Far as we know, Johnny hasn't even reported the guy's injuries, much less his vitals, and yet he might be the one getting the IV.

But before any IVs get started, and unfortunately even before the air tank gets lowered down the pipe, there's a rumble and another cave-in inside the tunnel. Johnny's unhurt, the unconscious guy is unhurt, but the less-injured one has aggravated his already-broken leg. Things look grim, but after a brief search Johnny finds the HT buried under all the loose dirt and things are looking up again.

By the way, is there a reason they actually tied up the yellow blankets to get them down the pipe? Why not just drop them down??

Also, I wonder what poor Stoker's doing during this whole thing. They got to the site about 5pm or so, and it's full dark when the trapped men are brought out. I imagine Mike tackling a couple chapters of War and Peace while he sits in the engine.

* * *

> Due to the size of the fire engine, it is hard to see to the rear of the engine even with mirrors. Backing accidents are

the most common type of accidents in the fire service. This is why firefighters stand on the tailboard of the engine so they can be the "eyes". Communication during the 70s may have been hand signals, visual with the firefighter or some engines have a button at the back of the engine. This sounds [a buzzer] in the cab. Depending on how many times the button is pushed will determine what the engineer needs to do. One push may mean stop. Two pushes may be back up. Three may be forward or some other combination the department has in place. Nowadays, voice communication through a headset can be used if equipped. Firefighters should not be on the back of a tailboard when the engine is moving but, unfortunately, it still happens. Usually, it is not during normal driving operations. It is usually during backing operations. Firefighters have fallen off the tailboard while the engine is backing up and they are run over. Firefighters should be on the ground where the engineer can see them in their side mirror but that does not always happen.

That makes sense. I didn't think it would be a visibility issue because I was pretty sure the jumpseat guy wouldn't obscure the engineer's view in the mirror, but I guess it makes sense that a rear-view mirror might not be too accurate for a long engine. And yes, I only see it on this show when vehicles are backing up. Thanks for the insight!

6.6 Rules of Order

Or, "Johnny's Worst Nightmare Comes True: Brice is in Charge." Okay, so that's not quite how it goes, but close enough.

Firstly, hats off to Bob Belliveau for his first (and only?) appearance on TV. (And I think he did better than some others I could mention who appear more regularly.) Of course, not only was he a real-life LACoFD paramedic, but he was THE paramedic, the very first one trained and certified. He then served as a script consultant and technical advisor for the show, so obviously Kevin and Randy knew him pretty well by the time this ep was filmed. (Although, to be honest, I'm not sure I can imagine him doing all the rappelling, climbing, and diving that "our" paramedics have done. But I've been wrong before, so maybe he did.)

Also, this episode was written by James G. Richardson, the actor who plays Brice.

~ Sometimes I have to wonder if Randy got all his daily nourishment on-set, in front of the camera, as in the past ten or so episodes we've seen him eat quite often. Not just nibbling or "pretend" eating for the sake of the take, but actually *eating*. Good thing he had a pretty high metabolism.

~ I liked the power pole rescue; that was interesting. And for some reason I was put in mind of Mr. McBeevy from an episode of The Andy Griffith Show. But it was good, just complicated enough to be interesting. And mentioning the creosote irritating the skin and stuff was a nice touch of realism later at the hospital.

~ Has Johnny ever worked with Brice? I don't think so, not that we've ever heard about, and even Roy commented that *he* had to work with Brice for two weeks. (But he said it was while Johnny was "sick," when in reality it was while his leg was broken; either poor continuity by the writers, or Kevin just misspoke.)

~ Did you see the hair on one of the other so-called paramedics? It was as long as, if not longer than, Johnny's, and bushier to boot. Good thing Chief Houts didn't see Gage and this guy standing together. And speaking of hair, I wonder if Chet's wild 'do would have set off the Chief's radar? Of course, Chet's hair wasn't so much *long* as it was... *big*.

~ Still talking about the 'other' paramedics... Larry Manetti's character name was Charlie, and later Roy mentioned "Dwyer." Apparently that was in reference to Manetti's character, and if so, then he's the *third* actor to play Paramedic Dwyer. Although in the other instances Dwyer's first name was Tom, not Charlie. Even more confusingly, the show's credits list the Manetti character's first name as Bert. Which makes me go "huh?" because more than once he's called Charlie.

~ The rescue of the climbers on the side of the building: Take note of the building, folks, as we'll see it again next week. (I bet the producers/directors had a certain number of days when that building was available for filming, and they took advantage of it.) Now, I'm not a climber, and I don't play one on TV, but I wonder if there was a reason why they didn't just use the woman's rope to pull her up from the get-go? Maybe they only trust their own ropes, or maybe she didn't leave enough rope at the top for three or four men to pull? Ah well, I like the rescue anyway.

~ ~ ~

We all know that this episode features the infamous Craig Brice. And was in fact written by the actor who plays Brice, James Richardson. The premise is simple, and guaranteed to spark the ire of one John Gage: Roy and Johnny hear that the Powers That Be are setting up a paramedic advisory committee. This is figurative music to Johnny's ear as he is always thinking of ways to improve the paramedics' job and the processes they follow. In any case, when learning that the committee might already have been chosen—and he and Roy not invited—Johnny actually drops his sticky pastry and says, "Boy, that really...." He doesn't finish the thought, but you can practically *hear* the next words: "pi$$es me off."

The rant is interrupted by a call to a car accident. I like this rescue... it features a car (driven by the hoity-toity Mr. Hoover) which managed to hit a power pole and injured the man who was working on the pole. Have to admit, I think the victim's position is kind of strange; why is his back somewhat arched? You'd think his body would be more limp rather than bowed backward. In this rescue we hear someone say "d@mn," but it isn't Johnny—it's Mr. Hoover. Anyway, even though it isn't 'our' guys who are actually up there on that pole, I like the rescue, and I like that it's complicated enough that both paramedics have to ride with the victim to Rampart. (Note: we do see Randy climb up the pole and deal with the victim, but I'm pretty sure that once "Roy" joins him—and Johnny climbs up even higher—at that point they're both stunt guys. I wonder who Kevin's stunt double is these days, as it doesn't look like Hal Frizzell.)

So they get the guy down and he has trouble breathing, a collapsed larynx or something. I wonder how that happened? It's not like he got hit in the throat. Anyway, those sure are some interesting sound effects when the doctors are doing the suctioning. Ewwww!

At Rampart, Roy and Johnny run into Brice and his partner, Bob (played by Bob Belliveau—and we all know who *he* is, I'm sure). They also learn that Brice and Bob are on the paramedic committee. Which has Johnny's shorts in a bunch because he doesn't like Brice to begin with; as they're leaving, Johnny makes a fist behind his nemesis' back. But no sooner do they pull back into the station (with Johnny ranting through the whole drive, apparently, about not being asked to join) than Cap tells them that *they* got called to be on the committee too. And, perversely, like an emo 15-year-old, Johnny says, "I'm not sure I want to now." (Yep, just like a moody teenager.) Cut to the next scene (next shift) and now he's talking non-stop about being on the committee—big surprise, huh? Anyway, I love this scene, how Roy just goes about his business, getting coffee, wandering over to the bulletin board to see what's new, picking up the newspaper, etc., and just letting Johnny talk and talk and talk. And talk. Roy sure knows his partner! But before he can sit back down and actually enjoy a sip of coffee, they get a call for a man down.

As they're riding down the road, their call gets cancelled. Which makes me wonder what the point of the call is to begin with, except that while they're out, the other six guys on the committee arrive at the station for their first committee meeting. (Really? That was quick.) The whole point of the first meeting is to flummox Roy and John, especially when, after hearing about Robert's Rules of Order, Johnny asks, "Who's Roberts?" Of course, Brice's answer doesn't enlighten Gage in the least ("The *Army!*"), and confusion and exasperation ensue.

At Rampart, Dixie asks them how the meeting went (Brice said it was good, although our guys obviously feel differently), and something she says gives Roy an idea, so next time we see them at the station, Roy's reading Robert's Rules of Order and says he now has a plan to deal with Brice. But before he can fill his partner in, the tones go off and the station is called out to a rescue.

I think we discussed last time around that the building in this rescue is used again in another rescue in just another couple of episodes, so take note. And the guy they're rescuing, I call him Raggedy Andy, because that's who he reminds me of because of that shirt he's wearing. Also, I love the fact that there's a guy selling ice cream there at the scene, or some other vendable treat, to all the gawkers and onlookers. And again, I'm quite sure that's neither Randy nor Kevin hanging down the side of that building. (Although I have to say, for the most part this show does a pretty good job of making us think it is, especially if one doesn't pause or zoom in, etc.)

Another 'also': I may not have ever mentioned this before, but I noticed it in this episode, so I'll mention it here: I love watching Cap walk. He's so purposeful and has such a nice, long stride. On a similar subject, I like watching Stoker run. Cap's walk, Stoker's run… both very fun to watch.

In any case, Roy's big idea on how to deal with Brice works, and all the guys on the committee seem glad to see the World's Most Perfect Paramedic get flummoxed, and the committee goes on its merry way to do its job.

6.7 The Exam

So the paramedics have to do a recertification exam. I can understand why that might be necessary, and yet… nurses don't have to be recertified? Doctors don't? Fire captains and engineers don't? Hmmm.

Also, small detail, but the timing of the exam was off. When the show begins, they mention they're taking the exam "tomorrow." And Johnny says at one point it's a heck of a way to spend a "day off." If they get off shift at 8am, it's not really a day off, now is it?? Then, when they return for next shift, Cap asks how the exam went "yesterday." Even if John and Roy really did have a full day off and took the exam, that's still just one day off between shifts, when (I thought) the usual shift schedule was one day on, two days off. If so, they messed that up. (Even worse, when they learn the exam is rescheduled for Tuesday, I assume that meant Tuesday would be when "*A*" *shift* paramedics would take it. Because there's

May Fair

no way *all* the paramedics in LACoFD could take the exam on the same day. Who would be available to run the squads??? Same question applies to the test they just took... everyone can't take it on the same day, or nobody would be working.)

~ What about Molly.... First off, I'm not crazy about Molly. I don't care for the actress who plays her. (Fun fact: the actress starred in a show with another E! guest star, Bobby Sherman. The show was Here Come the Brides.) Anyway, I just couldn't muster any liking or sympathy for her and she seemed like a helpless wimp. Also, I hated her very dated hair style. (And I know whereof I speak, as I wore my hair the *exact same way* at the time. So yeah, I don't want to see the style on me anymore than I did on her.) Also, Roy tells Johnny that her husband Dick did "everything" for her, he would "even go shopping." I dunno, call me crazy, but something about that just seems off. I understand that Dick must have done all the usual "husband-y stuff" around the house, and would troubleshoot any problems encountered, and I'm all for men helping out with the so-called "women's work" chores, and taking their turn at cleaning, groceries, etc., but why would the husband do all the shopping? I'm going to believe he was just a super nice guy who helped his wife out *too* much, and thereby inadvertently turned her into a helpless woman who didn't know how to do squat around the house.

~ And by the way, apparently Molly later began hanging out with Dr. Varner, as both are characters who were supposedly well known to our "core" characters, yet we never heard of them before, and haven't seen or heard from them since.

~ Leaving Molly's house, Johnny gets in the squad and then we see him reach for his helmet... just *before* the radio beeps them a tone. He must be psychic!

~ The football fan: was he watching the USC-Stanford game that Roy and Johnny worked at? Kinda looked like it. Also, I didn't know the guys on the engine could "patch in" a victim before the paramedics get there. What equipment do they have that they can do that??

~ Did we all notice the odd way the ambulance pulled in to Rampart when they brought the little girl in? Instead of coming through the tunnel, they used the tunnel to do turn and back in to the emergency entrance.

~ The return of the soapy music!! I know I heard it when Roy and Johnny were leaving Rampart and they were thinking about the girl. Johnny said "I get a knot in my gut when our victims are kids," and yet he doesn't acknowledge how much worse that feeling must be for Roy, who actually *has* kids. Then he says "I don't want to go back to riding on the engine. That's why I joined the paramedics in the first place." That made me go "hmmm" because he went from feeling sick about little kids being hurt to saying he doesn't want to be a firefighter and that's why he became a paramedic. That's at least three different and distinct thoughts in about two or three sentences... and some of them seem to contradict each other. Or contradict what we know about Johnny.)

~ Did anyone notice what looked like a newspaper clipping with pictures of a number of nurses in the Rampart break room? I wonder what that was IRL.

~ Last rescue: Angie got burned up!! Poor guy! I know why Cap stopped Roy from going to the car (he knew the two guys were dead), but it almost looked as if he was trying to protect him or shield him from seeing two bodies ("crispy critters"). No reason for him to try to protect Roy, of course, but that's what it looked like.

~ Also, after the car exploded Cap called for an ambulance, another engine, and a "mobile aid unit." And the call went out from LA for Mobile Aid 9 and Medic One. What's a mobile aid unit, and what's Medic One? At first I thought Medic One might be an ambulance, but Sam also said "ambulance is responding." A minute later we did see vehicle (not a squad) arrive, and we also saw another paramedic at the scene (stiff and goofy looking), so maybe some paramedics drive mobile aid units instead of squads?? (And Medic One is/was the name of the paramedic/ambulance service in Seattle, which we heard and saw in the E! movie Most Deadly Passage. I assume that's just a coincidence.....)

* * *

First question: No, we weren't supposed to know who Molly was. Just a case of them mentioning someone they supposedly see regularly but of course we've never seen or heard of them before. As for her late husband Dick... no, I don't believe it was a reference to either Dick Friend or Dick Hammer, both of whom were very much alive for another couple decades after this episode. But you bring up a good point and you'd think the writers could have come up with a unique name, one we've never heard before. Reggie... Brian... Dan... Marty... there are a hundred names they could use. But instead this show already has two Mikes (Stoker and Morton) and I believe the name Charlie was used for both the mechanic and someone else. For Hollywood creative types, these writers didn't always display a whole lot of imagination.

Second question: I have no idea what that truck was in that rescue, I assume it was the mobile unit. As I mentioned in my long-winded thesis—er, comments, I don't think we've ever heard LA dispatch Mobile Unit before, or Medic One. But there definitely were other paramedics on scene, so.... Maybe depending on where the movie studio was, other systems/jurisdictions were called in. (Yeah, I'm just guessing at this point.)

~ ~ ~

Watching EMERGENCY! Seasons 4-6

I agree... this is definitely a sub-par episode. And Molly—don't even get me started on her!! Oops, too late, I'm gonna go off about her anyway. First I had to laugh at Johnny's line about the needy woman: "With Molly, it's all the Hindenburg." And then Roy says that her now-deceased husband "did everything for her, even the shopping." Now, I can't be the only one who thinks that sounds wrong, right?? Not sure what kind of husband would do *all* the shopping for his wife, but chances are it's not the kind I'd want to meet. I know I usually rail against the 1960s and 1970s stereotypes that woman should stay home and concentrate solely on hubby and kids, but in that scenario, at least the wives are *capable* of doing their own shopping (and capable of other stuff, too). Additionally, Roy continues, "Now she's had to hack it out alone for the last year." Really? She's got a daughter to raise and no husband? Well boo-friggin'-hoo! She's not the first, last, or only woman who's had to go on after losing a husband—or in some cases never had a husband to begin with.

Anyway, it's interesting that, in this case, it's John who thinks something should be done about her repeated calls to Station 51. Hurray for Gage! And he's prescient, too: you can see him in the squad reach for his helmet to put it on, even before we hear the dispatcher's call to them.

That call is another football fan who suffers health issues while watching a game. (I think the game we briefly glimpse on the TV is the one from, oddly enough, The Game.) Engine 51 is already at the scene when John and Roy get there, and the victim gets agitated at being interrupted while watching the game. I do find it interesting that apparently the engine carries a set of "patches," as Chet told the paramedics they already got the guy patched in. I think we've seen that in another episode as well. And I have to say, I felt bad for Roy, having to get the respiration on this guy... I kind of cringed when he put his hand on the man's big, sweaty belly.

May Fair

So, about the titular exam.... The paramedics have to take a recertification exam. This test results in another one of those crazy conversations at Rampart in which it's implied that Roy and Johnny are the best paramedics in the world, possibly the only ones who are competent and capable. Dixie refers to "the boys" taking the test, and wonders if they could fail, and says "they're two of the best paramedics who ever went through training." Well doesn't that just s.u.c.k for people in the rest of LA County, who aren't in 51's jurisdiction!! Those citizens are obviously getting shoddy, second-rate paramedic care.

Anyway, apparently the eight-hour test is "tomorrow," and J and R are studying dutifully at the station. Inexplicably, they're wearing their blue jackets again. When was the last time we saw the guys wear them?? And I was wondering, why didn't they just split the two tables up again, like they were in the first season? One could be the study table, and there'd still be plenty of room for the six guys to eat. The paramedics get called out while the engine crew eats dinner, but it's a false alarm so they return. Again they try to eat, and by the way, obviously Marco doesn't have the monopoly on chili, as Cap makes chili, too—and apparently so does Chet. Anyway, no sooner does Johnny try to put some chili in his bowl than the station phone rings and it's Misfortunate Molly calling about her latest disaster. "It's for real," Cap says, and both engine and squad rush over there.

We all know about this call: child falls off five-foot ladder and hits her head... she's unconscious... blah blah blah. They get her to Rampart and everyone's concerned about little Jeanine. I noticed that, in the treatment room, the X-ray guy comes in, Early tells him what X-rays to take, and then Joe, Mike, and Dixie leave the room. But the other nurse stays in there. She's not wearing a lead nurse's dress, either; I bet she glows in the dark now!

As Roy and Johnny go out to the squad after this, we get that awful soapy music they usually play when Dixie takes someone for coffee and one of her patented heart-to-hearts. Instead Johnny tells Roy that every time they get a call that involves kids, he gets a bad feeling, a "knot in my stomach." Really, John? You're telling a guy who *has two kids* how awful you feel when a call involves a hurt child? Good thing you explain it to Roy, because otherwise I don't think he'd have *any* idea how bad it feels. (Yeah, I know, that's an overreaction, but I find Johnny's comment just a tad ironic.)

Next scene is back at the station. One thing I find funny here: Roy asks if there's any juice, and Cap says no, C shift drank the last of it. "They were here all night," he says, which I take to mean they were in the *station* all night, with very few runs. Roy says "Must have been a full moon." This confuses me; I'd think that if it was a full moon, they'd have a *lot* of runs, and be crazy-busy. If that was the case, they'd have been too busy to drink the juice. Second thing funny.... At the beginning of the episode, the exam was "tomorrow." In this scene, the exam was "yesterday." This isn't the first time it's happened, that something that happens off-duty "tomorrow" is referred to as "yesterday" on their next shift. Maybe one instance was when John and Roy went to look at that house for sale; another one might have been when Johnny was thinking of going into the rodeo with roping. In any case, it makes it sound like they work every other day, and on a regular basis, to boot.

Anyhoo.... on the plus side, Dixie finally tells Molly flat-out that she's using the guys at the station as crutches. Not a coffee cup in sight, and no soapy music needed, she just flat-out says it. And thank heavens, too. We also see the set-up for the next call: we're apparently seeing cops chasing a bad guy, but actually it's just a movie scene being filmed, with one Angie DeMeo driving the "getaway car." But accidents happen, and one happens here too, resulting in the car being flipped over on what looks like courthouse steps. Our guys are called out and just as the engine is arriving on the scene, some idiot with a bright idea is approaching the car with a blowtorch. Before Cap can say "bad idea," the guy and the car both go up in flames. (The man might have some burns, but that's the least of his problems... he might be going to jail for manslaughter.)

I think I asked this last time, but what's a Mobile Aid Unit? Cap requests one, and LA dispatches Mobile Aid 9, along with Medic One. No idea what those are, I don't think we've ever heard call-outs for them before or since. Incidentally, we do see another pair of paramedics, from 36s. Are they considered Mobile Aid? Medic One? And that one PM from 36s... he's slimmer than Johnny and shorter, too. Kind of scrawny, actually.

Last scene is at the station, when Cap tells Roy and Johnny what happened with the exam. He even uses his favorite epithet: "some twit punched the wrong button." And we all know what that means for Roy and Johnny's eight-hour exam.

6.8 Captain Hook

~ So as far as I know, Captain Hookrader (or Hochrader, depending on where you look) was first mentioned in the episode that introduced Henry. (Cap said Hookrader didn't know where Henry had come from, either.) So that's actually a tiny bit of continuity—a character being mentioned, and then actually being seen.

~ At the rescue of the girl with heatstroke (polar bear costume), I think Vince messed up his lines. When Roy and Johnny very first arrive, one of them says "Hi" to Vince, and

Vince replies "I don't know, I just got here myself," which doesn't make any sense. Then a minute later as they reach the victim Roy says "what's the problem?" and Vince says (again), "I don't know; people say he just dropped in his tracks." So I get the feeling Vince was supposed to say something else the first time.

~ I got the impression that Bobby Troup was reading from a TelePrompter as he was giving 51 instructions for the girl.

~ I've noticed a number of instances, in the past few episodes, in which the scene doesn't break (for commercial) naturally, but ends with a freeze-frame. I believe it happened in this episode, too, when Johnny discovered the 'polar bear' was a young woman.

~ By the way, does it mean anything that nobody mentioned that she was an attractive, well-put-together girl with a cute body? Obviously our guys are professionals and victims are victims first and all attention is given to that end, but later on, we didn't hear any comments about her (or suggestions about collecting a phone number). I'm going to take that as a good thing; Johnny, especially, is making progress.

~ Ah, we got to see Mama's Family. What a bunch of weirdos.

~ I like the final rescue of the helicopter pilot. Another one that likely couldn't really be rehearsed, and which also presented actual danger to those involved. Because, after all, those were real rocks out there.

~ Scenes from another episode (On Camera, I think, with the camera crew) were used in this one when Mike was using the engine to bring up the first chopper guy. But not when they brought up Johnny, Roy, and the other victim. (By the way, Cap was already starting to collect the ropes... did he forget Chet and Marco were still down there??)

May Fair

~ Speaking of Stoker using the engine to haul them up, I still find it hard to believe the engine doesn't have some sort of winch on it, even a manual one.

~ ~ ~

Well, this is awkward. No idea why this ep aired today (Oct 31), unless someone thought Captain Hook was some sort of scary character who ran around fire stations clawing firefighters on the shoulder. (And they'd be half-right.)

Anyway, I skipped almost all the station 51 nonsense because 1) we just saw this one a while back and discussed it then, and 2) I find the Captain Hook retirement party storyline to be silly and borderline mean.

There are a few things that I don't think I've seen mentioned before, or even that I didn't notice before. For example, at the girl-in-the-costume rescue, after Roy leaves in the ambulance, John is packing up to drive to Rampart and he gathers up some of their trash (good boy, Johnny!) and he stuffs it in the front seat of the squad. That totally makes sense and is a natural thing to do when they're in a hurry, but we never see the flip side, when they're at Rampart, or the station, cleaning out the junk they tossed into the squad. (Also, here's an odd thing I noticed: the girl isn't listed in the after-show credits, but if you look on this episode's imdb page, *two* girls are listed as "girl in polar bear suit.")

I like the rescue of the guy injured at the auto garage. Having him 'bite his lip' from the pain is a pretty good touch, I thought. But the other guy, Mike, for some reason he reminds me of someone I've seen on TV within the last few years... I think he looks like one of the guys who used to be on Extreme Makeover: Home Edition.

This is the episode with "Mama's family," isn't it? I hate that segment, so I just skipped it. Bleah, it's unpleasant all the way around. But when J and R get back to the station and are talking with Cap next to the squad, Chet calls to them from the other room, and Roy yells "What?!" I thought that was funny, and it's also sort of out of character for mild-mannered Roy to shout (or bark) like that.

At the helicopter rescue, I couldn't figure out what the point was of tying off the 'copter, since it slipped into the water anyway. Seems to me either they did it wrong to begin with, or they shouldn't have bothered doing it and wasting the time. Also, am I seeing that correctly—does Captain Stanley go down the cliff? When the first (uninjured) guy is brought up, the view we see from the bottom is of the stokes being pulled up by itself, and yet from the top we see Cap and some other FF being pulled up by ropes *with* the stokes. So how far down did Cap and the other guy rappel? And both of the chopper's occupants, as they were brought up in the stokes, both were totally wrapped up, from head to foot... almost looked like they were dead bodies instead of living people.

Anyway, once everyone is back topside, Johnny says, "we should write this up for the Fire Department journal; something like this has never been done before." What does that mean, what's never been done before? Rescuing helicopter victims? Bringing victims up a cliff? Helping out a fellow public servant (sheriff's office)? I don't understand what John meant by that.

Edit:

An observation: after having watched a S2 episode yesterday and a S6 episode today, I have to say that John Gage (Randy) looks significantly different (more, uh, 'mature') in the later seasons. Which isn't necessarily surprising; when the series began he looked quite young, 21 or so, but now, in the final season, he definitely looks like a 30-year-old. On one hand—again—that's not surprising, as that's how old he is (was) at the time. But the change takes place, quite noticeably, over just four or five seasons. And I don't think it's just his longer hair that makes him look older. I don't know, I hate to suggest it, but I wonder if his smoking habit had anything to do with it; it's well-known that smoking can 'age' people. Meanwhile, Roy looks pretty much the same in Captain Hook (S6) as he did in yesterday's Syndrome (S2), except for his hair color. Am I crazy for thinking Johnny/Randy looks that much older (i.e., his actual age) in these later seasons??

* * *

> every interview I have heard he says when the show started he was a 20 year old kid. I always want to shout, "No, you were 27 and that's not a kid!" But I guess in his mind he realizes he was really immature and that is how old he felt?????

I think Randy sometimes, um, 'encourages' the belief that he was closer to 20 or so when he started the show. He's been known to be pretty cagey about his age, so it wouldn't surprise me if he muddies the waters by claiming to be a "20-year-old kid" in the beginning, effectively shaving a significant number of years off his age. Eh, who can blame him… I know I'd love to shave a few years off my 'real' age, too!!

* * *

Here's a tidbit that might be of interest. I can't take credit for noticing it, but in the scenes at the station in this episode, Randy's left arm (more likely, shoulder) seems to be hurt. He's very careful moving it, or rather trying *not* to move it. During the rescues, he's fine, not a problem, it seems to be just the station scenes. (And maybe Rampart; he doesn't move his left arm much in the one Rampart scene he has, either.) Anyway, I guess he injured his shoulder somehow and had to do his best to hide it; he spends more time than usual with his thumb hooked into his belt buckle, trying to look natural.

For anyone who has The Book, can you check to see if anything is mentioned about this? I don't know if the same thing holds over to the next episode. Anyway, it kind of illustrates what we all know already: that all "set" scenes are filmed probably on the same day or consecutive days, and then location scenes are shot separately. And I imagine that some rescue scenes didn't always end up in the episode they were originally shot for

* * *

Oh yeah, I remember those scenes of Johnny obviously favoring his shoulder. Guess The Book doesn't explain that. Also in this season there's at least one episode (maybe two or three) in which we only see Johnny at rescues. He's not in any "casual" scenes at the station. Could be that Randy was filming some other project at the time and they just scheduled around him.

As for Mama... what was the original call-out on that? Woman down? Unknown-type rescue? If it was an Unknown Rescue, I can see why the engine was called out, but if it sounded like a medical thing (woman down, possible heart attack, etc.) it would fall into the category of "why did the engine go on that one?"

* * *

> I must say that since Henry arrived, every time I see him hanging off the couch, which is most of the time, I wonder how his nails don't ruin the leather.

Hmmm, good point!! Plus, I wonder if a dog's natural body oils or skin or fur or whatever might affect the surface of the couch. Or maybe it's not real (remember 'pleather'??). After all, a fire station is a lowly county facility after all.

6.9 Computer Terror

Somehow I think this episode was more interesting for possible screen shots than it was for storyline purposes. Even Johnny's incorrect paycheck fails to seem as dire as they made it (although I know that back in the day, paper paychecks were the only option, as opposed to direct deposit, and not being able to deposit a paycheck every two weeks was a Big Deal). But even that freeze-frame at the end of the first scene, with Johnny looking directly at the camera and shrugging was more interesting than *why* he was doing it. Also, there was very little of Rampart in this episode. Aside from the base station, and one conversation at Dixie's desk (about the aforementioned paycheck) we saw very little of our favorite medicos.

~ Calling Rampart from the junkyard, Johnny identified as County 51. Very early in the series (first season or so) it was Rescue 51, then somewhere along the line it became Squad 51. I think County 51 might become more prevalent here in season 6, we'll have to see.

~ Paradoxical breathing. Sounds like a mispronunciation, doesn't it? But it's not. It's when the chest expands on the outtake of breath, and falls in on the intake of breath, which of course is the opposite of normal breathing (and hence the name). Apparently it occurs with flail chest, which we also heard on this junkyard rescue.

Watching EMERGENCY! Seasons 4-6

~ Okay, dumb question: what is that thing on the guy's chest? It doesn't really look like either a scar or a wound. Or is it, and am I missing something obvious??

~ I guess it's a mystery as to *when* Johnny could have taken his check out of his shirt pocket and put it into his wallet. You'd think he'd remember deliberately doing something like that, it's not the kind of thing you do without thinking about it.

~ Okay, I just have to say it: that whole "dog by the pool" scene was just ridiculous. I know our guys are nice and it's their job to serve the public who pay their paychecks, but come on, they should have said at the outset, "Ma'am, we can't treat your husband until that dog is either tied up or put away." Surely they could've said that, and she could've done it. I have no patience for brainless people like that woman, and, naive though I might be, I find it hard to believe that someone would actually act the way she did. (Yeah, I know, I know: it happens in real life.) Anyway, while the situation annoys me I did get a kick out of a couple of things. 1) watching Roy try to walk with the dog biting his pant leg, 2) the little grin Johnny gave as he was talking to Rampart on the biophone and the woman told the dog to "sit next to daddy," and 3) seeing Roy get out of the pool soaking wet. Yeah, that third thing—er, those *three* things pretty much made that rescue bearable. *wink*

~ The scaffolding rescue. See, I told you we'd see that building again this week. But as I think I mentioned way back when, it looks like they tried to film it from different angles to cut down on the similarity (and of course back in the day when the show aired originally, it was probably a month or more between episodes). Anyway, I had to laugh when Cap said "it's too tricky to rappel down from the top." Because that's *exactly* what they did last time (say wha—??).

May Fair

~ The final scene back at the station, my favorite part was when Johnny, thinking he had "put one over" on the Payroll Department, was sort of gloating and smugly relishing the moment as he's telling the story to the other guys. Roy flat-out tells him, "Don't milk it." **Ha!**

~ ~ ~

This one opens rather oddly, with Chet and Johnny discussing the chances of winning for the LA Rams. Of course, this was back when the Rams actually played football in LA. In fact, it was when *anybody* played in LA. Hard to believe that the 2nd largest city in the US doesn't have *any* football team now. What's up with that?? Buffalo has a team. Heck, even Green Bay, Wisconsin (hardly a major metropolitan area), has a team. And yet LA? Nothin'. (Disclaimer: I know the city is trying to woo a team, so that might happen at some point.) Anyway, not only did Chet and Johnny make some random, generic, very vague comments about the Rams, but Chet mentioned sacking the quarterback and said "that's what's gonna happen to Harris." Incidentally, the Rams had a QB named Harris at this time, so it's interesting that they actually mentioned him, as this show doesn't usually get very specific. (Witness the awful TV broadcast of the gymnastics competition in The Girl on the Balance Beam.)

Anyway, the episode gets to the title issue quickly, as Cap comes into the dayroom handing out paychecks, and Johnny gets a big surprise. Or should I say a big $urpri$e. A computer error added a zero to his salary, making a check that should be in the hundreds to one in the thousands. (He has better luck than me: I once got a paycheck for $0. And yes, that was an error too.) In any case, it doesn't take a Rhodes Scholar or a crystal ball to know what happens with this storyline: the same thing that happens five or ten or other times in this series: Johnny goes overboard, doesn't listen to sound advice from anyone, and thinks he can be cleverer than everyone and easily attain whatever result he's looking for. And of course it *never* works out that way. Gotta love his enthusiasm, but dang, Gage, I'd think you would eventually accept the fact that it wouldn't kill you to listen to other peoples' opinions once in a while.

Getting back to the meat of the show, the first rescue is set up when we see cars getting flattened in a salvage yard. (I don't recall the name... was it the same one from the Billy Hanks episode?) But I like this rescue and, again, everyone pitches in in some way. It's a little odd to see Roy deal with the victim and Johnny hang back, contact Rampart, set up the equipment, etc. Usually Johnny is the "active" one and Roy is the "detail guy," so it's interesting to see the two switch roles, so to speak. (I'm not implying that Johnny does *all* the active rescues, or *always* works the equipment or handles the victims, etc. But it happens often enough that this was noticeable. To me, at least. YMMV.) In any case, after Mike uses the Jaws to open the smashed doors, and Roy asks that the crumpled roof be opened as well, he's finally able to access the victim enough to tape—of all things—sandbags on his torso to treat flail chest. (That's apparently when part of the rib cage breaks off, and there are broken [jagged] ribs floating inside the victim.) Not sure how sandbags were supposed to alleviate this condition in any way, but that's what used to be prescribed. And by my use of the phrase "used to," you can guess that sandbags are apparently no longer preferred treatment for flailed chest.

By the by, I think I mentioned this last time, but Johnny called in to Rampart as County 51. A sign of things to come?? I think they do that more often this season.

Next call is for a "person injured." This isn't one of my fave rescues. Well, *rescue* isn't quite the word for it, I guess I should say not one of my fave *calls*. It's one of those times when I think the guys just need to be firm and adamant:

May Fair

"Ma'am, please put the dog in the house; if you can't do that we'll call the sheriff's deputies to keep him out of our way." I know the guys wouldn't want to do that, but there are times when you have to put your foot down in order to be able to do your job... especially when someone's health/well-being/safety is at stake. Having said that, I will also say that that was a beautiful dog. (Tangent alert: must be strange for a dog to be trained to attack or bite or whatever, and have 'people' yell at him, shake him off, etc. Until the director yells "cut," at which time the 'mean people' become nice and friendly. Confusing much??) Also, I thought it was odd that we didn't hear Rampart's part of the transmission over the biophone. Usually it's audible, to us and the paramedics—and people—at the scene.

Last call is for an "accident with injuries." This is the same building we saw three episodes back, in Rules of Order. The director tries to make it look different (different address on the call-out, different building name, different filming angles), but it's definitely the same. And despite the fact that last time, the guys were able to rappel down from the top, this time Cap says it's "too tricky" to rappel. Yes, another way they try to make this rescue different from last time.

So this time, instead of rappelling down from the top, Johnny goes up from the bottom by pulling a Miley Cyrus: he rides a wrecking ball. Okay, so it's not a wrecking ball, but it's a close-enough approximation, in my mind. And yeah, Johnny does the "active" work and Roy mans the biophone, so I guess they balanced each other out in this episode.

Back at the station, Johnny strolls in acting like the cat that ate the canary, and revels in everyone's interest in how he "solved" his paycheck problem. He admits he doesn't have a check, but says he did get his money, and then grins enigmatically. Roy says, "Don't milk it," and Johnny divulges what he did... and soon learns why he shouldn't have. John,

Watching EMERGENCY! Seasons 4-6

John, John.... perhaps if there had been a seventh season, maybe he would have finally learned something. (Maybe??)

By the way, this episode is very Rampart-lite. I think we only see Dixie and Brackett on the line with the paramedics, and then Dixie and Early at the base station talking to the guys. No treatment room scenes, no Morton, no Brackett demanding something be done "stat!"

* * *

Re the bumping into people at Rampart... I think I did notice a couple of them, but I guess the light bulb didn't go off for me that there were so many. I guess the message is that Rampart was very busy that day. Also, I recall seeing Morton in the green scrubs in a very recent episode (The Exam, maybe?). But since I didn't watch Captain Hook yesterday and we didn't see him today I didn't think about it being an ongoing 'thing.' I'll have to keep my eyes peeled going forward.

> My only explanation for that was that the scaffold was hung from the top of the building, which may have impeded rappeling from the top.

My money is on the powers that be purposely not having them rappel down in this episode, because it would be too much like the Rules of Order rescue: same building, same strategy, probably same camera angles, etc. So they had to come up with a different way to rescue the victims, and since the snorkel truck is so... ordinary, they decided to find a different way. And in the process Johnny got to have a little fun.

(I know there's a coarse joke in there somewhere, which I forced myself not to think about or type into the above paragraph. Something about what Johnny was sitting on [*cough*bigball*cough] and where it was [*cough*betweenhislegs*cough*]. But NO, I told myself *not* to type anything like that because I went to Catholic school and I never, ever, ever think along those lines. Now, if you'll excuse me I have to get someplace where lightning can't strike me. ⚡)

6.10 Welcome to Santa Rosa County

The very first scene of this episode was unusual because... well, there *wasn't* a first scene. It's a cold-open, right into the intro, which was a little jarring. We see the guys at the station, ready for their vacay, and then bing-bam-boom! they're in Santa Rosa County, which is made evident by the twang of country music. Because after all, anything outside of LA County is automatically western-music listening, boot-wearing, hillbilly-accent-speaking, apple-pie-cooling-in-the-window country. Funny how that works, no?

At the lake, I had to wonder how long Roy and Johnny had been fishing. No cooler of drinks (or fish), no snacks, no chairs, nothing to indicate they'd been there longer than about fifteen minutes. They were *standing up,* for god's sake. Now, I don't fish, but even *I* know it takes time and patience, and you might as well make yourself comfortable—bring a folding chair or two. Also, they were very nicely dressed and clean-shaven, which violates another rule of a well-earned vacation.

And it seemed a little like Opposite Day. Usually Johnny is the impatient one and Roy is the "keep calm and carry on" one. But that's not how it was. And of all people, Roy told Johnny, "You're too trusting, that's your problem." Now, when has Johnny ever been too trusting? Roy, yes, I'd buy that in a heartbeat. But not Johnny.

On to the rescues. I thought it was funny that at the site of the climbing accident, the bystander 'happened' to know what was in the climbers' van. "You need rope? Sure, they've got rope in here, along with a bunch of other stuff I don't need—er, you might need. Don't mind the scratches on the door lock."

Later, when the fishing couple's boat blew up and John and Roy went out to them, they were swimming rather oddly at first, as though they weren't really swimming at all. I wonder if they were in maybe three or four feet of water and only pretending until the water got deeper.

And at the clinic, when you're looking for the drug supply and time is of the essence, wouldn't the locked cabinet with the big red crosses on it be your *first* thought, rather than your last?? But Johnny(Randy) had to draw it out as much as possible so he looked in random drawers and opened all the other cabinets first, I guess.

Lastly, I think whoever gave Roy(Kevin) that cowboy hat ought to be thrown into Santa Rosa Lake.

* * *

> why is Roy spending his vacation with Gage instead of with his wife and kids?

You know, I didn't even question this, oddly enough. I guess I figured it was just a "guys weekend" kind of thing rather than an actual vacation. To be honest, the old "TV characters going on vacation together" thing is such a well-known TV trope – one that I hate—that I didn't even question it. (I know: shame on me!) And by the way, I can't imagine Roy and Johnny spending a week's vacation together and still be speaking to each other at the end of it.

~ ~ ~

Must say, I like this episode, even though it has its weak spots. I applaud the writers for doing something a little different here.

May Fair

No squad, no engine, no structure fires or car accidents. Also, no biophone or drug box or even a stethoscope. Aside from Roy and Johnny (who are in every single scene except one--the one filmed at Rampart's base station), the rest of the regular cast probably got most of the week off, only coming in to film their brief scene(s).

As I mentioned last time, this episode is different from the very first second, as it starts with a cold open, immediately jumping into the opening sequence. From there, we get a brief scene at the station at 7:30am, when Roy and John are looking forward to having 4 days off, and going on a fishing trip. (I assume that at some point there was another 4-day-off cycle when Roy stayed home with the kids and Joanne went off to Vegas with some girlfriends. After all, fair is fair.) Anyway, as they discuss their trip, Cap says "Don't bring any fish back here 'cuz I don't want to have to see it or smell it." Meantime, while he's talking, Johnny steals part of Cap's donut. Big surprise, right??

Very next scene is the peaceful and idyllic Santa Rosa County, where we see our guys fishing in a lake. Now, I don't fish myself and don't claim to know a lot about it, I'm pretty sure that what we see isn't how fisherman actually fish. People spend hours fishing; wouldn't they be sitting rather than standing? Wouldn't they have a cooler or something to keep the fish in? Or maybe—at least—some beer? Anyway, when they start discussing their lack of luck, I kind of have the feeling that Johnny and Roy have switched personalities. Roy complains about the fishing location, Johnny says hey, the guy told us this was a good spot, and Roy says, "you're too trusting." That doesn't seem right, does it?? *Roy's* doing the griping? *Johnny* is too trusting?? What is this, Opposite Day??

Anyway, as they're leaving that spot in search of another one, they pass a couple who's bent on doing some fishing themselves, and Roy wishes them good luck with that. On their way out, the guys follow the wailing siren of a sheriff's car (probably by instinct) to the side of the road next to a big cliff, where two climbers have fallen. (I have to fight the urge to say, "I've fallen and I can't get up!!") By the way, did anyone notice that when Johnny puts his fishing rod in the back of his Rover, the end of it is sticking out one of the windows? I noticed it when he put it in there, and then Roy sort of "moves" the end of the rod when he gets out of the Rover at the site.

So the guys volunteer to climb up the cliff to the injured climbers, using equipment that they just happen to find in the trunk of the sheriff's car. And let's not forget the Nosy Nate who somehow, mysteriously, knows what's in the back of the climbers' van. Hmm, Sheriff Blaine might need to keep an eye on that guy, ya know? But our guys free-climb up the face, although right at the very end, Johnny's using an existing rope that came from—well, I'm not sure *where* that came from. As much as we talk about "lost equipment" on this show, in this case, they *find* some. E!-magic at work again?? I'm pretty sure it doesn't belong to the climbers they're trying to rescue. In any case, it ends up taking a while, but the Johnny and Roy doppelgangers get the two injured men down the hill, but they don't have any drugs or supplies with which to treat them. So we get a hell-for-leather ride in the back of a pickup truck to the nearest medical facility. No Doc Frick here. In fact, we don't see anything that happens inside; when the guys step outside the clinic a while later and meet up with the sheriff, we learn that one of the climbers didn't make it.

Over lunch (chili, coffee, and milk) Blaine picks John and Roy's brains about setting up a paramedic program in Santa Rosa County. This serves as a bit of a PSA for us (viewers) as much as for the sheriff himself. He's so grateful for the boys' help so far and impressed by them, that he insists on taking them fishing. Guess where they go? That's right, the same place the guys weren't having any luck earlier. The other couple they had seen is out on the lake in their boat, and before Blaine can get any lures out of his tackle box, their boat blows up and Mister Camper is on fire. Needless to say, the paramedics are in the water lickety-split to rescue the Burning Man and his wife. (Kind of looked like they were only pretending to swim. Maybe that's not the case, but I have the feeling that *something* was going on. We all know that Kevin is like a fish in the water, yet he seemed to be having trouble and Johnny got to the injured couple before Roy did, which doesn't seem natural.)

In any case, they load the injured man (burns on his back) into the camper and Mrs. Camper drives as they make another run to the clinic. (Heck with a paramedic program; Santa Rosa county could use roadside First Aid stations.) Anyway, I like this part of the episode. I like Blaine and his "act now, deal with consequences later" attitude. The guys need to get into the clinic—he breaks a window and unlocks the door to get them in. They need to be certified in Santa Rosa County—Blaine makes a phone call and gets them certified (and will deal with the paperwork in about another week). Johnny needs to find the MS which is probably locked up—the sheriff breaks yet more glass and gets him into the hard meds.

Back at Rampart, in the one scene filmed there, Joe tells Kel where the guys are and of course Brackett is as incredulous as Early was: "They can't treat the man! They're not certified! Blah blah blah!" Joe says, "Just want to let you know, Kel, I'm gonna go ahead and treat him, and worry about the legalities later." Kel's response: "I don't know, that might get messy. Let's both do it." Ha, gotta love it; it just sounds a little funny to me, like Brackett doesn't want to miss out on any fun and/or dangerous stuff.

Long story short, the paramedics do what they're trained to do and the victim gets handed off to the doctor, who's conveniently in the ambulance, by the way, meaning that neither paramedic has to ride to the hospital with the patient, which would put a serious crimp in Blaine's dinner plans and conversation.

Over that dinner, the guys suggest that rather than a paramedic program, maybe Santa Rosa County should train EMT-1s, which would go a long way to solving the problem and be a lot easier and less expensive, to boot. Plus, Blaine talks them into one more try at fishing.

Final scene: at the station with Johnny waltzing in with some newspaper-wrapped fish. Cap wants no part of it, and neither does Henry. Can't say I blame either one.

This 'n' that:

~ Yes, that was a good call about the guy I call Raggedy Andy (from Rules of Order). That maroon and yellow rugby-type shirt was back in this episode. No word on whether the wearer is the one who died or the one who didn't.

~ Johnny's license plate is (~~redacted~~). I wonder if the prop guys put a prop plate on his Rover for filming, or it was his 'real' plate? Are there any risks or legalities or dangers to showing your real license plate on TV??

~ Another episode without Dr. Morton.

~ The 'clinic' looked like it might have been part of some sort of summer camp.

~ The climbers were using some dark orange or red rope. Wonder if it's the same rope that Johnny'll test out for his friend in an upcoming episode??

~ We don't hear what the guys ordered for dinner, but it sure doesn't look very appetizing. Looks kinda bland, actually.

May Fair

~ This episode is also known for something else: *not* Johnny's best hair day. He must have left his comb in LA County.

6.11 Paperwork / Paper Work

I didn't like that the dad whose car ran into the fire hydrant told his kid, "Do you wanna get smacked?" Grrr. Speaking of the hydrant, I don't think Cap ever sent Mike or anyone to fix it or turn it off or whatever it is they do to stop them from gushing. I guess he'd call the city water department? Anyway, I didn't hear a word about the hydrant once they got to the scene. I realize the kid's situation came first, but one person could have been spared to make the necessary call or whatever.

And the guy who was doing the yard work and who inadvertently started the whole thing.... did he really need a chain saw for that little limb he was dealing with? I've taken care of limbs that small with a saw or even just by breaking them. Chainsaw, pfffftt… what a wimp!

When the kid was defibbed, I think he 'jumped' a little too early, and then had to 'jump' again once he heard "clear!" and felt the paddles.

When Brackett was saying he wanted X-rays on the kid, he told the nurse "call X-ray to come down immediately." I have the feeling he forgot the nurse's name and therefore just pointed at her. (Maybe that's not what happened, but it sorta looked that way to me.)

Re the Supply Nurse... Roy brought up a good point: would Johnny still be nice to her and be eager to give her a second chance if she didn't look the way she looked? (Roy's words: "You wouldn't say that if she was 50 and overweight." Gee, thanks.) And then Johnny says, "A girl who looks that good can't be all bad." Hmmm. I assume that at some point John Gage learned differently. At least, I *hope* he did.

Anyone else think that, back at the station, Marco acted really unrealistically by just grabbing up all the papers on the table and shoving them on the couch with Henry? I don't think anyone in real life would be quite that clueless. At least, nobody *I* know. (And if somebody I know *did* do that.... I can guarantee they wouldn't do it twice.)

So the paramedics responded to a call on a college campus, and what did they do? They left the squad not only unlocked, but *compartment doors open.* Yeah, right in the middle of campus. Recipe for disaster, fellas!

I liked the last rescue and fire scene. Roy and Johnny were first on the scene, with Engine 51 not far behind. I love when John and Roy told the Cap what was going on. Cap had just put a yellow clamp on one of the lines, and he turned and gestured to Marco (who was at the hydrant) to open it up. Then he had to kind of hop over some other lines from the engine. It was just cute and (to me) realistic all the way around. I just love those little details that are so small and a lot of people don't even consciously notice them, but they go such a long way in adding realism to the show.

Don't know how I could have forgotten, but I have to mention a scene that actually made me laugh out loud, something I rarely do, even with this show.

Picture it: Los Angeles, 1977. Roy and Johnny standing in line to see the Supply Nurse Ratchet. Roy's grumbling, but Johnny's trying to calm him down, confident that he (Johnny) can smooth-talk and sweet-talk the woman into compliance. "Let me do the talking," he says. "Don't antagonize her," he says. "She's only doing her job," he says.

Two minutes later Johnny's not feeling quite so sanguine anymore about the supply nurse. As she explains her by-the-book rules, you can practically see Johnny's temperature rise. (And not in a *good* way.) Then she tears up his form and hands him another one. He's just about to blow his top and tell her what she can do with her $#@$ forms when Roy grabs Johnny's arm and says "Don't antagonize her, alright? The lady's only doing her job."

Watch Roy right after he says that, repeating Johnny's own words back to him, and also Johnny's reaction. Pure gold! I don't know, maybe it's late, or maybe I'm tired, or both, but I found that to be so hilarious it makes me giggle just thinking about it. Johnny looking wrathfully at Roy, while Roy looks innocently away, an absolutely angelic look on his face. Too funny!

Okay, it's official. I need to get a life if a single scene of this show makes me so silly.

~ ~ ~

I like this episode. There are some quibbles, but overall I like it. It begins at Station 51 with the guys doing various tasks. Roy's cleaning the ovens, Chet and Johnny are doing stove duty, and Marco is inexplicably inventorying the fridge—in Spanish. I'm not sure why it even needs to be done in English, much less any other language. Anyway, Johnny pauses long enough to wonder about Henry and his "dog's life" just as Cap enters with the watchword of the day: paperwork.

At the scene change, we get an unusual transition, with the new scene literally "wiping" the old one off the screen. Have we seen that before on this show? That type of transition occurs about two or three times in this episode. Anyway, the set-up of the first rescue is sort of annoying, with a negligent handyman and a father who won't be winning any parenting awards. I could say something about the kid too, but hey, he's a kid, he at least has an excuse for doing something stupid. Oh, and the dog. Did you see the dog when the handyman finally went into the street and corralled him? I expect a disclaimer at the end: "no animals were harmed during the filming of this episode." (I certainly hope not!)

But back to the kid.... He manages to fall into the storm drain and Handy Manny can't pull him out so he tells a neighbor lady to call the fire department. (Question: who, exactly, did the *father* run 'around the corner' to call after his little accident, his insurance company??) Anyway, Station 51 shows up in record time and immediately gets to work helping the kid, with everyone pitching in. Except Stoker, who seems to be MIA in this rescue. Literally— MIA; in fact, I'm not even sure how the engine got there. A couple things of note here: 1) At no time does Cap say anything about getting the fire hydrant taken care of, despite the fact that it's spewing like a Disney theme park fountain. And 2) where the heck was the phone that dad went to use, anyway? While he's gone, this happens: his kid gets in trouble... someone calls for help... the fire department arrives (with sirens blaring)... and the guys manage to extricate the kid and start treating him, including *two* defibrillations. That all has to take at least fifteen-twenty minutes, right?? Still no dad. (The kid 'jumped' a little early on that first defib.) In the end, however, they get the kid back and into the capable hands of Rampart's doctors. (By the way, in the treatment room, I kind of get the feeling that Brackett was going to call the nurse by name, and then didn't; maybe he realized he didn't know her name.)

This is when Johnny and Roy meet... the supply nurse. They learn about her from Dixie and Mike Morton, and it doesn't bode well for them and their needed supplies. Johnny, however, remains confident: "Dix, I can get along with anybody." (Oh, really?? I think history might prove otherwise.) And when he gets a look at the supply nurse...

then he's *sure* he can get along with her, because hey, she's attractive, and therefore a 'given' that said young woman will conform to all of John Gage's preconceived expectations. Right? Well, not so much. The supply nurse is about as pleasant as a fungal infection, and Roy gets fed up pretty quickly with her stringent rules and procedures for supplies. Johnny sticks to his guns by rationalizing. "She's new on the job. And she's efficient, let's give her the benefit of the doubt," etc. Roy comes back with a classic: "You wouldn't say that if she was 50 and overweight." (As if there's something wrong with that....??) But Roy's right: Johnny's only being tolerant because the nurse is attractive. Meanwhile, the other guys at the station have their own paperwork to deal with, and after Chet carefully organizes the papers that Cap gave him to deal with, Marco callously comes in and jumbles them together as he clears the table for lunch. (Yeah, I call bogus on Marco doing that. Wouldn't happen.)

The next call for the paramedics (after another one of those transitions) is the college dude who drank some ancient Mycenaean wine. Yeah, that's one for the books. Or should I say 'for the scrolls'? Anyway, he now has severe cramps which aren't helped any by his professor boss trying to hold a bag over his mouth in an effort to catch his vomit. Both the victim and the wine decanter are taken to Rampart, followed closely by the professor, who's still anxious to get a specimen of the wine. But then he too is felled by cramping, and—funny story!—come to find out the culprit isn't the wine at all, but a chicken salad sandwich gone bad.

Meanwhile, back at the supply station, Nurse Picky Patterson is ringing a peal over the heads of two hapless (and nameless) paramedics, while Roy and Johnny wait for their turn. DeSoto's disgusted and seething, but Gage is still preaching patience. He's confident that he's got his ducks in a row and paperwork complete. "Don't antagonize her," he tells Roy; "She's only doing her job." So their turn comes and she remembers that they're County 51; Johnny turns on the Gage charm, which falters slightly when she calls him DeSoto. "No, I'm Gage; he's DeSoto." I half expected her to look at him and say, "Are you *sure?*" Anyway, things really go downhill fast after that, and next thing you know, Johnny's got steam coming out of his ears, defending their need for two bags of D5W: "We don't drink the stuff, you know!" And then comes the coup de grace, as Roy cuts him off in mid-rant, saying "Don't antagonize her; she's only doing her job." Roy's innocent and artless look is priceless, and so is Johnny's double-take as he realizes what Roy just did. Hoist with your own petard, Mr. Gage! I have to say, I rarely laugh out loud when watching this show, but this scene almost always makes me laugh every time I see it. It's a classic!

Back to the rest of the show.... The next set-up is some generic warehouse storing acetone, nitromethane, and other volatile, flammable materials. Aren't there ever any accidents at places that produce dish soap or mayonnaise? In any case, the foreman guy is jerky and careless, and bing-bang-boom, we've got an accident and a fire and of course the requisite explosion. With—you guessed it!—people trapped inside. Roy and John get the call while they're in the squad (and Johnny's pressing hard on his supply request form to make five copies) and they're the first ones at the scene. The engine isn't far behind and when they get there we see Cap doing the Cap things we love to see (at least *I* love it): he puts the yellow clamp on the hose as Johnny tells him what's up and he also signals to Chet to hook up the hose from the hydrant. Gotta love watching that man work! In any case, it's a good rescue as Roy hacks into the back of the building and they climb down into the office from above, with the help of another engine company. It's one of those times when the 'rescue' is not so much a medical rescue as an actual rescue, which always provides some nice action.

May Fair

Lastly we discover that Dixie solved the Nurse Patterson problem. She gummed up the works by messing with the supply inventory. Not that that would work so easily in real life, but Roy and Johnny sure are glad that Dixie got involved.

Quick bits:

~ Maybe it's not surprising that Picky Patterson is so naggy... I'd be unpleasant too if I was named Wilma. (No offense to women named Wilma, but it must be tough going through life named after Fred Flintsone's wife.)

~ I saw some other, non-Station-51 firefighters take the second ladder off Engine 51; I assume Cap knew about that.

~ Speaking of that last fire, is there any reason why the FFs couldn't just move those barrels out of the warehouse? They can't explode if they're not in there with the fire, right?

~ I saw a couple other nurses wearing pant suits, but most still wear the dresses. And aside from Dixie, most also still wear the caps.

* * *

> Did anyone else notice the dog sticking his head between the man's legs from behind, then the man struggling to get off of him? Thought that was cute.

Actually, if you watch the dog closely, you'll see that his tail was between his legs, and he was sticking very close to the handyman, practically trying to melt into him. I think the poor mutt was petrified; I don't think he wanted to be there. (I mentioned this in the screen pics thread, too.)

* * *

I've often seen (on TV, movies, etc.) people smack the ambulance doors twice once they're closed. But on this show it really didn't seem to be necessary, as one or the other ambulance attendants is usually there when the doors are closed. I think I've seen Johnny tap the door with one of the attendants right next to him, and the attendant then walks around to the passenger side of the ambulance. Hopefully the driver would *not* drive off once he hears the slap, as he'd be leaving without his partner. In any case, I don't think it's an official signal to the driver, but maybe just a double-check. But then, I don't really know, so I'm just guessing.

* * *

Yeah, the characters staying wet when they should be wet is sometimes an issue. Same thing happened in Welcome to Santa Rosa County.

One thing I've often wondered is about the guys tramping through Rampart's emergency department after coming from a structure fire or brushfire. They must smell awfully of soot and smoke, yet nobody ever seems bothered by it or even mentions it. Heck, I can tell within 100 yards when someone in my neighborhood is using their wood-burning fireplace, and if that homeowner was standing next to me, it'd be very obvious. Now and then they should have had Dixie shoo the guys away, saying "whew, you smell like smoke, get out of my hospital!"

6.12 Loose Ends

For this episode, I'll just mention a few items that I thought were noteworthy... most of them relating to dialogue.

May Fair

~ I always think it's funny, on this show and also on Adam-12, when a character says something along the lines of, "Sure, I'll give a statement. I'm a responsible citizen." Some people are so careful to mention how 'responsible' and 'upstanding' they are. Anyway, we were treated to an example of that in this episode with the Brackett accident.

~ Speaking of Brackett, he called a candy striper "honey." That wasn't really a big deal back in the day, I guess, but I still bristle whenever I hear it.

~ When Early suggested Johnny talk to the little girl (accident victim whose father died) to see if he could find out anything about her, he said, "She's in the room right next to Pediatrics." *Next to* Pediatrics? What, she couldn't get a reservation or something to actually get *into* Pediatrics?? Is it an exclusive, restricted floor? And wouldn't a child, of all people, qualify to be on that floor?

~ Roy and Johnny told the guys at the station about their 'caper' with the undercover police officers, and they all said how exciting it was. And Roy said, "It was a little like Police Story." Nice little plug of a sister show on the network, writers!! As long as they didn't do a cross-over with Police Story, like they did with Adam-12.

~ Ever notice when there's a big call-out, with lots of engines, trucks, etc., Station 51 is always listed first??

~ That scene with the broken fan belt was funny. Johnny looks around to see some guy run past and get yelled at by cops. Then he hears Roy call out to him and he turns to see what's up. He starts running toward him, but Roy tells him to bring the drug box, so Johnny stops short and does a 180 toward the squad. Just then the dispatcher calls out for a status. Johnny really looks like he doesn't know which way to look or what thing to do first.

~ Lots of stock footage in this episode, including in the final call-out, when we actually see Engine 8 drive out of its station. Anyone notice anything interesting about that scene? A familiar figure in the jump seat??

* * *

They've been saying County 51 for a few episodes now. I think I mentioned it a few eps back. Not sure exactly why the change. When the show first started they were Rescue 51, then it changed to Squad 51, which they were for a long time, until now. Anyway, someone once suggested that as the paramedic program grew, maybe LA city introduced paramedic squads as well, so our guys had to identify as County 51 to Rampart, so they wouldn't be confused with Station 51 in the city....? (I don't know how likely that is, but it's a theory; I just looked up LAFD, and the city does have a Station 51, which I find interesting. It's right next to LAX, but still, I wonder if anyone ever confuses it with the LA County Station 51 from the show.)

~ ~ ~

So what exactly are the "loose ends" referenced in the title? There don't really seem to be any loose ends to take care of. And, for practically the first time this season, there's no drama at the station involving paychecks or computer reports or vacation plans. There isn't even a John-and-Roy-centric storyline as there is in The Game or Santa Rosa County. Maybe the "loose end" was the writers trying to come up with a title for this episode.

Episode begins at the station with the guys just jawing. Actually, Chet was telling a story about a troupe of "little midget mimes," which I have the feeling was something that Tim came up with on the spur of the moment as a gag, maybe to see if he could get the other guys to crack up. Anyway, we don't hear any more of that, as the story is interrupted by the arrival of Dixie, who comes to the station to meet Henry. (This is just before 5pm; how often does she work 'second shift'??)

In any case, the guys have to run out on her as they get a call for a traffic accident. They get to the scene, where the sheriff's deputies are putting out flares (during the day? seems odd) in really crazy/unnecessary places. Two vehicles involved: one has a man and child, and the other is crushed so that the FFs can't get into it right away. Johnny's good with the little girl in the first car, and when he realizes that her father is dead, he gently rests the man's head against the steering wheel and turns his attention to Tina. Just like the accident in Snake Bite, I'm not sure why the kid is riding in the back seat. Anyway, while Johnny's dealing with that, the deputy is dealing with the onlookers and one guy indicates he saw the accident. Why, yes, officer, I'll be glad to give you a statement, because "I'm a responsible citizen." Love it! That line always kills me.

Meanwhile, Roy and Chet are working on the second car. Roy finally manages to force the passenger-side door open and tilt the driver's head up, only to discover... it's Dr. Brackett. (Dun-dun-*dun*.) He's got a small gash over his right eye and a hint of a bruise on his left cheek. So what does Roy do? He bandages the *bruise* to within an inch of its life. Yeah, Brackett ends up with a bigger bandage on that bruise than on the wound that's actually, you know, bleeding. Johnny calls Rampart and tells Early that the second victim is Dr. Brackett. "Would you repeat that?" Early says. Really? You need him to repeat it? "Yeah, I said the second victim is Buddy Hackett." If I was Dr. Early, *I'd* repeat what *I* heard and have John confirm it. In any case, Morton has to break the news to Dixie; not only does he (apparently) call her babe, but Dixie's so thrown by the news that she forgets the caller she *just* put on hold.

Not surprisingly, the doctor makes a very bad patient, right from the minute he's brought into the treatment room. One thing I thought was odd here: once they got Kel in the treatment room, it sounds like Dr. Early shoos John and Roy out of the room, so he could ask Kel a couple questions. Later on I turned on the CC and that has Early telling the guys to wait outside so he could ask *them* a couple questions. That makes more sense than sending them out of the room so he could ask Brackett questions, but still, why do they need to leave at all? They often help out in the treatment room, and there's nothing the paramedics can say that the victim (Brackett) wouldn't be able to hear. Not to mention, heaven knows there's the magic acoustics at Rampart that allows doctors to have conversations five feet away from the patient without the patient hearing a thing.

Anyway, the car accident leads to a ridiculously unreal situation in which nobody knows the little girl's name, where she lives, who her relatives are, etc. Um, hellooo... anyone ever heard of license plates and car registrations? Yeah, I know, the story is more dramatic if the girl is referred to as Jane Doe. This does give Robert Fuller a chance to do some emoting as he talks to Tina/Jane Doe; it's nice to see this side of Dr. Kelly Brackett. (Sort of ironic when he tells the girl about his love of horses; too bad he didn't say that he always wanted to be a cowboy in the old west, y'know?) But the scene was also a nice contrast to the depiction that Morton gave earlier of Brackett: *indestructible,* and *so in control.* Thank heaven Morton didn't see the 'crusty' Kel Brackett on the verge of getting emotional as he talks to Tina.

Meantime, Roy and Johnny stumble into an episode of "Police Story," which I guess was the mid-'70s equivalent of Law and Order. Pulled over to deal with a minor technical issue, Johnny's trying to fix the squad's fan-belt and Roy's in search of some food when a police stake-out results in bad guys fleeing every which way. One cop does a dramatic (and hilariously cheesy) jump in front of a getaway car, gun drawn, and I half-expect him to yell "Freeze, sucka!!" Another guy gets chased on foot right past Johnny, who literally doesn't know which way to turn with everything that's going on. Cars screeching, people running... he's totally confused, and watching him when Roy adds to the confusion by yelling for him is a hoot: turn this way, turn that way, do this—no, do that first, etc. Kind of funny, I thought.

Last call is for the fire at the freight yard. This one kind of reminds me of that other episode when they're at a rail yard and Roy gets overcome with smoke and Chet "drives" a train car, etc. But I like this rescue, it's kind of cool to see the engines stick a hose into the ocean and suck up water. We also got a good look at the deluge truck, including the bar that the operator uses to help him move positions. And of course—this *is* Emergency!, after all—there are two people stuck inside one of the rail cars who need rescuing. Heaven forbid John and Roy should man the hoses while Chet and Marco go after the missing people, y'know? Come on, Cap, mix it up a little bit with the assignments once in a while, would ya?? And once the people are rescued, that's the cue for the Battalion Chief (or even Cap) to get on the HT and declare "this fire is under control." Happens. Every. Time. But I did wonder why, after the damage this fire caused and the materials involved, why the Chief said all units out 30 minutes. I'd think it would take longer than that to do whatever it is that they do once the fire is out (cleaning up, making sure the location is secure, getting hoses back on the rigs, etc.).

Stuff:

~ Why is Dixie in street clothes when she stops by the station before work? As far as I know, most nurses wear their uniforms to and from work.

Watching EMERGENCY! Seasons 4-6

~ Even though Johnny identifies to Rampart as County 51, LA dispatch still calls them out as Squad 51.

~ We get a glimpse of alt-reality Johnny on Engine 8; he looks nice and cazh with his leg propped up. That Randy is such a ham when he knows he's on camera!

~ A bit of real injected in the fiction: at the freight-yard fire, there's an announcement in the background from Dispatch. It says "Battalion 7, squad 36 is 10-7 at Harbor hospital." We all know that Harbor is the 'real' version of Rampart, so I'm betting that was a 'real' call.

~ I want to know what happened with the little midget mimes.

* * *

>Okay, let me just say, I loved the fact that Johnny wanted the waterbed instead of the Vegas trip. Ok, enough said.

At the station, when Johnny says he wants to win the waterbed, Chet and Marco kind of look at each other knowingly, almost as if to say "Uh-huh, we know why he wants *that*." It was funny.

I too noticed the annoyed look Johnny gives Tina when she says she wants to go to the carnival. Selling a ticket for her would put Johnny in the lead in the ticket-selling contest, which he didn't want. I agree it was a bit mean-spirited of him.

I don't usually turn on the closed-captioning (Netflix) unless I specifically want to find out what someone said. They do occasionally mix something up, but for the most part the CC'ing is pretty good. On Adam-12, there are (or were) entire sentences that are different. They might be *similar,* but different. (Example: We hear "Okay, buddy, come on out slowly, hands where I can see 'em" but CC says "All right, mister, come out and make it slow, hands up.") If I didn't know better, I'd almost think that the CC comes directly from the actual show script, and the variance in the dialogue would be due to the actors somewhat ad-libbing a little.

So compared to that, the E! closed-captioning is far more accurate.

> Also during this scene, we hear Sam say, "Paramedic calls in a false alarm. All units cancel". What???????????????

I like to try to hear what's going on in the background of these scenes when I can, but I missed this one. My assumption is that maybe the paramedic notified dispatch that it was a false alarm (i.e., when the squad got there they realized it).

6.13 An Ounce of Prevention

~ This was a PSA-laden episode, with both Roy and Johnny's presentation on the TV show being a PSA, as well as the familiar parathion thing. I think at least every second season the writers have a parathion storyline.

~ Once again we see Roy reading a book. Couldn't tell what it was, though, but it definitely didn't look like any sort of fire department manual.

~ A rescue involved a man who was ill on a malfunctioning amusement park ride. I'm guessing that wasn't Kevin who climbed on the 'double' Ferris wheel. (Is that what they're called?) We never got a good view of him during the climbing sequence, and when we did see Roy, it was more of a close-up which could have been edited in. In one of the scenes (as they're lowering the boy down) it's kind of a faraway shot, and it doesn't quite look like him up there. But, I could be wrong.

~ Once again, while Johnny and Roy are climbing the heights and doing the exciting stuff, their "ground crew" is safe on terra firma, watching the action and doing not much other than holding the occasional rope.

~ So a man was ill on the ride, and a young guy stupidly got out of his own chair to try to help, and of course he got stuck. My question is what would have happened if the man had died while Johnny and Roy were dealing with the kid? How awful would that have been? They could have gotten to the man 10 minutes sooner if they hadn't had to deal with the would-be Good Samaritan.

~ Don't you love how they always call Cap over when the victim's family member is getting in the way? I wonder if the captain's exam has a section on "Tact 101."

~ I'm going to say again that when they got the call with the little boy, the original call included Engine 36. They must've gotten lost, though, because the engine never shows up. Even when R and J went back to the house to check out the garage, Engine 36 was still a no-show.

~ In the final rescue at the TV station, I think there must be a scene we don't see. That host Tom Jensen of course asks nosy questions when the guys are very busy working on the real-life rescue, but he said something about a live wire and "did you put it out with a block of wood?" And Roy answers yes. We didn't see that, did we?? That would've been interesting, but I only saw J and R picking the guy (victim) up and moving him—and even that, we didn't see very well, because of the lights and other equipment being in the way. So I feel like I missed something and maybe there was a scene that didn't make the cut.

~ ~ ~

May Fair

The meaning for this episode title is very evident, very quickly, as in the first scene we learn that "headquarters" wants Roy and Johnny to go on a local talk show to do a fire-prevention demonstration. "But we have guys for that," Roy protests, looking Not Happy At All, "so why us?" "Because I went down there and talked to them," Gage answers, as if that explains everything. Yep, folks, John Gage, he who, just a few seasons ago, froze in front of a camera like a sloth in daylight, now wants to go on live TV and do a demonstration. And Roy, Mr. Cameras-Don't-Bother-Me, is mildly panicked about it—if not panicked, at least definitely annoyed. Go figure.

This news comes after we learn that Chet is working with Henry on developing his ESP, by the way—Henry's ESP, not Chet's. Just thought I'd mention that little tidbit.

First call is to an amusement park for a man who's ill, and oh yeah, he's stuck 100 feet (??) up on a malfunctioning Ferris Wheel. What the station 51 guys don't know yet is that a young man unwisely got out of his own Ferris Wheel car in an effort to try to help the older man, and of course *he* fell and is now stuck and injured himself. Isn't that always the way? Anyway, this rescue bothers me in a couple of ways. First is the decision to have both paramedics go up on the Wheel and deal with the young man, and lower him down to the ground first, before tending to the other man, the *original* victim, who is still unconscious and whose condition is totally unknown because nobody is in any condition to communicate it. But anyway, that's what the paramedics do: they hook up a pulley (I didn't see anyone climb to the top to hook that up, by the way) and get Young Guy secured and send him down. (I have to chuckle... even though we know the close-up scenes were filmed much closer to the ground than the long-shot scenes with the stunt guys, Roy still looks like he's holding on for dear life when dealing with Young Guy.) Never mind the fact that the Older Guy could be dead or dying while the guys deal with Young Guy; I'd think they should at least check on Older

Guy first so they can accurately triage their victims. Anyway, after Young Guy's taken care of (we saw the same actor a few weeks ago in Captain Hook), John and Roy turn their attention to the other, original, victim and his now-traumatized wife. We don't actually see them get the unconscious man out; that would have been a real trick (i.e., ordeal) in real life, so I guess the PTB just figured it would be easier not to show that part. Once he's been extricated, Johnny moves in to deal with the wife, and he ends up having to slap her lightly to snap her out of her fear. Then, to add insult to injury, he accidentally bops her in the nose with his elbow after he fastens the belt on her. (And he didn't even apologize!) He also said "Good girl" to her. I wonder if he said "Good boy" to her husband?

Anyway, this leads me to the second thing that bothers me about this rescue. We've mentioned before that for some reason the paramedics seem to be the *only ones* who ever go after people who are stuck someplace or other (even when they can't render any meaningful medical care at the time), and this is another instance of that. It's bad enough that Older Guy had to wait to be dealt with until Young Guy was on terra firma, but even once they got Older Guy harnessed in and lowered down, there's *no* paramedic on the ground who can begin treating him. Nooooo, both paramedics are still on the Ferris Wheel dealing with TraumaWife. Older Guy on the ground could be dead or dying, and while Cap and Chet and Marco can do *some* things, they're not trained or authorized to do the more complicated things which might have been necessary to save Older Guy's life. The man could have literally died while the only trained medical personnel within five miles were busy getting an hysterical woman out of a Ferris Wheel. So, that's my beef with this rescue: paramedics need to be where they're most critically needed, and if that means one or both of them waiting on the ground while the other guys do the 'heavy lifting' once in a while, then so be it.

On the plus side, I'll give the show props again for the illusion that those guys we see climbing on the Ferris Wheel really are Roy and Johnny (Kevin/Randy). Not that we can't tell it's not them, because we can if we're observant, but the audio of them calling out or saying this or that usually matches what we see quite well. And the audio doesn't sound obviously dubbed, either; it sounds as natural and similar in tone/volume/whatever to the rest of their dialogue. This rescue also gives us a mention of Cheyne-Stokes respiration, which I don't think we've heard before, at least not that I recall.

At Rampart, Roy's still stressing about having to go on camera, thanks to his best pal. And back at the station *we* have to watch a very awkward (and rough) run-through of their spiel. This rehearsal, both the first part with the wood and sawdust, etc., and the second part, with the aerosol cans, serves as a back-door PSA to viewers about household safety. Especially if you use AquaNet hairspray, apparently.

The demonstration is cut short by a call for the paramedics. They, along with Engine 36, are called out on a "sick child" call. (Although we never do see Engine 36 show up at the scene; did they take the scenic route to get there??) I do like this rescue, as it's obvious that the guys can't begin to guess what's wrong with the boy. I sort of cringed, though, when the mom asks "Is Corey going to be all right?" and Johnny replies, "I hope so." Bad, Johnny! Also, at Rampart, Drs. Early and Brackett note the dust on Cory's jeans and decide to get it analyzed, and yet.... they don't bother removing the jeans but instead go ahead and treat him while he wears them. Yeah, the stuff might be toxic or whatever, but let's leave it on him! Great idea. In any case, after the paramedics enjoy a nice stroll back at the Phillips' house (and Engine 36 *still* isn't there) we find out that among the crap-load of toxic stuff the dad keeps in his (unlocked) garage, is... guess what? *Parathion!* It's probably been a couple whole seasons since we had a parathion scare on this show. Guess the Powers That Be felt we needed a story that would hit us in the gut. But anyway, now that they know what the problem is, Brackett gives the parents a Stern Talking To and then says they can go visit their son, who's going to be fine.

Next scene is John and Roy as they're getting ready to do the TV show. They're wearing their dorky ties and Roy is actually sort of looking forward to it. At the TV station, they're each true to form: Roy barely takes a sip or two of coffee, while Johnny insists on stuffing a doughnut in his mouth. Powdered, no less. Needless to say, the horribly awkward interview is as horribly awkward as we all knew it would be (and as bad as Chet and Cap say it is), and to be honest I fast-forwarded through most of it. At least until the hapless worker-bee inadvertently causes an explosion off-stage and gets burned. Then we see the 'real' Roy and Johnny, as they spring into action and take charge of the situation without hesitation. (It would have been interesting to see what the viewers saw of this whole thing, too.) But I wonder about two things: 1) Apparently Roy put out a "live wire" with a "stick of wood." Huh?? Did we see that?? And 2) the timing: almost immediately after getting the victim away from the fire, Roy says he'll go out to the squad for supplies, and by the time he's coming back into the studio, the engine is there, responding to the fire. That has to be the Quickest. Response. Ever. Seriously, you'd think Cap had the engine lurking right outside in the parking lot the whole time. Also, I like Johnny and Roy's responses to the host, Jensen, as they were working on the victim: "I don't have the time," "not now," etc. Yay for them!

Final scene, at the station: the paramedics are commiserating about how badly they flopped on the TV show, and they don't want to see a TV camera again for long time (all the while actually facing one, of course). But Cap has other news: headquarters has gotten a lot of positive feedback about the "incident" at the TV studio, and the Tom Jensen producer has called to invite the boys back on the show. The guys, however, are having none of it. Johnny's philosophy is "quit while I'm ahead," and Roy agrees, mentioning the First Rule of Show Biz: "always leave 'em wanting more."

And, yes, Roy. We do.

* * *

> Did [the TV host Jensen] think there wasn't enough room for his annoying facial hair and super dated newsreel speak?

Ha, yeah, him and his garden growth on his face. It *was* annoying, wasn't it?? And the newsreel speak—nailed it! He sounded like those old movie newsreels that sometimes play on M*A*S*H. You're also correct that yes, the host's job is to keep things smooth and conversation moving along on TV, no matter what.

Now that you mention it, great point about people in real life not freezing up in front of a camera. I guess I've seen interviews in which people just respond monosyllabically to interview questions, or don't speak loudly enough, but you're exactly right: I've never seen anyone actually freeze up. In fact, in the past 10-20 years or so, most people seem eager and anxious to be on TV (waving and saying Hi, mom! in the background, etc.). Maybe the proliferation of cameras everywhere has conditioned us to be more used to it these days and it's not such a rarity anymore. Who knows?

6.14 Insanity Epidemic

Episode directed by Randy... his second one. (And this time Johnny didn't have to get hit by a car!)

Watching EMERGENCY! Seasons 4-6

~ Chet trying to 'train' Henry. Yeah, like that's gonna work out. All Chet has to do is listen to the tuba music and he'll know that Henry's gonna do what Henry wants to do. Which is: stay on the couch!

~ When Cap comes into the dayroom, we *see* Roy say something, but don't hear anything until Cap apparently replies to him, saying, "We just got a new battalion chief, that's all." I'm no lip-reader (though I wouldn't mind trying in this case, ifyouknowwhatImean, wink-wink), but I think Roy asks cap what's wrong. But I wonder why we don't *hear* it??

~ I hate the set-up for the gas station rescue. Both the man and woman were acting like jerks and being stupid, and I don't want to see that. And the gas station attendant... did we all recognize him? He's been in two other episodes, in one on which he plays a very memorable character.

~ At the hospital, Dixie and Brackett were griping about a new administrator, Elgin. What happened to O'Brien, who was played by James Shigeta? Good thing Dixie didn't take that job he offered her or she'd be working for a worse jerk now.

~ At the scene of the father/daughter married couple (*shudder*) I like the line that Roy has... as he's putting the tape on his leg (yay!) in preparation for setting up an IV, and he has something in his mouth that he's talking around (lucky thing), he says something about putting the IV in the lower arm "in case they want to start an antecubital later on." Just a throwaway line that didn't impact anything we saw, but it's another small detail that lends an air of realism to the scene.

~ And I had to laugh when the ambulance attendant brought the O2 to Johnny... I'm guessuming the guy's name was Sonny, because when Johnny thanked him, I assume (I *hope*) he said "Thanks, Sonny," instead of "Thanks, honey," which is what it sounded like.

May Fair

~ The ice-skating scene, which I mostly fast-forwarded through... it was at the Pickwick Recreation Center. Which is interesting because earlier in the episode, as the squad and engine are driving to the gas station, we see a sign for Pickwick Western Stores. Is/was Pickwick a big name in LA County?? Two instances of the name in the same episode kind of makes you go 'hmmm.'

~ I like the last rescue, kind of complicated and not easy. But when the tones went off, dispatch said only "Freeway accident, Orange Street off-ramp." Pardon me, but in LA County weren't there multiple freeways running through their jurisdiction? Identifying the location simply by the name of the off-ramp doesn't seem to be very specific, does it??

~ Once again, at that last rescue, I thought the sequence of events of getting the girls out of the car seemed a little strange. But oh well. And how did the guys know to run when they got everyone out of the semi? Everyone hurried away and seemed to know the truck was about to blow, but I don't recall anyone mentioning that they were working against the clock.

~ Also, I have to smile.... for some reason I love watching Stoker run. It's so cute!! We saw it briefly when they first got to the scene.

~ ~ ~

This ep was directed by Randy... and his character didn't have to break his leg this time. I do wonder, though, when someone is slotted to direct an episode, if they get the opportunity to choose which ep to direct, or if it's just assigned to them. Either way, Randy's ep had a good bit of silly going on.

In the opening, Chet's determined to get Henry off the couch and into the new doghouse that he procured for that purpose. Of course, knowing Chet, and knowing this show, nothing will happen as expected, and of course, it doesn't. Hmm, just yesterday, in Ounce of Prevention, Chet was working with Henry to develop his ESP. (Henry's ESP, not Chet's.) And today is more of the Chet 'n' Henry show. I guess maybe Tim Donnelly wasn't joking when he said working with the dog would get him more screen time. (Meantime, I wonder if Marco's getting jealous.)

Cap comes into the dayroom and suddenly, seemingly from out of the blue, says, "We just got a new Battalion Chief, that's all." This announcement took me by surprise (as it did last time, too), so I ran the scene again, and if you look closely, you can see that Roy actually says something to Cap as he walks in, but for whatever reason (bad mic? edited out?) we don't hear Roy's comment. Based on Cap's response, though, I assume Roy says "What's wrong?" or "What's new?" or something along those lines. In any case, this sets up the premise of the episode: McConnike becoming the new Battalion Chief, and Cap apparently freaking out about it. But of course, nobody knows why.

First rescue is at a gas station, with a very unpleasant couple with whom I feel no empathy whatsoever. They're both jerks and I don't really care what happens to them. (Mean, aren't I??) But they're only part of the scene at the gas station. Apparently Ed Marlowe did everyone a favor and quit the LACoFD and became a "hose-jockey" of another sort: a gas hose-jockey. He watched the accident happen and actually did the right thing right away, the result being that Engine 51's guys were breezing along doing their jobs (which, curiously, includes washing gasoline directly into the sewer system, as we've noted on previous viewings). In any case, Marco's doing something or other that Cap told him to do, but suddenly, the station owner decides it's time to turn the power back on, and zzzzzzt— Marco goes flying and the remaining gasoline on the ground starts burning. This is mostly bad news, but the upside is that we see Stoker actually handling a hose again. Since Marco's incapacitated, Mike and Chet have to handle the hoses. Interestingly, Johnny says very little throughout the whole scene with the injured couple (Roy does most of the talking to the victims) and yet J-man is the one who lets out a loud and dramatic "Nooooo!" as he sees the station owner turn the power back on and thus endangering Marco. Director's privilege, I presume?

At Rampart, while Morton (again wearing scrubs, as is customary this season, apparently) is checking out Marco's hands, we learn that the hospital is dealing with a new administrator, Elgin. No word on what happened to O'Brien, the administrator who offered Dixie a huge promotion a few seasons ago. Anyway, other than some angry bluster from Brackett, the Elgin storyline doesn't really end up going anywhere. And Kel's remark about Dixie's "great idea" about breaking a telephone to order a new one, well, that doesn't get explained, either.

What does go somewhere is Cap's irrational paranoia about Chief McConnike. He thinks McConnike is "out to get him" somehow, someway, but nobody can figure out why he believes it.

Next rescue: Daisy Mae Yokum, looking young and fetching in her "hot pants" and red/white gingham checked shirt, accidentally *nails* her sugar-daddy husband (heh) in the chest. When Roy and Johnny get there, they're taken aback by the lack of blood (apparently only a third of a ketchup packet) until Roy carefully cuts the man's shirt away and they find out (somehow) that the nail hit the dude's pacemaker. Other than the wife saying "he has a pacemaker," I don't know how they figured out he had one. (And don't you think that's the kind of thing the paramedics would need to know, like, up front?) In any case, Daisy Mae is a concerned wife, although I think Dixie was a bit surprised to learn that she *is* his wife. Nurse McCall is even more surprised (among other things) when Daisy Mae says of her husband, "He's almost like a father to me." Ummm, okay. Yeah, nothing weird about *that*. (eyeroll) By the way, when Joe Early's at the base station talking to the guys at the scene, this is one of those times when I get the impression that Bobby Troup is reading off a TelePrompter, or cue cards just out of camera range or something.

Back at the station, Captain Stanley is still stressing about McConnike, who's due to stop in at 51's anytime. He has the guys going crazy trying to make the place perfect, but when McConnike does show up (and we get another Keystone Kops routine with the guys frantically running around, trying to find their hats), all McConnike does is introduce himself and meet everyone and remind Cap about some drill coming up on Friday. The FFs are all commenting that the Chief seems like a nice guy, and when Cap comes up and says something, Johnny gets startled and jumps.

Fast forward to Friday and the drill, which is held at a movie studio back lot. Everyone has a job to do and Cap's standing with the Chief, ready to observe. Next thing you know, a charged hose bursts and water explodes everywhere, mainly on Chet, Cap and the Chief. Cap apologizes profusely and is somewhat taken aback when McConnike shrugs off the accident, saying, "It can happen to anyone." Somehow, Cap takes this even less well than he would a tongue-lashing.

Next scene is at the station, with Cap sulking and Johnny making some stew recipe he got out of a magazine. (Who knew Penthouse included recipes??) But before anyone can try out the dish, a call comes in and off they go. This is the rescue at the ice-skating rink, which is *not* one of my favorites. Too silly. And it has that stupid clown music. Ah well, we can't pick and choose the calls the guys get. The best part is the very last scene of that rescue, when Cap is watching the craziness and just kind of gestures with his hand as if to say "Bah! Forget it!"

May Fair

Once again we see the station's dayroom (really, there's an awful lot at the station in this ep) where Cap is trying to memorize everything that was ever written about firefighting, apparently. To impress the Chief, don'tchaknow. The alarm goes off for a vehicle accident: a car has run off an overpass and into the trailer of a truck that's carrying something deadly and lethal. (Maybe if the car had been going just a little slower it would have landed in a semi carrying throw pillows or cute stuffed animals. Ya think??) But I like this rescue, even with the predictability of the hazardous material. The truck driver looks familiar, but I don't know who he is. In any case, there are complications in the truck that mean they can't simply hose down any leaking gasoline, so John and Roy have to wear air masks and hope nothing ignites before they can get the car's occupants out to safety. Oh, by the way, Director's Privilege also extends to using the Jaws to pry the truck's door open, apparently. Also, did I miss something? How did everyone know for a fact the truck was gonna blow? Once they got the second girl out, everyone hustled away, apparently aware that it was seconds away from igniting, but I don't think anyone actually said the words to that effect, did they?

Final scene: back at the station—again. The guys are trying to cheer Cap up by telling him what a great job Station 51 did at the accident scene, and all due to Cap's leadership. But he's still paranoid. And Chet.... He's still trying to get Henry into the doghouse, which is now on the couch. Except now Chet has resorted to actually putting a doggie bone in his mouth (ewww!!) and getting into the doghouse himself. Needless to say, the doghouse falls over with Chet inside it, but not before Henry, in all his 'male' glory, goes inside the house, tail a-waggin', and gets his bone back.

~ Why does this show credit characters in such a way that you can't tell who's who? The credits (and imdb) lists an actress as "Instructor." Instructor of what? I assume they mean the ice skater who talked to the guys at the rink (?), but I didn't know she was an instructor. And other characters in this ep are mostly nameless, so there's no way to tell who plays any particular one. Grrrrr, it's so annoying.

~ Upon arriving at the accident scene, it looks like Stoker was about to rear-end the squad with the engine, as he was approaching it at a fair clip; but at the last second he pulls around the squad.

~ The guys should chip in and buy a GoPro camera to put on Henry. Then they can finally find out what that hound does all day, not to mention find out how he eats and 'does his business.'

* * *

> At the car/semi accident scene, I wondered why they didn't use cervical collars or backboards on those victims. If they didn't have a spinal injury before they removed them from the car, they certainly did afterwards....During the gas station story, The Book says that Mike Stoker actually had his eye brows and eye lashes singed.

Yikes! Did they explain why/how he got singed?

And good point about the cervical collars. Roy had a time getting the one girl out of the vehicle-inside-the-trailer. Of course, half the time when they do use cervical collars, they flop the victim's head around so much in order to get the collar on, it probably causes as much injury as it prevents.

* * *

Yeah, I don't know if this episode is particularly bad, or if it occurs regularly, since I don't always check imdb for each one, but Insanity Epidemic really was a bad one as far as crediting the actors/characters. I think the lady with the older husband did have a name (Foster, maybe?) but half the people listed in the credits, I have no idea who they were. The writers should either be sure a character is listed by name, or not name the character at all, and credit them as "blond ice skater, or "shrew at gas station," or "jerk-face husband," etc.

6.15 Breakdown

~ The call-out for the first rescue gives us a fine example of Sam saying "Warshington."

~ Charlie asked if they were going to give an IV to the gas line and "debrillitate" the battery. I guess he was mangling the word defibrillate, but I had to put the captions on to understand what he was *trying* to say.

~ At the weaver's house—er, shack... um, abode? after Johnny looks at the tapestry-slash-blanket, Roy points to something and says, "this is nice." I went, "Huh??" It looked like a giant macrame owl. Not exactly high art, imho. (But I confess I don't have any expert knowledge of crafts.)

~ Anyone ever notice Roy when he's checking a victim's pupils? He doesn't even lean over the victim half the time. Johnny will lean directly over the victim and moves in pretty close to check the eyes, but Roy doesn't display that much energy.

~ At the water park for the final rescue, usually Roy and Johnny are with Cap when they arrive at a scene and "someone" is explaining what happened. But this time they were standing off to the side, by the squad. That just seemed odd to me.

~ The height of that spire was terrifying. I think it was mentioned 240 feet? Yikes. Does The Book mention how that was filmed? Couldn't have been a chopper, or there would have been a killer downdraft or whatever it's called. So I wonder how it was filmed?

~ In the previous discussion of this ep, we discussed the bizarre musical score during the rescue scene. Sounded more appropriate for a love story than an action sequence. And then, once they get the victim down to safety, *that's* when the score gets more dramatic. Go figure!

~ I think it was pretty obvious this time that it was not our fave actors, Randy and Kevin, up there on that spire. Actually, the illusion worked pretty well until they were ready to lower the victim down and the camera moved in closer. Not only did we not see either face clearly (and of course we know the rule of thumb), but when the camera moved in, it became obvious that "Johnny" somehow packed on a good 20 pounds between the station and the water park.

~ This being the case, I'll say again what I've said before (but can't remember where or how long ago): when stunt doubles are used, they do a good job of having Randy and Kevin dubbing in dialogue. It doesn't sound spliced in, as if it was recorded in a nice sterile studio, and it does match what we see. For example, if "Roy" reaches for a line, we hear Kevin say "let me grab the line; OK, I'm ready now," or something like that.

~ Oh, and the obligatory "Johnny eating" scene. Twice. I think the second one was ice cream. He seemed to be polishing the spoons at the same time, though; I didn't quite get that.

~ ~ ~

The reason for this episode's title is pretty evident, as the squad tends to quit on John and Roy at very inopportune moments while they're on runs. I won't go into the mechanics (physics? logic?) of the fact that some rogue part only affects the electrical system at certain moments and the connection gets "broken" when the squad door slams. Suffice it to say that that's the story, and we're sticking to it. If nothing else, it introduces us to Charlie, the LACoFD mechanic, he of the hard nose and Brooklyn accent. After he finds a medical bandage on some hose or other under the hood (instead of electrical tape, which the paramedics *should* actually have in their arsenal) it's funny to hear him say "If it wasn't for me, these guys would probably give an IV to the gas line and debrillitate the battery." I assume the mispronunciation is intentional, although Kevin looks like he's trying not to smile at it. (Note: on Netflix, the closed-captioning gives the correct word, defibrillate).

Once the boys fix the squad—or think they do—Cap sends them out on a call about overgrown weeds. They end up at a little farmhouse/shack that apparently has no running water or electricity, and a yard full of various livestock. Good times! The guy who lives there is Gerald, who, along with his wife Jane, is living the simple life long before Paris Hilton ever thought of it. Jane is sick with bronchitis and Gerald is weaving and pumping water, tending to his wife, etc. Roy admires an ugly macrame owl (I *think* it was an owl) and Johnny points to something else and says, "That would look great on the wall over my TV." Umm, what TV, Johnny? I thought you gave yours to the station? Anyway, when the guys see how sick Jane is (coughing, hacking, etc.), they offer to help her, but Gerald thinks he can handle it. No sooner do they get back to the squad, though, when Gerald runs out to flag them down. "She's coughing up blood. That's bad, right??" Yeah, Gerald, coughing up blood is definitely not a good thing. So the guys end up treating Jane anyway and of course she has to go to Rampart. Turns out Jane's cold-turned-bronchitis is actually bronchitis-turned-pneumonia-turned-anthrax. And, worse, her mother's in town. (Another dysfunctional relationship. Wasn't too long ago we had Rab and his superstitious wife who had parental problems. And before that wasn't there the girl who was pregnant and her father shot her husband, not knowing they'd gotten married? Not to mention Nail-Gun Nelly, who apparently married her father. As we've remarked before, this show just doesn't know how to write healthy, normal relationships.)

Moving along....

More stuff with Charlie at the station, as he gives the squad a thorough once-over. His veiled accusations of a practical joke rile the paramedics, especially mild-mannered Roy, who's understandably exasperated at Charlie's doubt. "There are two other paramedics who drive that squad," he reminds Charlie. Really, Roy? Only two? I realize he probably meant one driver for each of the other shifts, but still, he should have said *four* paramedics, as maybe the other guys actually take turns. Anyway, relief ensues when Charlie finally finds the problem and, his criticism of Cap's coffee notwithstanding, everyone's happy and satisfied. Cap, Johnny, and Roy walk the mechanic out of the station, via the Mystery Door which we discussed in some detail a year or so ago.

This is where the final call comes in, when the station is dispatched to Oceanland Park to rescue a guy trapped in the most inconvenient place imaginable. I think I mentioned this before, but it did strike me again: usually R and J join the Captain when they arrive on scene and listen to what the person there has to say. But this time they were standing apart, which seems odd to me. In any case, they have to ride up to the top of the tower and spire to rescue the workman. It's a relatively routine rescue, except for the unusual location. And except for the crazy musical score that doesn't fit the scene AT. ALL. It's more suited to a 1970s family drama or love scene than a dangerous and exciting action show. By the way, I wonder how they filmed that? We don't see any rotor downdraft or shadows anywhere. At least, I don't think we do;

May Fair

I assume we would have noticed shadows if there were any. In any case, when the firefighters leave that top level and climbed back down to join the others, Chet goes last, and he leaves the hatch open. Also, when he's on the phone with Rampart, Johnny tells Dixie that the victim has a "possible broken right femur," and to stand by for vitals. Um, Johnny, doesn't it strike you as odd that someone who "only" has a broken leg is unconscious? Wouldn't his lack of consciousness be worth mentioning to the hospital, because maybe, just maybe, there's something else going on? Eventually, though, they get the victim down and rejoin Stoker, who's been waiting in the engine and catching up on his Penthouse Forum reading.

After the ambulance leaves, Cap asks Johnny how the squad has been since Charlie gave it his magic treatment and Johnny says "fine." "Good," says Cap, "because I don't want to talk to Charlie again." And that's the cue for Mike to say "Uh, Cap...." Yikes! Poor Cap—he does his crucifixion impersonation, asking the Big Man Upstairs, "why me???"

This 'n' That

~ Speaking of pronunciation of words, we get *two* examples of dispatcher Sam saying Warshington.

~ For some reason, with the woman who has anthrax, I kept wanting to hear the husband say "Jane! Stop this crazy thing!!"

~ Only two rescues in this whole episode: Anthrax Wife and Oceanland Oscar. All the rest of the ep is drama about Jane and Gerald, or the Mystery of the Stalling Squad.

~ Brackett's got some funky brass wall sculpture in his office. At least, I *think* it's new; I don't recall seeing it before.

~ I assume Johnny was eating vanilla ice cream in that scene in the dayroom. Either that or it was a big ol' bowl of mashed potatoes.

~ A previous episode had the guys at Oceanside Park. This one is Oceanland Park.

* * *

Good point about the imported wool. I was under the impression that Gerald, aka "Mr. Anti-Establishment," *did* shear his own sheep and make his own wool.

And yeah, Cap can say a lot of things about Roy and (especially) Johnny being goofy and playing tricks, but there's *no friggin' way* they'd endanger a victim or mess around on a call just to play a trick. *Ever.* Especially since they didn't want to call Charlie to begin with. (I always think of Charley with an -ey as being the female version, and Charlie with an -ie as the male version. No idea why.)

I echo the RIP for Richard Bakalyan, who died in early 2015.

6.16 Family Ties

~ So Chet misplaced his badge. How does that happen? It's supposed to stay attached to the shirt you're wearing, and you change it when you change shirts. I wonder if they can get two badges, or if there is only one assigned at a time per person?

~ Funny, the conversation about "mother-in-laws." Sounded odd each time someone said it, which was about five or six. Later on, Johnny got it right: mothers-in-law.

~ I think I mentioned this last time, but I thought Roy's hair looked great. "Swept to the side" is a good look on him.

~ I had to laugh when Early told Brackett, "You always get the fun part of playing doctor." Really, Joe? You're saying that

May Fair

Kel likes to "play doctor"? Better be careful who hears that or he might be brought up on charges.

~ Am I the only one who gets the feeling there might have been a scene or two we didn't see? The dad injured in the car crash made a point of telling his daughter "Stay in school, become a doctor." And then when Early asks if she's a doctor she kind of pauses dramatically and then says "I'm in medical school." Maybe there was going to be a storyline that she'd wanted to quit med school, but this accident and the dedication and care of the doctors (blah blah blah) inspired her to stay on or something. I dunno, it just seemed like there was a piece missing.

~ The Acapulco Challenge... Brackett and Early each insist the other should attend the conference in Mexico. Early has fond memories of the food there, and Brackett remembers the great tennis and getting a tan. And I'm so glad Brackett told Joe he could play tennis anywhere, because playing tennis should not be the major deciding factor for going to Acapulco, since LA has great courts too. And if I'm not mistaken, the same sun shines in LA as in Mexico.

~ The fire in the patient room at Rampart... didn't the woman have a call button next to her bed? Especially if she has to wear a mask, I'd think the call button would be made pointedly available. Also, Roy got the fire extinguisher, but it shot out a stream of ...water? or something else that looked like water? Anyway, it sprayed like a weak garden hose. If it was water it wasn't a big stream, so not sure how helpful that would be in a lot of situations. I wonder if there was a reason Rampart didn't have a CO_2 extinguisher; I don't believe there's any reason why they couldn't, I think hospitals do use them.

~ And where was Johnny during that whole situation? Roy had already been looking for him before the fire, so it was a little odd that Johnny was MIA for so long. At least he had the handy-talkie so he could rush back and get Roy if they got a call.

~ I like the final rescue but there are a couple of odd or interesting things. I think last time this was on we discussed the illogic of bringing the victims out through the attic window rather than sending Roy and Johnny up there to carry them out through the house. Later, when Chet got blown into the tree, I think Cap says "babe," again. And earlier, when the first victim was brought down by the firefighter, the scene was a long shot, no close-ups, but in the audio we hear Johnny address the guy who was carrying her as "Fireman." Obviously Randy didn't know this guy from Adam, but it did make me wonder how one FF addresses another FF he doesn't know. I guess "fireman" is about as good a way as any, though.

~ Also, after Chet gets out of the tree, they walk him over to the paramedics, but both J and R are busy with the other victims, so Chet just sits on the curb. But a moment later when we see the huge hole in the attic, there's good ol' Chester B, up in the thick of things, back at work. Guess you really can't keep a good firefighter down for long.

* * *

> AND, did anyone see the girl's hand resting on Johnny's leg and him removing it and laying it on the ground? I thought that was hilarious. If I were her, my hand would have been there too.

Ha, I didn't notice that, so I just went back and rewatched that scene. Too funny!!! It looked like he rested her hand on his leg so he could take her pulse, but when he was done, she definitely moved her hand up. Can't say I blame her, either, can you??

May Fair

Also, in rewatching that scene, I did see Cap in the background sort of checking out Chet out to make sure he was OK. I'm embarrassed to say I *totally* missed that the first time around, and wondered why Chet had gone back to work without either Roy or Johnny looking at him.

~ ~ ~

I like this episode. It has good rescues and no extreme silliness. The underlying station storyline (Roy's mother-in-law coming to visit) isn't annoying, thank heavens, and the Rampart storyline (who's going to attend the conference in Mexico) is not a heavy-handed patient-related melodrama.

Scene opens at the station: Chet's looking everywhere for his badge (and he practically ignored Cap, which he *never* does) and Roy's on the phone with his wife. (By the way, remember that funky white phone we see Roy using back in Election? That's gone and we now have a standard black-and-silver pay-phone.) And of course whatever conversation is taking place between the DeSotos, Roy's not coming out on the winning end of it. After hanging up, Roy confesses that he has a problem: his mother-in-law is set to fly in for a visit, and he's not looking forward to it. Cue up every mother-in-law joke or stereotype you can think of, and I bet the writers tried to cram it in this episode. But Cap knows the tune Roy's playing: "I'll spot you my mother-in-law against your mother-in-law, and five points." Too funny!

First alarm is for a traffic accident, with a car that rear-ended a truck carrying all sorts of wire or whatever the heck that stuff is. The adult daughter is more or less fine, but her dad's hurt and his door is stuck. Roy takes care of the girl, which is simple enough, and Johnny deals with the dad, who's getting agitated. No sooner do daughter and Johnny get him calmed down when Cap comes over with the prybar and starts pounding on the car door. Uh, Cap, don'tcha think it might be wise to give the nervous and excitable victim a little warning before banging around with his car door? Also, again the paramedics are very 'kind' when it comes to a victim's age. The man is 45?? Ummm.... okay. Maybe that's not fair of me, though, to judge how people looked *then* based on how people look *now*. In any case, I like this rescue.

Back at the station, Johnny is inexplicably looking at mail (Really? Firefighters get mail at the station??) while Roy is inexplicably making a list of some sort. And of course Chet is still looking for his badge... in the same places he looked in the first scene, no less. Chet asks what's wrong with Roy and Johnny tells him (much to Roy's irritation), and thus ensues a conversation in which the incorrect term "mother-in-laws" is used not once, not twice, not even three times, but *five times*. Later on, though, Johnny does get it right (mothers-in-law).

At Rampart, this is where the Brackett-Early Conference Conundrum takes root. Only one person can go to the Acapulco conference, apparently, and both Joe and Kel insist on being noble and letting the other one go. And each also refuses the honor and insists the *other one* attend. After a little bit of male stubbornness, Dixie manages to solve the issue, as usual. And it doesn't involve even *one* cup of coffee!!

By the way, the scene in which this issue is finally hashed out and solved is funny: Brackett is in his office, standing at the bookcase, when Early walks in, "tells" Kel to sit down—in a guest chair—and Early himself sits at Brackett's desk. Not only that, but he proceeds to put his feet up on the desk. Then, when Dixie knocks at the door, it's Joe who says "Come in." Like he owns the place! Kel just gives him a look.

Speaking of Rampart, a woman brings her father in to Emergency; dude looks like he was the inspiration for ZZTop's famous facial hair. This is a cute scene, and of course it's Joe Early who treats the man (he always gets the unusual ones). But the best part is when Dixie grabs the man's britches and says "You'll get your pants back when you do as you're told." Ha, too funny! In any case, it turns out that the man has some form of lead poisoning, from either his job, or from Sister Duncan's miracle "compound." Yes, this does come across as a bit of a PSA, which makes me wonder how often people in the mid-'70s drank random "elixirs" that were sold to them on street corners by complete strangers. Hmmmm….

Next comes a rescue at Rampart. A candy striper has just finished giving a woman an alcohol rubdown (I kinda doubt that's in a candy striper's job description, by the way) and through an accidental set of circumstances, a small electrical fire begins. The panicked woman tears off her respirator and tries to unhook herself from everything so she can escape, but apparently can't breathe without the respirator (duh!) and quickly passes out. Luckily an alarm is set off at the base station (but, oddly, not those funny lights we see in every episode, and which have never been explained) and Morton goes to check out the alarm. As soon as he sees what's up, he yells for Roy and the two of them proceed to deal with the emergency. Mike wheels the patient bed out into the hallway while Roy grabs a fire extinguisher and goes to work on the fire, tearing down the curtain that's aflame and watering it thoroughly. Back in the hallway, Mike and a nurse are working on the patient, joined by Brackett and another nurse, and when he's finished in the patient room, Roy does what he can, as well. It's only when all the drama is over and the smoke has cleared does our friend Gage wander over and say "Hey, guys, what's up?" Uh, Johnny, first of all, did you not hear the alarm and announcement for "Code Red, Emergency"?? Secondly, where were you that you *didn't??*

Next, cue up the last rescue, which features a kid—who is assuredly not the class valedictorian—testing a rocket in his attic. Younger sister protests mildly, but Baron Von Stupid insists that he knows what he's doing and lights up said. Needless to say, we do *not* have liftoff; what we *do* have is a small explosion and resulting fire. I like this rescue, it's another good one, and again Cap gets to issue orders to the other engines that are called out. Couple things I thought were odd, though. For one thing, when Chet went up to ventilate the attic, wasn't he worried about flashover or whatever happens when they open a door (or, in this case, a window) and let a rush of air in to where the fire is? Secondly, why didn't Cap just send the PMs up to the attic from inside the house? Would have been much easier. And thirdly (or maybe this is secondly-2, since it's related to the prior item), shouldn't Chet and Marco have been wearing air masks when going into a room that had, you know, an actual fire in it? You'd think, wouldn't ya?? (Oddly, Roy and Johnny join the group at the side of the house, and they're wearing air masks, yet the two guys who are actually inside the burning building... aren't. Go figure.)

On the plus side, we always wonder "why is it always the paramedics?" and this time it's actually two of the other guys who do the rescuing. (Yay!) Chet hands the girl out to another FF (a real one), and Marco takes the second one down the ladder by himself. Once the victims are on the ground, Chet has just started down the ladder himself when the attic blows, sending the ladder falling backward. Luckily it puts Chet into a nearby tree, and he's not hurt badly, but it does lead to a cute/funny exchange: As Cap helps Chet down to the ground, he asks if Chet's all right. "Oh yeah," Kelly replies, "it was a hell of a ride, though." To which Cap says "It really was."

Also, on at least two separate occasions in this rescue, we hear FF address another FF as "Fireman." First Marco yells it out the window, to call one of the FFs up the ladder to take the victim. Then Johnny says it to one of the "real" firemen at the scene as well. (Just occurred to me: both Marco and Johnny say it, and I *think* it's to the same guy, the same FF from 116s who carried the girl down the ladder. Hmmm.) Additionally, twice Johnny called the girl "Hon." I know he was trying to comfort her, and the times were different then, but still, it seems a little... questionable, for him to address a young woman that way.

Lastly, final scene at the station. Roy is frantic because he's running late to pick up his mother-in-law, and is running around with his deep-V t-shirt on—for which we are deep-V appreciative. Suddenly Joanne calls and while he's trying to apologize for being late, she tells him that her mother is no longer coming to visit. Yay! Reprieve! Since his replacement is already at the station, Roy decides to take his wife out on the town. As he's walking out, Chet walks in, and he's relieved as well. He finally found his badge. Trouble is, nobody's interested in listening. Poor Chet!

Quick bits:

~ Johnny's not in all the station scenes. He's in the one with the mail, and also—very briefly—in one other one, but other than that... he's not. Combine this with the fact that Johnny wasn't at the Rampart 'rescue,' and the fact that Roy and Johnny didn't perform the rescue at the house fire.... Hmmmm.

~ At Rampart, we hear a page for "Dr. Shapiro, Emergency area," but no idea who Dr. Shapiro is, or if we ever see him in the emergency department.

~ I know we mentioned it last time, but I'm still intrigued by the paper that falls out of the squad when Roy pulls out his turnout coat. Johnny picks it up and puts it back. In my imagination it's a page or two of script that got put into the squad for some reason.

~ After Chet got blown off the ladder, Cap checked him out and then Chester B went right back up there, back to the attic. Good man, Kelly!

6.17 Bottom Line

Yeah, Cap's remark about the baseball bat [for the naggy wife] made me wince a little. (Especially considering what's been going on with the NFL. Yikes!) And I particularly wondered why the engine was called out on the call with the bad back. No rhyme or reason to the calls, I guess. (And at the other scene, with the hyperventilating man with the shrew of a wife, Morton actually prescribed the 5mg diazepam first, and, after Johnny questioned it, *then* he added the D5W.)

Did anyone notice? It seemed as if everyone was pronouncing it *diazepan*, instead of *diazepam*.

Funny how they hadn't had the least whisper of an issue with Morton for the past two or three seasons, but suddenly he's a "problem." Go figure! (In other words, nothing but a plot device.)

> I really was wondering why Stanley continued CPR on the victim once he was in sinus rhythm.

Hmm, I didn't notice that the first time I watched, but yep, you're right. And that's a no-no. What I *did* notice was that Roy yelled "clear!" before Johnny even started the count-up to the 400 watt-seconds. So all in all, I think the scene was filmed a little sloppily all around.

Anyone notice the horrible, inappropriate music was back? I think it was during the back-patient scene.

May Fair

Johnny got to swear again. "He damn near shot me with this thing." Where was the other officer during this little set-to, I'd like to know? And I know Roy felt bad about saying Vince was "OK," but really, what could he have done? Taken pulse and BP... what would that have told him? Even if he felt a knot on Vince's head, he (or anyone else) couldn't have predicted what would happen. Maybe they should have mentioned a Sheriff's department policy—that any officer involved in an accident should have his weapon removed, just as a precaution.

I do think Rampart has some questions to answer. The back-pain guy was brought in via ambulance—with paramedics as escort—and then what happened? He lay in the hallway for a couple of hours. Did his IV run out? Did anyone check on him periodically? If Morton thought he was important enough to warrant "constant supervision," maybe he should've "constantly supervised" and attended to the guy sooner. And the little baseball player—did the admitting nurse really do anything wrong? (Other than stick the parental permission slip into some random folder, that is.) People have to wait in Rampart's Emergency waiting room all the time. Unless, apparently, they come in yelling, in which case they get whisked to a treatment room right away. But even if the nurse had looked at the boy closely, she couldn't have known how badly the kid was hurt. He didn't even have any symptoms when he first got there.

Anyway, this episode pretty much points out (with a few awkward twists and manufactured issues) that we can't always tell how serious an injury is right away. I guess that's the "bottom line."

Two other things...

~ I think I mentioned not long ago how Johnny and Roy always call out to Cap when a family member is being bothersome. That didn't work with that one lady today, unfortunately (the shrewish wife). Luckily Vince stepped in and took the lady off their hands. And I think she knew it, too.

~ I know someone mentioned this last time around, but I do hope Roy or someone did something with Vince's gun after Johnny put it on top of the squad. Can you imagine that flying off the squad as it speeds down the street?? Another detail that would have been good (and easy) to deal with properly.

~ ~ ~

Another good episode. Not surprisingly, it's an Issues episode; those tend to appeal to me more than the 'gimmicky' ones. Although I have to admit, some of these Issues episodes (depending on the Issue Du Jour) tend to be alike, with Johnny and Roy grousing to each other and eventually working their way up to Righteous Indignation. But I guess that's the nature of the beast. In any case, I like this episode, with one caveat, which will be mentioned shortly.

Action starts at the station, and jumps right into the Issue of the Day: Morton ordering IVs on non-critical victims who almost certainly have nothing seriously wrong with them. Morton's reasoning is "better safe than sorry." Roy and Johnny's reasoning is "if we have to set up and IV and follow-up to the hospital with a non-critical case, we're not available for potentially serious, time-critical victims who *do* need our help."

First call for our guys illustrates this point. Station 51 is called out for a "back injury." (Really? The engine, too?) The victim in question has severe back pain, but Roy and Johnny discover the man's vitals are normal, meaning nothing 'seems' to be truly wrong with him. They wonder whether he's faking... although, to be honest, I wouldn't necessarily have thought that. There's a big difference between having a sharp pain that doesn't end up being serious, and simply faking it. In any case, the paramedics are satisfied to pack the man off in an ambulance and let Rampart figure it out. And that's exactly what's about to happen, until.... (dun-dun-*dun*) Morton gets involved. He figuratively shrugs and says, "what the heck, let's start an IV on the guy," thereby committing the paramedics to spend an extra 30 minutes or so out of service. Needless to say, our guys are not thrilled with this, and the matter is far from over.

At Rampart, before that ambulance arrives, a man stumbles in, delirious with pain and saying his arm is on fire. He's quickly rushed into a treatment room (see? no waiting!) and Brackett explains he's suffering from white phosphorous burns. Now we get a mini-PSA about white phosphorous, effectively conveying the "Kids, don't try this at home!" message.

We now see the ambulance arrive with Backache Billy, escorted by Johnny and Roy. Apparently business at Rampart has "ramped up," so Dixie intercepts the group and tells the ambulance guys to "leave him outside Room 2 until something opens up." Which is ridiculous on the face of it; an ambulance ride with lights and siren, not to mention the accompaniment of a paramedic along the way, and the guy's just gonna be left in a hallway? Yeah, some "emergency!" If his case was important enough to warrant the precautions Morton prescribed, then he should be important enough for a doctor to check on him right away. Anyway, even though I understand Johnny's frustration with the situation, I do like that Dixie more or less told him "talk to the hand," and shut him down there in the hallway. I think Johnny's query of "what is (Morton's) problem?" was a little uncalled for, and I think he should know that carping to Dixie isn't going to do anything to solve the situation. Dixie knows this and rightly suggests they bring their concern to Brackett. Which they do, as the dapper doctor happens to arrive at the base station at that very moment. Brackett more or less tells them the same thing that

Dixie did: Morton's the doctor and his word goes. Obviously, Roy and Johnny are less than satisfied.

Meanwhile, down at the other end of the hall, a baseball coach brings in his young player, who was hit by a pitch. The coach has a piece of paper from the boy's parents authorizing him to act on their behalf if something should happen, and he gives it to the admission nurse, who tucks it into a random folder and says of the boy, "he doesn't look too badly injured; just have a seat and wait." Yeah, it does sound callous, but honestly, I don't see that the nurse really did anything differently than any other nurse on this show. She mentions that cases are triaged as they come in, so that would lead me to believe that someone else must have looked at the boy (or *should* have looked at him) to gauge his condition.

Next call is for a "man down." Again, I have to wonder why the engine is called out with the squad, although as things turn out, it's a good thing it is. The "man down" is a hen-pecked husband living with yet another version of the shrewy wife. Just looking at the poor man, a casual observer could tell he probably just needs to keep a paper bag on hand to breathe into (and, as Cap says, a baseball bat—whoops, did I say that out loud?). And yeah, as soon as Roy gives the guy a bag, he starts to breathe more easily and they're able to get vitals on him. Johnny calls it in to Rampart and guess who takes the call? Yeah, you guessed it: Morton. And yes, he prescribes an IV, much to Johnny's disgust. (Note: both Johnny and Morton pronounce the word *diazepan* instead of *diazepam*. A total of three times between them. They're supposed to be the professionals, no??)

However, in an ironic twist of fate, that "unnecessary" IV may indeed have saved a life. Rather than just loading the hapless husband immediately into the ambulance, the paramedics have to take the time to set up the IV on him. By the time they accomplish this and are finally ready to take him to Rampart,

May Fair

there's a scream for help from next door, and it's discovered that a man has passed out and about to drown. This is where Chet and Cap shine, and together they manage to get the man out of the hot tub (I guess that's what it was?), and the paramedics do their thing once again... this time on a *real* emergency case. Roy calls in and asks permission to send Hapless Husband in the ambulance without accompaniment so they can stay behind with the drowning man. Brackett vetoes this and says "hold the ambulance to take both victims." Yay, the voice of reason and sanity! Or two of them, I guess. So the paramedics treat drowning dude, including having to defib him. (Is that safe to do on someone who's wet? Although I guess the point of defibbing is to shock/electrocute them anyway, isn't it?) Long story short, in effect, that five minutes it took for the guys to establish Hapless Hubby's IV meant they were nearby and 'available' to save Drowning Drinker. Irony, thy name is Emergency!

In any case, when they get to Rampart, Roy and John run into Backache Billy. Almost literally run into him, as the poor man is still lying on a gurney in the hallway. (Shameful!) Some emergency, huh?? If his case was that important and dicey, Morton should have taken care of it by now. Which is exactly what the guys tell Mighty Morton just a few seconds later. Not surprisingly, neither side budges in their opinions.

Back to baseball boy... he more or less passes out in the waiting room and of course Dixie has him whisked into a treatment room; I guess that's the standard of treatment at Rampart: you either have to be brought in by ambulance or fall over onto the floor in order to be seen right away by a doctor. Anyway, the kid's "endocranial pressure is building" and he needs surgery (stat!) to relieve it. Sadly, the surgery isn't successful and the boy dies on the table; Brackett goes on a righteous rampage, as if that's going to do any good or be of help to anyone.

Watching EMERGENCY! Seasons 4-6

In the hallway, the paramedics and everyone's favorite resident are getting into it, in a very public way (and with a cop and some other dude watching, by the way). Brackett swoops in and ushers them all into his office where the debate continues. *Playing it safe because 'you never know'* vs. *common sense and don't tie up the resources.* Bottom line is... there's no definite bottom line. The scene plays out as if Brackett agrees with the paramedics, but A) he doesn't control the policy, and B) nothing was actually agreed upon as far as a change of tactics. So I gotta say that while this Serious Issue was nicely laid out for those of us at home, there was no actual solution and it didn't really seem to affect anything long-term. (And the problem with Morton that has been so serious and egregious in this episode disappears after this, never to be heard of again.)

I do have to say, though, that I do have an additional concern. I think it was very unprofessional of Johnny to mention Dr. Morton by name and discuss their unhappiness with the issue—in front of victims, ambulance attendants, police officers, etc. Having a beef with the doctor—or with the policy—is one thing, and is certainly his right. Bringing that beef up in public in front of strangers who aren't involved... that's not cool, Gage. Not cool at all.

Anyhoo.... The final rescue. This is the one that gives me pause, and diminishes my enjoyment of this episode, albeit not by too much. So Deputy Vince was pursuing a couple of bad guys, bad guys swiped a parked car, fishtailed, crashed and rammed into Vince's cruiser, trapping him. One of the baddies is DOA and the other is seriously hurt. Vince seems to have suffered a bump on the head, split lip, etc., but after the FFs get him out, Roy gives him a once-over, and goes to help Johnny. Yeah, this is where the wheels fall off the wagon. Roy *did* drop the ball when it comes to Vince, but he's definitely not the only one. First off, I'm not sure what BP, pulse, respiration could have told him about Vince's condition (although checking his eyes might—might—have provided a clue). Anyway, Roy asked Chet to watch Vince. Cap, in his capacity of being 'in charge' at the scene, should have kept an eye on Vince, and most definitely the other cop dropped the ball, as the minute he realized that Vince had any type of injury (especially a head injury) he should have A) taken Vince's gun, and B) called in to his superiors, who would certainly have ordered Vince to the hospital for a complete check-up, and C) taken Vince's gun. Yeah, I know I already mentioned *taking Vince's gun,* but it's pretty much a no-brainer for law enforcement when an officer is injured that his weapon is surrendered, for everyone's safety. Also, I don't understand why Johnny didn't call for Cap (or the other cop) a little sooner when Vince aimed his gun at him. I guess that can sort of be chalked up to his being startled or not thinking clearly in a situation of extreme stress, but on the other hand, Johnny's a trained rescue man/fireman/paramedic; stress and danger are part of his daily routine. He should be better equipped than most to handle it.

Notes:

~ Henry eats chili?? From what I hear, basset hounds are odoriferous enough on their own, without Marco's spicy cooking added into the mix.

~ That final call is listed as "corner of Olive and Devonshire," but the street we see at the end of the episode is Ethel Ave.

~ Did anyone hear Roy honk the horn of the squad? It was right after they get called to the final rescue, as Johnny is responding "10-4." I thought it was kind of unusual.

* * *

Re Brackett feeling the arms and shoulders of Baseball Boy (Randy Sherwood)... I assumed that he was looking for bumps or other sensitive/sore areas that might indicate additional injuries.

> I noticed that Johnny was wearing a small button or pin on the right side of his shirt, a few inches over his name badge. (I had never seen that before, which doesn't necessarily mean it wasn't there). Later I saw that Roy had one, too, almost right on his name badge. Speaking of name badges, Officer Vince was wearing one with his real-life last name Howard on it.

I think this matter came up a while back (either in an old thread, or a thread that's gone, can't remember). The pins are pins from the paramedic program, which is why only paramedics have them. Usually it's right above the name badge, but yeah, Johnny's was affixed a little higher than usual in the scene in Brackett's office.

And yeah, funny that Vince got to use his 'own' name. Good for him!

6.18 Firehouse Quintet

I'll just come right out and say it—this isn't one of my fave episodes. In fact, it's probably in my bottom ten, if not five. But just because I don't care for it overall, doesn't mean there aren't parts of it that I like.

I like the first rescue, for example, at the generically-named International Industrial Corporation. (Yeah, what do they do, exactly? Build industries?) And incidentally, in the call-out, Sam called it Industrial International, rather than International Industrial. Either Sam's script was wrong, or the sign was; not that it really matters. Either way, it's a silly name.

May Fair

At least once, but maybe twice in that rescue, someone referred to Chet as Kelly. Which is fine, since that's his last name, but usually his own guys call him Chet rather than Kelly. After all, Marco is always Marco, and never Lopez. Also, it was cute that both Roy and Johnny (but Roy first) spoke ungrammatically. "I can't see nothin'." "I can't see nothin', either."

So yesterday (the previous episode), Morton was a pain in the paramedics' butts, but in this one, there was no problem, and they chatted with him like they've been friends forever. At least this time, when they called him about the theatre guy with the broken clavicle, he didn't order an IV. (Maybe he learned his lesson?)

And Dixie apparently works seven days a week, as she answered the biophone when B-shift called in to Rampart from the gym.

In the scene at the station when everyone's in the breakroom and Cap's going over basketball strategy, a few interesting things happen. For one thing, we hear the phone ring, and Mike says "I'll get it," and he disappears. Guess it's just one of those things that happen, like in real life, and it doesn't necessarily mean anything and we never see/hear anything more about it. The second thing is that Roy says, "It's been a quiet night, I hope it stays that way." Which is a dead giveaway that—bam!—the tones are gonna go off. And the third thing is, after the tones go off and we see the speaker and hear Sam's summons, everyone is leaving the day-room, and suddenly Roy's carrying the drug box. He hadn't been holding it earlier, it wasn't on the floor next to his chair... it hadn't been *anywhere* in sight, but suddenly he was just carrying it from the day-room, for no apparent reason. Go figure!!

The unnamed paramedic who took over from them at shift-change is listed as the ubiquitous Dwyer. Is he the only other paramedic at Station 51?? It looked like the days fluctuated from John and Roy's shift to Dwyer's shift. What about the third one??

I'm not gonna say much about the basketball game, as I think it was just plain silly. Not the least of which was the fact that the team was made up of a single six-man shift. That's crazy... IRL wouldn't it be the whole station on one team, with a max of 18 guys, so there would be an actual second string? Ah well, it's over now and I can move on.

* * *

> What annoyed me also with this game was the benchwarmer who sat with Chet. Why did they show so much of that guy?

Good question. I guess I assumed it was just to reiterate the fact that Chet had to stay on the bench—as the other guy says, "yeah, they won't let me play, either." Which is laughably funny, because he's a good six inches taller than Chet.

Anyway, I'm just glad they didn't have Johnny make some awful bet against the other team, like he did with the baseball game. I thought the basketball stuff was painful enough to watch as it was, without everyone being mad at Johnny.

~ ~ ~

I've already talked about my general dislike of this episode—of the running theme of it, that is—so I won't belabor it again. I will note, however, that this ep was written by Christian Nyby, he whose name might be more familiar as a director, as he directed a couple dozen episodes of E! Turns out he's written two episodes, this one and The Game, another one of my non-favorites, and one of the movies—and not what I would consider one of the 'better' ones, either ('better' being a relative term in this case; *very* relative). Christian, I love ya as a director but... well, 'nuff said.

Anyway, action opens at the station, in a scene without either John or Roy. Our beloved A-shift (I assume these guys are A-shift) somehow made it to the finals of the basketball league. Even though they apparently only played a total of five games. (Not gonna go into the idiocy of each shift being a separate team, as opposed to the whole station being one team.) So, anyway, there's the setup.

First call is to a fire at the imaginatively-named Industrial International Corporation. And it's worth noting that when the alarm sounds at the station, Roy and Johnny emerge from Cap's office. Maybe doing some of that invisible paperwork that we never see? Anyway, at the scene, we learn that the fire started in the cafeteria and (of course) there are people trapped. However... Cap is told that four people are trapped, yet I think I only saw three come out. Maybe the guy was counting that big slab of beef as a person? (Just kidding!) In any case I think on two occasions someone called Chet by his last name, Kelly. That doesn't usually happen on this show, not with Chet, anyway. In any case, after both Roy and Johnny make the non-grammatical pronouncement that they "can't see nothin'," they discover the missing people taking refuge in the freezer. No mention of the people being cold, although I imagine that the surrounding flames nicely offset the bone-chilling atmosphere of the freezer, and one guy is having heart issues. I'm a little surprised that they didn't use the 'fireman's carry' on the guy; instead, Roy and Johnny awkwardly carry the man out, one at his head, one at his feet. Later on, when they were patching him in for an EKG, I thought the man was wearing an odd, furry t-shirt, but it turns out his Carpet of Virility is apparently of the shag variety. (Yikes!)

At Rampart, the guys are trying to drum up a team against which they can practice before their playoff game. They're directed to Dr. Morton who played on an intern team at Rampart (and with whom there is now absolutely no residual 'attitude' from the previous episode concerning his annoying habit of ordering random—and often unnecessary—IVs) but unfortunately that avenue is a dead end so the A-shift team has to practice on its own. Which leads us back to the station where John and Roy are chatting with Mighty Morphin' Power Dwyer, who has apparently undergone a little plastic surgery since his earlier appearances on this show. (He's still the same LACoFD-approved "type," though, so it's not a jarring change.) Anyway, Dwyer must be partnered up with the Invisible Man, as we don't see anyone else with him as he conducts a start-of-shift review of the squad's supplies.

We see Johnny's Land Rover pull up to the basketball venue, and he parks behind the butt-ugly vehicle that apparently belongs to Chet. I wonder if it was Tim Donnelly's real vehicle? I admit I hope it wasn't. Anyway, I also admit I fast-forwarded through the basketball practice scenes—just not interested, and to tell the truth, I'm a little embarrassed for the guys when I see it. I have to wonder if they actually enjoyed filming this ep.

In any case, I started watching again when the cute blond gymnast screamed and her b.f. was down for the count, bringing the off-duty firefighters running. (Fun fact: the blond gymnast was played by Joanna Kerns, who at the time went by the name Joanne DeVarona. As in, sister of Olympic gold-medal swimmer Donna DeVarona. Cool, huh? Another fun fact: Joanne herself tried out for the 1968 Olympics as—you guessed it—a gymnast. [Thank you, imdb.]) Okay, getting back to the man who got injured.... John and Roy do the best they can with what's available, which isn't much, and no sooner does Cap run off to call for help than we hear the siren of the squad, and Dwyer and his partner (who turns out *not* to be invisible) arrive to take over. Poor Dwyer's partner: he has no dialogue, and nobody at Rampart is likely to refer to *him* as "one of the best who ever went through the program." In fact, he doesn't even merit a name, apparently.

Next scene is the next shift, as Cap is sketching plays on the blackboard in the dayroom as the guys watch. They're all sitting around, except for Stoker, who's standing, perhaps just waiting for the phone to ring so he can answer it. Which it does, and which *he* does. And Roy must have been practicing magic tricks as he apparently makes the drug box appear out of nowhere. Not there when he's listening to Cap, but when we see the guys troop out when the tones go off, there's the drug box, in Roy's hand. It's E!-magic!!

The call is to a movie studio, which must have been a long drive for the squad and engine, stationed as they are on a studio lot (*wink*). Both vehicles drive right in to the soundstage (or whatever it's called) and I have to laugh when Cap tells Mike, 'Stoker, why don't you stay here." What, as opposed to walking the 20 yards to where the other guys are going to stand? Anyway, since this is a 'height' rescue, not surprising that Johnny's the one to go up after the injured man, who's dangling precariously from a broken beam. I do wonder, though, why Cap doesn't at least try to find *something* they could put on the floor in case the man falls before Johnny reaches him. Not sure what that would be, but surely the studio has cushions or at least the ubiquitous empty cardboard boxes, which might at least help to a small degree. Meantime, Johnny's doing his Johnny thing and climbing up to the crossbeams there, talking to the victim as he does so, chattering away as he always does. I'm quite certain the audio of what we hear was dubbed in, as I'm sure the real conversation was a little less paramedic-y and a little more safety-related. In fact, as the two are being lowered to the ground, I'm pretty sure we hear Johnny say something and yet his mouth isn't moving. (Not positive of that, though, as I had to watch on a non-Netflix venue, so quality wasn't as good as I'm used to.) Also, as the two guys treat the vic, it's funny to see the goof of Johnny taking his respiration twice.

At Rampart, Morton (who seems to now be the guys' BFF) offers them some coffee, but Johnny reminds him that they're hoping to get a good night's sleep before the game. This hope goes out the window when they get a call right then and there, which does not bode well for their prospect of rest and relaxation. (Is it just me? The dispatch voice we hear over the HT didn't sound to me like Sam. But that could be poor audio from my non-Netflix viewing experience.) That call comes in at 19:45 (7:45pm), and unless there was another call after that, this is one very looooong call, as they don't get back to the station until after midnight. Then, no sooner do they lie down for a little shut-eye than the station gets called out for a tire fire, and of course they're gone all night. When they return, Dwyer is there again. So apparently, there *are* only two shifts at Station 51, and only three paramedics: Roy and Johnny are on one shift, and Dwyer is on the other... by himself.

I can't imagine how they could even begin to think they'd be able to sleep at the station. Yes, they know they're off duty, but I would think that instinct alone would cause them to jump up automatically when they hear the tones go off. Not sure how you can get any rest like that.

And that, dear friends, is pretty much where I quit watching. Oh, wait, I did come back to see the final (non-basketball) scene at the station. In this one, Roy's up to his magic tricks again—watch for the Disappearing Milk Glass he gives to Chet. He sets the glass down on the table near Chet's elbow, and it appears and disappears at will, depending on the camera angle. Maybe A-shift should forget basketball and get a show in Vegas.

6.19 The Boat

Or, "Another Station 51 Plan Goes Awry."

~ Roy and Johnny walk into the day-room and nobody's there. What the heck was Roy talking about, sitting on the couch and watching an air-hockey game? Was that a thing back then, watching air-hockey on TV? Or does air-hockey mean something else in 1977 LA than it does to everyone else??

~ Any word on when this ep was filmed? I noticed Roy's hair was funky again, after having looked good for quite a while. (And it looked good again when it get messed up in one scene.)

~ I think this might have come up before, but I'd think that the US Coast Guard would have its own emergency/rescue teams. Also, I think (in my opinion) they spent too much time showing the helicopter flying. I confess I fast-forwarded through some of it.

~ The heart-attack bookie. How'd they end up getting the address? Cap tells the guy on the phone "you're the one who called it in, how come you didn't have the address?" So I wonder how they found the place, since this was in the days before GPS and phone tracking, etc.

~ Speaking of that heart attack guy, there was another minor flub when Roy defibbed him the first time. Roy has the paddles on the guy, looking at his rhythm, and when they see they need to defib, Chet squirts the lubricating stuff. Roy holds the paddles on the guy's chest and says "Clear!", *then* realizes nobody pressed the button on the machine, so he has to do that with one hand while holding both paddles in the other. Kind of an "oops!" moment.

~ By the way, I noticed they actually made a point of closing the squad doors when they got to the guy's building. Which is kind of unusual for them... they usually leave them wide open. This time they would've made Brice proud.

~ Love when Cap says to Vince, "Maybe you can tell me what's going on in this squirrel room." Thought that was a hoot! On the debit side, I do think that Big Alvie's actions weren't believable.

~ I also like the explosion at Rampart. Can't believe the plumber guy survived, though. I think it would have been more believable if he'd bit the dust.

~ Speaking of Rampart... the guys were only there to pick up supplies; did they really park in the emergency entrance when they go 10-8 there? Heaven forbid other ambulances and squads bring in victims. Also, I wonder how the show managed to get access to the parking area of the real hospital (Harbor General) to bring in all those trucks and engines. They must have cordoned off the area and rerouted 'regular' traffic for filming.

~ Lastly, in some of the establishing shots at Rampart (in general, not just this episode), the camera starts by showing the parking lot and emergency entrance, then pans upward to the left, to the third or fourth floor. But when we see the scene, it's in a treatment room in the emergency department... on the ground floor.

~ ~ ~

I like this episode. It was written by Hannah Shearer, who wrote at least one other episode and also, apparently, a number of the movies. But I won't hold that against her since we're not talking about the movies (thank heavens!); I'll just repeat that I like this episode and leave it at that. There are some good rescues and no real inanity. The title story about the boat doesn't get too silly, although even if you haven't seen this episode numerous times (like many of us) it's not hard to figure out what's going to happen.

Note about the mechanic: in Breakdown, in which we first meet Charlie, his character is listed as Charley, with an –ey. But in The Boat, both the closed-captioning and the credits list his name as Charlie, with an –ie. Which is fine, I prefer the –ie, so that's what it's going to be.

Returning to the what's going on at the station, Roy is apparently telling Johnny a story about a game he was watching on TV, and he mentions air hockey. Now, either Kevin fudged the line and added "air" before the "hockey," or they show some really unusual games on TV in LA County. I know air hockey is fun and all, and was probably very popular at the time, but as far as I know, it was played mainly in bars, basements, and college dorms. Showing air hockey games on TV? That seems a bit much. In any case, it's just meaningless filler as the guys walk out behind the station and see what the *real* story is: the boat. And while I have no trouble believing that Charlie could build a machine that fills the "need for speed," I do have trouble believing that that's the kind of boat he would have built for his wife to enjoy. But my opinion on this is neither relevant nor important.

As the guys are admiring the boat the squad gets called out to join the Coast Guard for, ironically, a boat wreck with injuries. So off they go and we get an extended view of Roy and Johnny in transit, first in the squad and then in the Coast Guard chopper. (Ho-hum, try to stay awake.) The rescue of the erstwhile boaters is brief enough, thank heavens, and pretty straightforward: get on the ground, check to see if the injured vic can wait until he's in the chopper for treatment (he can), and get in the little basket to be hoisted back up. I'm glad the rescue isn't drawn out, but on the other hand, it *is* really quick. In fact, more time is spent showing us the helicopter ride to the scene than is spent on the actual rescue with the victims. Go figure! Oh, and did we all see Johnny as he was pulled up from the island with the female boater? The two of them are obviously facing each other as they're both huddled in the basket, and Johnny keeps his hands on the woman's knees. Then she briefly puts her hands on top of his. Hmmmm. Are all Gage Girls jealous yet?? Luckily the return flight doesn't seem so long as we hear the guys communicate with Rampart along the way. We don't see anything in the chopper, but we hear them and we see Joe Early at the base station. I was a little surprised, though, when they land on the helicopter landing pad, that the "ambulance" is one of those old hearse-style vehicles, like we used to see in the first season or two. Ugh, I thought we had long since moved past those. Maybe they're only used to transport patients who arrive via chopper, since the ride to the Emergency Department is only a hundred yards or so. Also thought it was interesting that R and J wear their helmets when they first get into the coast guard chopper, and then take them off. But when they arrive at the landing pad, they're wearing the helmets again. Guess it's a good way to keep up with them: you can't accidentally leave the helmet anywhere if it's on your head, right?

We don't see any more of Rampart (I'm guessing the guys had to hustle back to the copter for their ride back to the Coast Guard station) and next is a scene that we rarely see: the squad backing into the apparatus bay from the open back bay door. (And did you notice how far Roy backed the squad? Usually it looks as if the squad is parked toward the front of the bay, not far from the garage doors, but here he pulls almost all the way back. The engine is parked pretty far back, as well.) Anyway, we now get more of the boat story, including a cute Johnny-and-Roy prank of pulling the boat's tarp over Chet and leaving him "tarped" in. That leads immediately to another station scene, although I'm not sure when this one takes place in relation to the previous one. But Chet has his Big Idea for his shift-mates: pool their money, buy Charlie's boat, and rent it out on days when they can't use it. (Does that plan sound familiar?)

The set-up for the next rescue is a heavily-locked room and a man juggling multiple phones as he jots things down on the surface of his card table. Yeah, he's a bookie and we see that he's feeling bad and having pains. Finally he tells "Sidney" to call... someone. He never finishes the sentence, but apparently Sid takes that ball and runs with it and calls the fire department. *Bing-bang-boom,* five minutes later Engine and Squad 51 roll up to the building. Once again Cap tells Stoker to hang back with the engine (duh) but once inside he contacts Mike on the HT and asks for a prybar and an axe. But not before Johnny stupidly takes a run at the locked door with his shoulder. (And when he lands in a heap on the floor, nobody helps him up.) But Mike arrives with the equipment and gets the heavy work done, then Chet follows up with the axe and does the rest. Inside, with the vic, everyone gets busy with pitching in, including Cap playing receptionist with the table full of phones. Seriously, though, I'm not sure why he bothered trying to answer them all, and I'm glad that Vince finally just knocked all the phones off the hook. Meanwhile, the boys have defibbed the vic twice, and finally Bookie Bob is back in the land of the living. (Yeah, I know, we only know his last name, Clinton, but that messes up my alliteration, so I'm giving him the first name of Bob.) By the way, I love how Cap refers to the crazy goings-on in "this squirrel room." Now if he would only have used the word "twit" in the same sentence, it would be over-the-top Cap Coolness. Also funny when Alvie comes in, practically delivering himself into Vince's custody (although why he didn't immediately turn and leave—quickly—the minute he saw all the uniforms in the room is beyond me). So, this being an awful long paragraph, let's recap here: Stoker does some cool fireman stuff with forcible-entry tools, Chet swings an axe, the paramedics get the victim's heart restarted, and Vince gets to take credit for a big gambling bust. It's a win all around! Also, I like today's entry to the Brackett Tie Collection, so we can add that to the win-column as well.

Yo-yoing back to the station, the guys are trying to determine who gets dibs on using the boat on their first day off. For a change, Johnny is the lucky one... twice, first with cards and then with drawing numbers. After his win, he and Roy go to Rampart for supplies, and it's lucky that they do.

Dixie goes to check the lab for blood test status, since some county inspector is checking for a possible build-up of sodium azide. Great idea, huh? So off she goes, and out the paramedics go, and next thing you know the lab goes boom! Guess Morton won't be getting his blood test results anytime soon. Not to mention the tests that Brackett ordered for Bookie Bob. Eh, what the heck, it's not like they need those results because they're in the middle of surgery or any—oh, wait. Darn!

So Roy and Johnny call in the explosion as a still alarm and are first on the scene in the basement. They find Dixie and the lab guy and Johnny escorts them out as Roy gets the nearest fire hose and drags it to the burning lab so he can work his way inside. Incredibly (and I do mean incredibly, as in unbelievably) he finds the inspector guy—alive!—and pulls him out. I mean, he just slung that man over his shoulder like he was a sack of potatoes instead of a full-grown dead-weight man. Maybe that Carpet of Virility also gives Roy super strength. Anyway, the next scene always confuses me a little, as Johnny runs back down to the basement. Did he even see Roy come back up with the explosion victim? I don't know, we don't see them run across each other, and at first I thought maybe Johnny's looking for Roy—although really, he must have passed him on the stairs. In any case, Johnny doesn't seem surprised not to find Roy down there in the basement, and instead he simply picks up the hose Roy had gotten and starts fighting the fire, so obviously he *wasn't* looking for his partner.

Meanwhile, Dr. Morton has enlisted the help of Johnny's former fiancée Valerie—oops, I mean Nurse Michelle—to start evacuating all patients and personnel. And Engine 51 arrives and Cap takes charge of yet another scene as other engines pull in as well.

I do have to chuckle with incredulity at Roy barging in to "O.R. #2" where the doctors are doing surgery… in the middle of a power outage and with a fire literally down below. And in walks Roy in his smoky turnout coat. Seriously, why does Rampart even bother having separate operating rooms (or a wing, or whatever) when Early and Brackett just perform operations right there in the emergency department?

Kidding aside, I do like this rescue. It's got a little bit of everything and I like how it plays out. Everyone does his job, and by the time the Battalion Chief gets on scene, the fire is more or less under control. Even though he does call in as "all units out indefinitely for overhaul." Usually they give a specified time for units to be out, such as one hour, two hours, etc. In this case I'm sure they had to run the fans for quite a while, at least. Otherwise I don't know what "overhaul" entails other than just making sure there are no smoldering embers or fumes or other fire hazards.

Last scene is at the station, and we all know what happens here: Charlie decides not to sell the boat, but instead to just "rent it out" to other FFs when he's not using it. The guys are disappointed and Johnny wants to know where Charlie got that idea. Guess what—for once it's not Gage's fault! Yeah, that's a nice change, that Johnny's not the butt of the joke; this time it's Chester B who's the culprit. And even Henry deserts him because of it.

Miscellany:

~ I know we often wonder why sometimes the engine is also called out on medical calls, such as "person down," etc., and even possible heart cases, but in the case of Bookie Bob it's a very good thing the engine *was* called out, as the extra manpower—and tools—really come in handy.

~ When Cap arrives at Rampart, I love how he flips the switch to prop the automatic doors open. Just another one of those little details that don't seem very important but really add to the realism of a scene.

6.20 Isolation

I know some people don't care for this episode. I don't mind it too much... it's outside the standard 'box' of episodes, which I find interesting. I think the final MVA is more or less what saves it—at least the guys get in *some* action. (Paramedic action, that is.)

~ I think I've mentioned before about how often we see Roy reading, and the opening scene of this ep is no exception. The book (catalog? magazine?) is about George Tooker, an American painter whose work was in the "realism" mode. I wonder where Roy/Kevin got that reading material—was it just laying around on set, or maybe one of Kevin's personal items?

~ Station 86. Not exactly luxury accommodations, is it? We only see the apparatus bay and the dorm, though; I wonder what the kitchen area looks like. Or maybe it was supposed to be at the other end of the dorm? I read that what we saw was actually station 65, 'playing the role' of 86. Whatever the station was, they sure liked Smokey Bear. Also, I wonder if they actually hosed down the road and driveway to make it look as if it was wet from rain.

~ Speaking of being wet from rain, the empty lot where the chopper landed was suspiciously *not* wet or muddy.

~ Meanwhile back at Rampart... a cop was hit by lightning. "He was picked up immediately by the ambulance," we're told. I guess the writers had to explain why paramedics weren't involved and he was instead transported by the scoop-and-runners.

~ So much for "It Never Rains in California." ("But it pours; man, it pours.")

~ When the psychiatrist is getting ready to help the guy with the head wound and Roy gets her the stuff she asks for, there's a nice moment when Roy touches her arm. It's brief, but very sweet. And he's also very sweet with the old lady who hurt her hip.

~ There was a mini-crisis in this ep, when the power went out at Rampart, and it was nice to see our guys take the initiative on treating the heart victim. Roy decided on lidocaine bolus and the consulting doctor concurred. (Although I always find it strange when she says, "It's a good drug." They're not looking for your opinion of it, doc, they just want your OK to use it.)

~ At Rampart, after making his phone call to the station, it was funny when Johnny turned and tossed the pen/pencil to Dixie. I wonder if that was scripted or just done on the fly. However it happened, he almost hit a nurse who was passing by.

~ Is it just me or did the location of that final accident seem familiar?? I know we've seen one of those "Positively No Smoking" signs before, and the scene of the chopper landing seems awfully familiar. Or maybe I'm just imagining things.

~ And I say again, I find it surprising that these engines don't have winches.

* * *

But now I'm wondering.... why did the show use one station but call it another one? If they were going to use the facade/building of station 65, why not have the script say that Roy and Johnny were at station 65?? Maybe it wasn't isolated enough? But how would *we* know that?

* * *

For some reason, when Roy parked the squad in the driveway, I had the impression there was another vehicle that belonged inside the bay but just wasn't there at that time. (Did Station 86 have a squad, maybe, that was stuck elsewhere? Eh, probably not. But it still seemed as if something else belonged at that station.)

As for the drug box thing.... other than the episode with Brice, I don't think we've ever seen them lock the compartments, have we? Heck, most of the time, they leave the compartment doors wide open when they're at a scene. And as often as they send other people to the squad to get things for them (other FFs, or cops, even civilians) I don't think they've ever referenced the compartments being locked.

Speaking of the squad.... If Johnny and Roy were stuck at 86s for three days, what did B- and C-shift at Station 51 do for a squad? I assume there were extra vehicles that they could borrow in the interim. (Actually, I'm sure there were, since Cap suggested getting a replacement in Breakdown, when the squad kept shutting down in the middle of their runs.)

* * *

May Fair

Once the paramedics went in the copter to Rampart with their victims, I didn't get the impression Johnny "chose" to go back to 86s. I don't think it was optional. I suppose they (LACoFD) *could have* assigned the next shift of Squad 51 to go to 86s via chopper to relieve Roy and Johnny, but that wasn't mentioned so I assumed they had to stay up there until the road/bridge re-opened. (Because, after all, they were the only medical personnel in that part of the county until the road reopened, so *somebody* had to be there.)

* * *

> And I'm not so sure if I had a date with a guy and he had to cancel I would just go out with two of his co-workers. I guess she knew them because she worked for the Department as the maintenance clerk, but isn't the purpose of a date to go out with a particular person? I don't know, I just thought that was all kinda weird.

I remember on the "old" thread mentioning that if I was the girl, I wouldn't just agree to go out with not one, but *two* guys I'd never even met before. Firemen or not, being out on the open sea with two 'strange' guys and no means of escape would definitely cause me to think twice.

~ ~ ~

So some people don't care for this episode, and I can understand that. But instead of dull or boring, as some people might describe it, I choose to go with the glass-half-full point of view and applaud the writers for trying something a bit different. Yes, it deviates from the usual show 'formula,' but really, how often can they have our guys respond to minor medical call, a "possible heart attack," and a structure fire at which they're told "there's someone still inside!"?? So I give them props for stepping outside the box a little bit, and, as it happens, putting our guys into a much smaller box.

Watching EMERGENCY! Seasons 4-6

To start with, I was a little disappointed to see the guys wearing their blue jackets again, but it turns out okay because not only do they need them later on, but also, I assume this episode takes place in winter (or whatever passes for "winter" in SoCal). Still, I have to admit that the "three days of solid rain" does strain the credulity a little. And the less said about the so-called lightning we see, the better. Also, I get a chuckle when, after Johnny mentions having a date the next day, Roy suggests looking in the paper, and Gage says "Yeah they do have a long-range forecast." Hmm, I never realized that "tomorrow" is considered "long-range."

First call is a "man trapped," and in addition to the squad, the engine gets called out in place of engine 86. But en route, engine 51 gets cancelled as 86 becomes available. An hour later R and J are ready to return to the barn, but the one-and-only bridge is out, and of course there is absolutely no other road in the whole county that can take them in any way back to where they need to go. Yeah, I know, one reason they stay at 86s in fictional Oakvale is to provide a measure of medical care to the isolated area. So... that's the set-up for the episode: two paramedics and a couple additional firefighters serve as hospital for the stranded part of the county. Oh, and to make matters worse, the phones are out. (This is mainly an issue only for Johnny, who can't call to cancel his date for the next day.)

Anyway, no sooner do the guys get to 86s than a woman drives into the station with two accident victims: a young woman with a gash on her forearm (not sure how that happened in a car crash), and a man with a cut on his forehead, with some glass embedded in it (much more believable for a car accident). And I was impressed with the amount of blood we see on his makeshift bandage, too—there's probably more blood on the bandage than we've seen on gunshot wounds and nicked jugulars on this show. This is another case of the guys applying a cervical collar only after the victim's head has been lolling around and turning this way and that for a while, but I guess it's better late than never, eh? In any case, the victims are taken into 86's dorm, which, I have to say, looks like just about every summer camp building I've ever seen. Except for Smokey the Bear, that is. In addition to the regular, smaller Smokey picture like the one Johnny has in his locker, this dorm also sports a life-size pin-up of the shovel-wielding grizzly. (Wonder if Johnny was tempted to filch it for his own?) Anyway, no sooner do these two victims get checked out than a third victim comes in: Jeffrey, a boy with bronchitis who was having an episode when a power outage rendered his vaporizer tent useless. So into the dorm with Jeffrey, making three patients for the harried paramedics. (I guess station 86 maybe has its own O2 set-up? Kinda seems that way.)

No sooner do they get the boy halfway comfortable when Captain Flynn comes in with bad news: choppers are grounded for at least an hour, so John and Roy are going to have to do the best they can in the meantime.

Meanwhile, back in civilization at Rampart, Dr. Joe Early is looking sharp in a nice pink shirt and burgundy tie with blue (?) or grey (?) stripes. And even Dr. Fashion Risk—that is, Brackett—is playing it safe with a solid-color shirt and one of his patterned ties that we've seen before. Anyway, they get a call that an ambulance is bringing in a cop who's been hit by lightning—no explanation as to why a paramedic squad didn't get dispatched to him—and thanks to Vince, the guy has apparently been receiving CPR almost since it happened. (Nice bit of detail: the officer's jacket zipper was fused together by the jolt, so Brackett has to cut the jacket off him.) In any case, the man is defibbed twice, and this is Rampart hospital, dammit, so of course they get him back to sinus rhythm relatively quickly and he's on track to make a good recovery. (Question: I thought it had been remarked that the hospital was very busy due to the storm—lots of accidents, etc.—yet all three doctors and a couple of nurses are in the treatment room taking care of *one* patient.)

Up at 86s, next up for treatment is Roy's new girlfriend. Well, not *new*, exactly, but new to him. She's a feisty little senior citizen who calls him doctor and hurt her hip in a fall. I get the feeling that once she's back on her (orthopedically-shod) feet she might even give Joanne a run for her money when it comes to the handsome DeSoto. At this time Cap comes in with some *good* news for a change: a doctor has arrived. Yes, she's a psychiatrist who hasn't done 'practical' work in ten years, but as Joe Early says, it's sort of like riding a bike: once you learn, you never really forget. While she's performing delicate surgery and taking the piece of glass out of car-crash-guy's forehead (can't believe she didn't ask for light; no idea how she could possibly see what she was doing), Roy goes back outside to see what the siren is about and brings in a man found in the road where he collapsed while trying to push his car. Yes, it's our Weekly Cardiac Case, folks; it just wouldn't be an episode of Emergency! if there wasn't at least one. The guys are treating him, and—good news!—a copter is finally on its way, when suddenly Cardiac Man starts arresting. Dr. Slade does what little she can, but it's up to Johnny and Roy to defib him. They get him back, but as soon as Johnny tries to contact Rampart for further instructions, the hospital has a power failure and the connection is lost. So Roy does that thing that Roy does so well, and tells Dr. Slade: how about we give the guy some lidocaine? She says "it's a good drug" (??) but isn't sure about the dosage. He tells her what the standard amount is and she says "go for it." Which they do. The man is stabilized and by the time Rampart comes back online, the victim is in much better condition. So basically even though *she* has the degree, it's the paramedics who more or less call the shots on this one. (Heh, shots.)

Finally everyone gets to Rampart. That helicopter must have been like one of those little clown cars at the circus that has a zillion people inside who all come tumbling out when the door is opened. Personally, I'm not sure why the first woman (car accident) had to go to Rampart. I'd think if I was her, I'd just wait and see my own doctor, especially since the chopper *was* so crowded. But at the hospital, the patients all are in good hands and Roy visits his feisty little girlfriend again. Best news: Morton's going back to 86s with them. Funny how he and the paramedics are bestest friends all of a sudden—no blowback from the "TKO" episode. Poor Johnny tries to call Debbie to cancel their date but can't reach her, so he calls the station and asks Marco to call her—but admonishes him "don't tell Chet." Of course, I envision that when Marco hangs up the phone at the station and turns around, Chet is standing right behind him, lol. They should have shown that. And what would Johnny have done if Chet had answered the phone? By the way, as Johnny says goodbye to Dixie and turns to leave, watch him toss the pen to her; he just misses a nurse who appears out of nowhere.

Once back at 86s, no sooner does everyone arrive at the dorm when the squad and engine get called out for a car accident. I like this scene. They actually did a decent job making it look like it had rained hard; the squad slid in the mud, and so did Patrol 86. And Johnny, too, I might add. The van that went through the fence has some drunken reunion guys in it, talking about their "old ladies," who are probably "swinging" themselves. (This is me, rolling my eyes.) Anyway, first job is to tie off the van so it doesn't go over the edge, and once that's done, everyone evacuates the non-injured drunk guys. But of course one person is trapped (big surprise!) and our friend Angie DeMeo is helping him out until professional help arrives. Roy's in the van with the victim and Johnny calls for the PortaPower as they work to free the man's trapped hand. Finally he's out, and just in time, too (of course!), as the van finally succumbs to gravity and falls into the ravine. (Question: it had been tied off. Did they untie the ropes super quickly, did the rope break, or did the engine get tugged down with the force??) Anyway, one of the reasons I like this one is because A) it's messy, and B) it's one of those rescues that can't really be rehearsed. Well, maybe A and B are related, but in any case it adds up to an enjoyable rescue, and maybe compensates a little for the relative 'dullness' (i.e., lack of action) of the rest of the episode.

Back at the station, we learn it's been three days since the guys first left. (What did the other shifts do for a squad? I assume they used an 'extra' fleet vehicle.) Apparently 86s has a washing machine, because Johnny's and Roy's uniforms didn't look filthy like they did after the MVA rescue. But of course Johnny's only thought is for Debbie... until he learns what happened in his absence. Which only reminds him that he was right to warn Marco: don't tell Chet!

This 'n' that:

~ No "live" footage of Stoker, and Cap's only in one scene, at the very end, with two measly lines.

~ I believe the Captain of 86s is an actor (maybe?) but I think the other FFs might be real.

~ Roy's a little touchy-feely in this episode—first it was Dr. Slade, and he also put his hand on the boy Jeffrey's arm at the hospital.

~ At the accident scene, what, exactly, does Patrol 86 bring to the party??? Nothing but maybe an additional pair of hands.

6.21 Limelight

~ Episode was written by the actor who played Brice. Just like the episode about Roberts Rules of Order was written by him.

May Fair

Interesting how that happens, isn't it: someone writes an episode that revolves around his or her character. Hmmm....

~ I get the feeling Randy's voice really was rough and scratchy during filming of this ep, so it just got written in.

~ First rescue, with the overturned tractor and the agitated father... I like how the scene was a little chaotic at first, with everyone talking at once. Also, for those keeping score at home, this is the *first* and *only* episode in which we actually see the non-paramedic FFs doing the 'rescue' of the daughter, while the PMs take care of the older gentleman. How often have we pondered why they're the "only ones" who can do a rescue, and here we see the other guys doing it. (And the odd thing is, this is one case in which I think it would have made more sense for at least *one* of the PMs to be down there at the tractor, supervising the proceedings with the daughter. Go figure.)

~ There were a couple of medical acronyms in this one. First, upon arrival at Rampart, Johnny mentioned an MICU form. I think it probably stands for Mobile Intensive Care Unit form (MICU is the official title of the paramedics)—in other words, this form was paperwork on their two victims: vitals, step taken, treatment administered, etc. We've *never* seen or heard of one of these forms before, and yet, here one is. Also, Brackett asked Early to check the patient's CNS, which I believe stands for *central nervous system*. Interesting to hear a little medical-speak that we haven't heard before.

~ Air pellet gun victim—first of all, again, no blood to be seen. Also, Brackett inadvertently said *thoractomy* instead of *thoracotomy*. He said it correctly the second time.

~ During that boy's surgery, Mike Morton referenced the Bird respirator. Also, after the nurse put all those nice folded sheets on the boy's chest, Brackett spread some saran wrap across the area, and I assume he cut through that. Is that to cut down on blood-mess, I wonder?

~ Morton called the nurse "dear," which while questionable today, probably wasn't too unusual back in the day. (In MASH Trapper John used to call the nurses "honey" during surgery.) Also, I saw Morton pick up an instrument, and then toss it aside and request another one.

~ This is also known as The Episode Without a Watch, in which Roy famously takes a pulse and respiration count while looking at his bare wrist. And yes, I got a cap of that scene... it's too famous not to.

~ Also at the scene with the babysitter/au pair, before he sat down to help the girl, Roy turned off the toy train that was running. I thought that was a funny detail. (Definitely something I would have done.)

~ Brice's bright idea about transcripts of paramedic calls... I don't get how that would be so helpful considering the time and effort involved in creating them. Someone would have to sit down to listen to the calls and then write them out, type them up, and then make copies. Or, should I say, make Xerox copies, because copiers and printers weren't nearly as ubiquitous as they are now; even a place like Rampart might only have one copy machine in the whole building.

~ At the final fire, it was kind of funny to watch Squad 51 blow past the Battalion Chief when they first arrived. Obviously they heard his instruction and were complying as they drove around the building to assist Engine 51, but it almost looked like they were gonna go support Engine 51 no matter what.

~ ~ ~

May Fair

Guess who makes another appearance in this episode? Yep, everyone's favorite, the "perfect paramedic," Craig Brice. (Insert eyeroll here.) And—surprise, surprise!—the ep was written by James G. Richardson, the actor who plays Brice.

Episode opens at the station and Johnny is hoarse. He blames it on "that last fire I was in." (Was he in it by himself?) Anyway, it's pretty obvious that Randy was hoarse for some reason so they just improvise a line or two to 'explain' it in the context of the show. In any case, the conversation is apparently about the paramedic review meetings, at which Brice annoys the $%^#@ out of everyone. Big surprise there, amIright? But at least it's a bit of continuity, referring to the meetings that appeared in a previous episode. (Fun fact: Johnny's not wearing his name badge in this first scene in the day-room.) Before the guys can grab some lunch and forget about the meeting, the tones sound and the station is called out to an "accident with injuries."

The accident is a tractor that's rolled over down an embankment. An older man is there, and Vince informs the firefighters that the man's daughter is the one who's pinned under the tractor (loader) and the father is pretty upset, giving Vince a hard time, etc. Roy and Johnny try to calm the man and take him back up to the squad so they can look at him, leaving Cap to supervise the extrication of the girl. I admit I always find this odd and a bit jarring. Even though Johnny reminds Cap to put a cervical collar on the girl's cervi—er, I mean neck, it still seems unusual that one of the PMs doesn't stay and at least take the girl's vitals, assess her condition, etc., while Marco or Chet assist the other paramedic with the father. But yeah, I get it: the story calls for them *both* deal with Frantic Father, so that's what happens. And as it turns out, the Father really is a handful. He's worried to the point of hysteria about his daughter and not cooperating with them by being still, and when the ambulance arrives, the thought of leaving his daughter behind causes him to go even crazier. (Yeah, that seems a little odd to me. There's a limit to how acceptably-worried a dad should be when his daughter is A] not in imminent danger, and B] being tended to by trained professionals. Kind of twigs my radar a bit.) Anyhoo, moving on.... Cap rounds up both Chet and Marco to assist him with something or another, so it's nice to see Mike Stoker do a few things other than his 'usual.' I notice that he pulls some lever (sounded like a generator or engine or something) and then he pulls the reel line, which also makes a fun sound, sort of a ratcheting type of sound. In any event, the paramedics end up having to "call an audible" and change the plan in an effort to keep Frantic Father as calm as possible, so they delay transporting him to the hospital until the daughter is extricated and ready to be sent to Rampart as well.

At Rampart, we already see that Brice is doing his Bricely best to be as efficient as possible; apparently the "annoying" part is just an unexpected bonus. When Johnny and Roy bring their two patients in, they're both put into the same treatment room... again, a little creepy/strange, imho. Dr. Early treats the daughter and Dr. Brackett checks over the dad, and eventually it's pronounced that both will be fine, because this is Rampart, after all. By the way, as they're bringing the victims into the hospital, Johnny hands Dixie a paper and says, "here's the MICU form." I think I remarked on an episode recently about an ambulance driver handing Dixie a piece of paper, so perhaps that was the MICU form as well. (MICU = Mobile Intensive Care Unit. In other words, paramedic. I think I can count on one hand the number of times in six seasons we've seen anyone hand over an MICU form... and still hold my ice-cream spoon with the left-over fingers.)

Also at Rampart, a woman frantically runs into the ED yelling that her son shot himself. Turns out the "son" is about eight years old and the gun is an air rifle. In contrast to Johnny's standard reply of "he'll be fine, he'll be fine," when the mother grabs Dr. Brackett's hand and asks if her son would be okay,

Kel replies, "It's too soon to tell." Yeah, *there's* an answer designed to soothe a mother's worried soul, right? (But, yes, it *is* honest.) The wound is (of course) on his chest, although when we see the kid with his shirt off, there's almost nothing to see on his skinny little torso. I will say this about this particular scene: my guess is that the medical technical advisor for this one had a little too much coffee that morning, as the medical jargon comes thick and heavy. Pulsus paradoxus... pericardial tamponade... pericardiocentesis... thoracotomy... asystole.... And that's all in one scene in the treatment room. Of course, while Brackett is checking the kid out, his condition deteriorates, resulting in emergency surgery, with Kel being assisted by Dr. Morton. (Ever notice how Morton can be a little, um, less than gentle when dealing with patients?) Anyway, the surgery goes well and the pericardiocentesis is successful, saving the kid's life. This surgery scene was interesting in a couple of ways: first, did anyone notice the funny sucking sound effects for the suction? It was kind of odd, sort of like the exaggerated bubbling sound effects we've heard in other episodes. Also, the way the surgery scenes are filmed is interesting because we never actually *see* anything, as the camera are trained on the actors' faces, and yet we still get (or at least *I* still get) the impression that actual surgery is taking place. Yeah, it's a little hokey and sanitized and totally PG—unlike today's shows—but they still make it seem dramatic. (That's how I see it, anyway.)

Anyhoo.... At the station, John and Roy walk in on the other guys watching a TV news segment featuring Brice. Apparently he took part in a perfectly routine call, but a news crew happened to be around and interviewed him, and his description of the scene is apparently riveting. I guess you could call him a "publicity hound"—oops, no, wait, that's Tom Wheeler. But Brice is close, always getting his face on TV and his name mentioned in the news. Next, the paramedics are at Rampart, waiting in the lounge for Morton to tell them something. While perusing the newspaper, Johnny sees a picture of—guess who?—yep, Craig Brice. A picture of him appears with an article about the upcoming firefighter Olympics. When Morton finally arrives, he hands them transcripts of base station calls for them to review in advance of their meeting, so they don't waste valuable meeting time—an idea come up with by Brice, no doubt. Anyway, this, along with Morton's other comments about Craig, sends Johnny into one of his little rants. "Brice. Rice. Mice. Lice." And he's off and running. Roy tries to tell him to calm down and forget Brice, but you know that the more you tell John Gage to "forget" something, the more he's going to obsess over it. And, of course, he does.

Next is the famous nanny/au pair call, which is interesting for a number of reasons, such as Roy's magic, invisible watch, and the dog that runs into glass doors, and the Pong game on TV. Even with all that fun stuff, though, I have a hard time making myself watch those awful kids. Maybe it's me, but I don't find that kind of wild, rude, out-of-control behavior to be amusing or entertaining. So I totally sympathize with poor Erika and I totally get why she agrees to be taken to the hospital. Roy asks how old she is while the camera is on Johnny, and when she says she's 27, I half-expect Johnny to look at her and have a light bulb appear over his head, as if considering whether she's a likely candidate for a date. After all, she's very pretty... sort of looks like Gwyneth Paltrow. And when Johnny realizes how quiet the boys are and goes outside—I bet he suddenly realizes that maybe Brice might be right about locking the squad's compartments. More trouble ensues when the ambulance arrives, and Vince also arrives. Johnny somewhat sneakily leaves Vince instructions to call the boys' parents—and apparently stay with them until those parents show up. If I were Johnny I would have said, "Consider this payback for pulling your gun on me a while back."

May Fair

At Rampart, the guys are going to one of their paramedic review meetings. Roy says something that's very normal: "I'm gonna get something to eat out of the machines." Yet where does he go? He goes past the Staff Lounge, and is heading toward Treatment Room #7. What kind of sense does *that* make? Wouldn't the machines be *in* the Staff Lounge? Anyway, the meeting doesn't go quite as Johnny plans, as first of all, he acts like a 14-year-old doofus on his first date, and second of all, Morton and Brice actually agree with his assessment (or defense?) of squad 51's call, which is not what he's expecting. But the meeting is cut short when Squad 16 (Brice and Bellingham) are called out (along with engine 51, among others) to a factory fire. Just before they get that call, I think Ron Pinkard kind of flubs his dialogue; he repeats himself and doesn't make a lot of sense.

We see engine 51 arrive at the fire and Cap speaks briefly with the Chief, who tells him to bring his rig around back. This leads to a funny scene which I don't think I've heard anyone mention: when engine 51 stops and Cap hops out to talk to McConnike, Chet steps down off the rig to put on his air tank and mask. Problem is, Cap has received his orders and is ready to have Mike move the rig around back, but Chet's still standing around working with his air tank. In the foreground, we see the captain of 16s tell McConnike about the crazy gamblers and how his men could use some help in getting them out, but in the background we see Cap apparently say something to Chet and Chet hurriedly hops back into the jump seat so Mike can drive away like he's supposed to. Chester B. is holding up the action.

At the station, Johnny's still griping about the meeting and how foolish he felt. And of course griping about Brice. But then they get called to the scene of the fire. And when they get there, who do they have to look for and rescue? Brice!

Watching EMERGENCY! Seasons 4-6

Brice and Belliveau—er, I mean Bellingham (*wink*)—had gone in after the gamblers but for some reason Brice hasn't come out yet with his victim. So guess who gets sent in to find them? Yep, our own fearless paramedics. At first I thought Bellingham went in with them, but I think it's only Marco and Chet with them. Inside, it's hot, it's fiery (duh), it's smoky, but eventually we hear someone call out: "In here!" And lo and behold, Brice and his gambler are huddling under a table, and we get a *great* view of Roy's perfectly rounded butt as he and Johnny pull the men out. Once outside the building, Chief McConnike has inexplicably allowed a news crew within ten yards of the fully-engulfed building, and of course they film the rescue party coming out, mentioning Brice by name and getting a comment from him in passing. Roy and Johnny don't see that, but they are quite surprised when Brice comes up to them and thanks them for coming in for him, and says he'll let the Chief know what they did in his report. (Which is great, of course, but they were just doing their job. And now that I think of it, why would Brice be in contact with the Chief?) Anyway, suddenly Johnny's feeling very charitable toward his erstwhile nemesis, saying, "you just gotta understand Brice and keep things in perspective," blah blah blah. What does Roy do? He does the walkaway.

Later, at the station, the guys are talking about Brice and the guys who'd been having a craps game in the building. Again Johnny defends Brice. Cap gets word that coverage of the fire is on TV, so they turn it on. Who do they see? The newswoman saying that the victims were "helped to safety by Craig Brice." And that's all she wrote, as Johnny's back to thinking of Brice as a "lousy jerk." The scene and episode end with Roy making a comment about Johnny's still-hoarse voice, and Johnny saying, "Ha-ha, very funny." Then he apparently looks directly at the camera and... freeze frame. I gotta wonder if he said or did something that caused them to freeze the shot at that moment... something, perhaps, that couldn't be shown/heard on TV? (Just kidding!)

May Fair

This 'n'that:

~ In Rules of Order, Brice is partnered with Bob Belliveau. In The Nuisance, we hear that Brice is going to be partnered with Bob Bellingham, aka, "The Animal." Here his partner is Bellingham, as in Bob Bellingham. Is Bellingham a reference to Belliveau?

~ Speaking of Bellingham, the actor who plays him is the same guy who played the FF from 86s in Isolation and Hypochondri-Cap. Also, the Captain of 16s in this one played the Captain of 86s in those same two episodes.

~ Have to chuckle when a call includes directions for someplace called Hilldale. Just seems odd to me, like something called Updown, or Rightleft.

~ Johnny made a comment about the paramedics reviewing the "backhoe incident from last week." I take this to mean the rescue of the Frantic Father and Darling Daughter. But if that was "last week," why is Johnny's voice still hoarse?

~ At the fire, we hear Brice calling out "in here," but when John and Roy reach the two men, and in fact as Johnny is pulling them out (and we're looking at Roy's butt, up close and *very* personal) I heard yet another call of "in here!" Perhaps the audio guy got a little excited and couldn't resist adding another sound bite?

~ Who is sixth man at the table in final scene? Presumably it's Mike, but we never see the person's face, just hands and arms. Could have been anyone.

~ In the scene with the boy who shot himself, I think there were some mispronunciations of that medical jargon. Brackett says thoractomy, and I think Morton says precardiocentesis, rather than pericardiocentesis.

6.22 Upward and Onward

~ Anyone else notice the lack of Johnny in this episode? He's only in the two rescue scenes, but not at the station at all except for the meal at the very end (figures: where there's food, there's a Gage). Roy and the other guys, even Mike, appear throughout, but Gage is MIA. I wonder if Randy had some other project going on the week this was filmed, so they wrote him out of non-essential scenes.

~ And what about Chief McConnike, showing up with a thermos to take all their coffee? Another reason this station needs to invest in a large urn or something.

~ Weren't we just talking about the paramedics having to deal with annoying people? At the TV studio, if I were John or Roy, I'd have told that producer guy to *BACK. OFF.* They shouldn't worry about trying to be so nice, as their politeness is totally lost on some people.

~ I noticed the 'pretend' doctor's hospital room had some artwork featuring large flowers. I guess it's appropriate for a hospital room.

~ Speaking of that hospital room and the scene with the TV people... Go, Brackett!! He's quite appealing when he gets riled up. Mmmm-hmmm!

~ The tale of two doctors—one real, and one not. If "Doctor Ned" had stayed in the hospital any longer he could have roomed with the real doctor, and maybe learned something.

~ Once again we see the footage of Engine 8 with John Gage riding in the jump seat.

~ I like the last rescue, with the paramedics and victim being stuck in the elevator. It shows another example of the unexpected things they face from time to time. Even though the 'elevator' was just a set, I bet it did get kind of warm for real in that enclosed area, and under the lights. I bet the guys' perspiration was real and not 'misted' on. I know I felt clammy just watching that scene.

~ I felt bad for Marco when he got up to the roof and Cap said, "We don't need the water, there's a fire extinguisher in here." He'd just lugged that heavy hose up about five flights of stairs, and it's not needed.

* * *

> I know I don't usually like the drawn-out scenes at Rampart but these I didn't mind. I liked Brackett's overreacting and strictness to the rules and Early's and Dixie's disregard for them. It just all worked for me.

I agree, this storyline at Rampart was quite entertaining, unlike a lot of others. And the way Joe and Dixie sort of played with the TV people was hilarious... like when Early said, "Why yes, I think I have heard of a laparotomy. Maybe in, oh I don't know... medical school?" And, "I could lend you some old EKG strips." Too funny! I do think, though, that Dixie was being awfully mellow about all this. We all know how she rules her department with an iron fist, and nine times out of ten she'd have shut down those shenanigans long before Brackett caught wind of them. But who knows, maybe there's a reason for her 'laid-back temperament' in this case.

~ ~ ~

So, this episode is notable for a number of reasons, one of which is the fact that it was written by Mike Norell. Guess that explains the Cap Craziness, huh? Also, Johnny is MIA is most of this episode. He's at both rescues (there are only two, although one is kind of long), but definitely MIA at the station. And the odd thing is, there's no mention of him. No offhand comment about him being in the dorm taking a nap or writing up a report or cleaning out the squad or anything. They could even have had Roy say something as he walks into the dayroom as if he's talking to Johnny in the other room. But no, there's no reference or mention of him at all, as if he doesn't even exist (even though you *just know* that he'd love to hear about the incident with Cap and McConnike's hat).

Episode begins with a cute scene of Chet using a soft, silky material to shine a hose nozzle; just so happens that the soft, silky material in question is Henry's ear. There's some mention among "the guys" about Cap being a little nuts now that he's studying for the Chief's exam, which is the running theme of the ep. Meanwhile, the squad gets called out for a "man down" at a TV studio (but I didn't hear the final 'tone'; did I miss it?), and thus we meet Dr. Ned. I don't know who the equivalent would have been at the time—Dr. Steve Hardy, perhaps, from General Hospital? Anyway, this is one of those scenes in which I think (or at least wish) Johnny and/or Roy would just get real and lay down the law with the spouse/relative/neighbor/bystander and raise their voice(s) to say "Get. Out." Seriously, they had enough trouble with the victim himself; they do NOT need to put up with stupidity from those around him, who are only making things worse by upsetting the victim. Dr. Ned is sure he has something fatal, and the TV people want him on-set to perform a laparotomy on Ellen Rockstraw's illegitimate son, Toddy. Love Roy's response: "You're gonna have to find somebody else to open the little fella up, you know what I mean?" (Side note: I wonder how many parents of kids watching the show found themselves explaining what "illegitimate" means.) Long story short, they finally get Dr. Ned calm and are able to transport him to Rampart. Unfortunately, that's not the end of the story of A Doctor Faces Life. (Yeah, what kind of title is that, anyway??) By the way, did anyone notice the ambulance attendant hand Dixie a piece of paper as they came into Rampart? I assume it's some sort of transfer paper (MICU form, perhaps?), the kind of thing that's probably really required in real life, but we almost never see it on this show.

One of the funniest scenes of this ep—of almost any ep, for that matter—is when Joe Early talks to Producer Arnie and Writer Jody, and the subject of Dr. Ned performing a laparotomy comes up.

Jody: That's where he opens up the abdominal cavity.

Early: Thank you very much. You know, I seem to recall hearing that someplace before. Possibly in... medical school.

Arnie: Maybe you saw it on television.

Early: Maybe I did!

Haha, too funny! Anyway, turns out Dr. Ned "only" has mono, so he can go home in a day or so. But that's still not the end of this story, as the TV people get a bright idea that *you just know* the hospital people are gonna hate.

Meanwhile Station 51 gets a surprise visit from Chief McConnike. He comes in to fill his thermos with coffee—can you imagine that? The station barely manages to have enough coffee for one or two cups at a time; how do they have enough for an entire thermos?? And then, Roy gets a cup for himself. How much coffee does that little pot make, anyway? The Chief is invited to come back later for dinner (Marco's Irish stew) and after he leaves, we hear the story that Cap, back when he was engineer for Captain McConnike, set fire to McConnike's hat. The 'why' of the incident... that's a mystery for the ages. And now Cap's stressing out about McConnike performing his review.

Back at Rampart, Producer Arnie is turning Dr. Ned's hospital room into a sideshow and satellite studio set, complete with writers, assistants, lighting people, etc. Arnie tells the network exec that the hospital "loves" his idea and there's a doctor, a "quiet, grey-haired type" who might make a cameo; he "reeks of empathy." When Brackett and Dixie storm in, Arnie calls him "dynamic" and says maybe Dixie could take a bit part, as she has a "fabulous bod." Needless to say, Kel doesn't take kindly to his hospital being turned into a three-ring circus, so he shuts things down and drives the money-changers out of the temple, so to speak. Joe offers to give Arnie some old EKG strips—"that could be very dramatic"—but it's too late, and off they go. (Just occurred to me: Kel is in charge of Emergency, but this craziness isn't taking place in Emergency, so technically it's some other doctor's problem.)

In Cap's office back at the station, Roy comes in and tries to ease Cap's mind by suggesting that maybe McConnike hasn't been a Chief long enough to evaluate Cap. Hank loves this idea and says, "I know just who to call." He calls someone named Chief Suggs... and guess what Suggs' first name is? *Charlie.* Seriously, how many people named Charlie have we had on this show?? Meanwhile, Roy asks Cap why he set fire to McConnike's hat, and Hank comes back with, "What would you have done under the circumstances?" Roy: "Well, I— huh?"

This is when the alarm goes off for the final rescue. And it's a doozy. First of all, this is two episodes in pretty quick succession in which the engine is called out for a heart case, and in both cases it's lucky that it is. The other day it was the multiply-locked door that the crew worked on so the paramedics could get to Bookie Bob; today another possible heart attack, and it's darn lucky that Cap and the others are there when Johnny and Roy get stuck in an old elevator with their victim. As it is, however, the paramedics do their best to keep the old doctor calm while Chet is on the horn to Rampart and Cap and Marco do what they can to get the elevator moving again. It's a tense scene, and even with all their equipment, Roy and Johnny are pretty much helpless. But all's well that ends well and the elevator is lowered to the ground floor by hand.

At Rampart, Kel is confronted by Joe and Dixie, who begins her speech with, "It's not my fault." Now, to me, that would indicate that she's going to present him with bad news, i.e., a problem. In fact, both she and Joe begin telling Kel about various infractions that Dr. Ned and his entourage have committed, but then... they tell him that it's all been solved. Why not just lead with that??

Finally, at the station, the Chief has enjoyed Marco's stew and gives Cap a bit of news: he's on the board for the orals of the Chief's exam. He even makes a joke referring to the burning-hat incident. Cap simply sighs and tosses his exam study books into the trash. D'oh!

~ The TV producer Arnie is played by Tom Williams, exec producer of Adam-12. And the actor who plays the retired doctor is the guy who also played the reverend on Little House on the Prairie.

~ Anyone notice McConnike's comment referring to Marco as a "broth of a lad"? I don't recall hearing that saying before, but apparently it means *lively* or *fine*.

* * *

And yeah, I can think of a LOT worse things than being stuck in an elevator with Johnny and Roy. Especially if they're all hot and sweaty. But, no cameras, please!

6.23 Hypochondri-Cap

~ First scene: Roy had a book. Again.

~ The guy who got his hand caught in his garage-door opener... was it just me or did the other fireman's flashlight lack, oh, I don't know, light? (I've seen the same thing happen in other scenes, and it's kind of a hoot.)

~ The woman who suffered unconsciousness due to aerosol can: the doctors didn't prescribe an IV, and yet it looked like Roy was going to go to the hospital with her.

~ The stunt guy with the new... rope, or rigging, or whatever. Seriously, what exactly was it the guys were testing? I guess it was a rappel rigging? Anyway, after Roy lowered Johnny down, and "Wally" came down, why didn't Wally just use Johnny's line instead of throwing down a new one?

~ Speaking of, the rope they were testing was orangey-red, and later on Roy and Johnny were using a rope that looked just like that. I wonder if there's any significance to that.

~ The refinery explosion and fire. I think that was filmed at the place that was right across from the (real) station. The address was Wilmington, cross-street Carson, and that's not far from Station 127.

~ I really like the last rescue, with them having to rope over from one tower to another. That in all likelihood wasn't really Kevin who went across there, but I still say the show does a good job of making it sound like it's really Kevin (or Randy) even when it's a stunt-man (i.e., good audio work). I did notice they didn't show Roy getting the stokes rigged up to send off to the other tower. I bet it would have been awfully difficult for one person to do, to lift and connect a stokes with a full-sized person on board (not literally a 'dead weight,' but you know what I mean). In any case, they skipped showing that part, as well as showing them treating the patient once they reached the ground.

May Fair

~ I thought it was interesting that Johnny told that one guy (Andy?) that he did a good job, roping across between buildings even though he was afraid, etc. The irony is that the guy was (I think) a stunt-man in real life, and normally he would be telling Randy that *he* did a good job on a stunt. Yeah, I know, that's kind of silly, but I found the role reversal sort of ironic.

* * *

> it shows Johnny's cockiness that "we are handy and can do anything" but then it shows that whole confidence implode and Roy saving the day. I just love the dialogue between them, "I know you're handy but do you need some help".

Yeah, Johnny's cockiness was funny. He talked about how highly trained he and Roy were and the stuff they can do, and Roy tried to bring him back to earth: "Just as well-trained as the rest of the guys."

And yeah I didn't mention it in my original comments, but Johnny was once again missing in a few scenes at the station. Not all, but some.

~ ~ ~

I think this is a pretty good episode. It has some "meh" moments but it also has some saving graces. It starts out oddly, though. Another thunderstorm? Really?? I thought heavy rain in southern California was unusual enough, but to have it feature in two episodes so close together? Add to that the fact that Johnny/Randy doesn't appear in the first scene, and you have to wonder. And there's another extended station scene that he appeared in only very briefly and with no lines.

So Cap is stressing again, except this time it's not about McConnike or even the Chief's exam. He's been a bear and the guys are starting to grumble. When we do see Johnny, he's very curious about what Cap's problem is. Roy is markedly less so. If Roy had his way, he'd play least-in-sight until Cap's mood blows over; he's not curious so much as he's practicing self-preservation.

The first call, which comes in during the "rain storm" (note the quotes), pairs the squad with Engine 86. If Cap doesn't start minding his manners at the station, the guys at 86s just might become Roy and Johnny's new best friends, since they've been spending so much time together recently. So the call ends up being for a guy whose hand is stuck in the works of his automatic garage door. When the power went out (due to the storm, don'tcha know) he tried to open the door manually, and, well, things got ugly and here we are. Johnny deals with the man and tries to determine if his fingers really are "off at the knuckle" (as the man fears), while Roy scopes out the chain and trying to disconnect whatever it is that's connected. When the engine arrives they have the guys bring in bolt cutters and a magic flashlight that shines invisible light. (Or maybe it just shines so weakly we can't really *see* the light; the jury's still out on that.) In the end, the man's hands end up being fine, if greasy, and all he had to do to open the door was pull some release lever that's probably in plain sight. So now he's got a broken garage door opener chain and his chopsticks are probably going to slip through his fingers for a week.

The next day (or next shift, actually) as Johnny and Roy are having their "Aren't you curious?" "No, I'm really not" conversation about Cap's problem, and the man himself comes into the dayroom and says he wants to talk to Roy… privately. "Well, I'm not done with my coffee," Johnny protests, but Cap shoos him out anyway. Umm, question—well, two questions: 1) if Cap wants privacy, why talk to Roy in the dayroom? He has an office! And 2) Johnny, your coffee mug has a handle on it… it's portable! This is one case when you really *can* take it with you. Anyway, Gage finally leaves (without his coffee) and Roy is looking sort of panicky. Cap hems and haws and indicates that he needs Roy's "professional and confidential advice," but before he can go further, the alarm sounds and off they go.

This call is for an "unconscious woman in a car," and that's exactly what they find. Vince tells them the woman lost control of her car and luckily the curb stopped it from going off the road. Vince also says that when he first opened her car door there was an odor that has since dissipated. "It smelled like some kind of spray." Hmm, really? I didn't know that sprays had any particular odor that pegged them as sprays. In any case, Roy finds a spray can in her grocery bag and it looks like the button has been depressed, perhaps by another grocery item in the bag. Other than being unconscious, her vitals are normal and she soon comes to. We never do find out anything more about this case, such as what she inadvertently inhaled or what the prognosis is, etc. Darn those chlorofluorocarbons, anyway!

Once the paramedics return to the station, Cap calls Roy into his office (see, he's getting smarter!) and has the door closed so they can continue their conversation. He has Roy look at his hands—how do they look, can Roy see any sign of anything wrong, etc.—and finally we find out why Cap be crazy: he believes has arthritis in his hands. Now, I confess to being a bit confused here. Is arthritis a 'death sentence' as far as firefighters go? Is it automatically debilitating or grounds for taking someone off duty? I'd think that as long as the person can handle the discomfort and/or pain (and can physically do the job, of course), it shouldn't be an issue. But what do *I* know? Roy urges Cap to see a doctor and offers to set up an appointment for him with Dr. Brackett, but Cap doesn't want to and they go in circles about it: "See a doctor, you'll stop worrying." "I don't want to be told I have arthritis." "You might not *have* arthritis." "They why see a doctor??"

Roy does call Brackett for advice, which goes exactly how you'd expect, and after hanging up, Brackett gets paged to go into Treatment #4, where Dixie is. He's standing ten freakin' feet away from room 4—all Dixie had to do is poke her head out the door and call to him. The patient they deal with is an unusual one: woman had apparently received some sort of el-cheapo, under-the-table cosmetic surgery including skin grafts of her neck and legs. It sounded like a PSA situation ("Folks, don't try this at home!") but it was just plain icky and unpleasant. But it does give us another glimpse of Nurse Michelle, who, after she quit dating Johnny, changed her name from Valerie and left her brood of kids to become a nurse.

Next we see Johnny and Roy at the movie studio to do Johnny's friend a favor. I admit I learned something this time around that I hadn't known before. On previous viewings I assumed that they were testing the *rope*; after all, the rope being used is noticeably different from the 'usual' rope we see the guys use (it's orange). But I must be wising up: I now think they were actually testing the little *harness thingy* that Johnny put on. It looked a little uncomfortable, and it didn't perform well when he went down the side of the building wearing it. This of course leads to a comical scene of Johnny being all higgledy-piggledy and hanging upside down and Roy zipping down to 'rescue' him (just a little ironic). At the risk of being shallow, the two of them looked pretty cozy being so, um, close to each other and with their legs more or less intertwined. Well, I don't want to start any rumors so I won't go into that any further. I do wonder, though: why did Johnny say he has "bumps and bruises" all over him and that he'd be "sore for a week"? He didn't really hit anything that would cause any bruising. Although based on the way that harness fit, he might experience some, um, er, 'fire down below,' so to speak, so maybe that's what he meant.

At the station, Roy keeps his word and won't tell the other guys what's bothering Cap, but Cap comes in and blurts it out anyway. He still doesn't want to see a doctor, but Roy says he already made the appointment.

Next rescue is a box alarm at one of the handy-dandy refineries that seem to be on every block in 51's area. It's being decommissioned but something went wrong and there's an explosion and fire and—well, you know the drill. This time the "people who are trapped" are easily visible, but not easily reachable. I do like this rescue… it's complicated and dangerous and there are lots of trucks/engines involved. Speaking of the vehicles, I love watching the engines that stick big hoses into water (ponds, lakes, ocean, etc.) and literally suck it in to fill the engine. Anyway, I find it interesting that this time Roy's the one who goes over to the other tower, but I'm glad he did. I think we mentioned last time that it must have been difficult for him to get the victim into the stokes by himself, and the stokes hooked up to the line. I wonder that he didn't have Andy help him at least get the guy into the stokes before sending him across. But all in all, a good rescue. By the way, did Randy forget one of his lines? After they're geared up, just before they start climbing, Johnny tells Cap "We're going to need a stokes with a traverse, uh...." And Cap says "I'll shoot it up there to you." I have the impression Johnny was supposed to—or intended to—say something after the *traverse,* but he just let his sentence trail off.

Quick bits:

~ Firefighter from 86s who's referred to as Joe is the same one we saw in Isolation. Apparently in real life he was a paramedic with LACoFD and also worked as technical advisor on the show.

~ Is it just me or does Johnny's hair look a little goofy in a few of these episodes? Looks like it may have been trimmed (although not styled).

~ Speaking of Gage, he did his "smack the door" of the ambulance thing after the last rescue. And it's a good thing he moved away after he did that, because the ambulance backed up. !!! It would have run him over if he'd still been standing there.

~ If anyone listens with headphones or has good hearing, listen to the scene with Cap and all the guys at the station. Right when Roy says "like I've been telling you to see Dr. Brackett," I hear a little buzz or beep or something. It's really not that loud—I'm surprised I heard it at all—but it's definitely there. Not sure if it's Netflix or something that took place on set or what.

~ Once again we see examples of Wardrobe making good use out of their supplies. Brackett's shirts and ties are repeats from recent episodes, although they've been mixed-and-matched a little differently, so it's not exactly the same. Except for the yellow shirt with the white (?) pinstripe—he wears it in this episode with two different ties on two different days.

~ Speaking of clothes, is this the first, last, and only time we see Mike in anything other than his uniform? (Except for the basketball game, of course.) I have a pic for the screen pic thread, which I'll get posted when I can.

* * *

Speaking of the shooting gadget Johnny uses to get a line to the other tower, every time I see them use it (which isn't often) I'm always, *always* reminded of a SuperSoaker.

Also, speaking of Cap, sometimes it surprises me when I think that this show was Mike Norell's first (and almost only) acting job ever, as far as I can tell. I always find it fascinating when people who've never acted before do so well in front of a camera. Other than E!, he did one episode of Police Story, and that's it for him in front of the camera. I guess he really liked the writing gig, as he went on to do quite a number of things on TV: a LOT of TV movies, The Love Boat (if you can believe that), and Nash Bridges. Far as I can tell, though, none of his E! co-stars were ever in anything else he wrote.

6.24 All Night Long

The last episode!! *sniff*

Last time around, I think I was the only one who talked about this episode. (Unless I missed some comments....) And yet, somehow I still have more to say on the subject. Big surprise, huh?

~ Episode was written by Kevin—yay! The first call is listed as "11876 Fishburn, between MacArthur and West 7th." I have no idea if there really is a Fishburn Street or Ave. in LA County, but it *is* Kevin's real last name, so that could be the reason for that street name. Also, I couldn't find evidence of either a MacArthur or a West 7th Street/Ave./Road in LA County. *However*...MacArthur Park is located on West 7th Ave in LA City. Maybe Kevin liked MacArthur Park and stuck the park name and its street in his script...? (Yeah, I know, dumb idea.... but in the past this show has used actual street names or intersections, but this time they didn't, and combined with the use of his real name... well, my imagination ran away with me. It's kind of an occupational hazard, I guess.)

~ Boo on the stock shot of the guys getting into the rigs, and Marco doesn't have a mustache. Also, at the scene of the old jazz musician, Roy doesn't have his uniform shirt on, just the blue jacket over his t-shirt (believe me, I noticed!). The same clothing situation was true later on, when Johnny was up late typing (fully dressed, darn the luck) and the other guys were in the dorm, but this call had come in much earlier, and Roy had been fully dressed when the tones sounded. (What did he do, take his clothes *off* for the run?)

~ Speaking of that old jazz player (and his friend, the familiar "Detective Crockett"), he was telling a story about someone in New Orleans and mentioned the guy's "hefty old lady." Then he said something that sounded for all the world like "I sure would hate to do it with her." I have a hard time believing that would actually be in the script (Kevin, you devil!!) but I can't figure out what else he could have said. Unless maybe it was "I sure would hate to duke it (out) with her," as in fight. Maybe??? (Since this ep isn't on Netflix, I didn't have the luxury of closed-captioning. Or the same picture quality. Grrrr…)

~ Anyway, in addition to the Fishburn thing, I wonder if the old jazz coot could have been sort of a tribute from Kevin to Bobby Troup and Julie and their jazz music days.

~ Kevin (Roy) flubbed one of his own lines, I think. At the station when Johnny tells him he's writing something, Roy shrugs and as he's leaving he says "This too shall come to pass." He probably meant "This too shall pass."

~ Johnny still = Prince Valiant. Roy = not the best hair. But I have to say Chet = looking good in this one.

~ Both Dixie and Sam (dispatcher) apparently work all hours as they were both 'seen' in the middle of the night. Dixie was talking to the old coot's friend and a clock in the background said 2:03am. Then cut to the station, tones going off, and Sam dispatches them to the car accident, and the "time out" was 1:50. So in addition to shrinking the hairstyles, apparently E!-magic includes bending time backward, from 2:03 to 1:50.

May Fair

~ Johnny seemed a little cavalier with the man from the car accident. He tried to get a carotid pulse in the car, and then when they got him out he checked again. He told Vince, "I can't get anything. Cover him up." I suppose (hope!) we didn't see everything he tried, but I know they don't just check once or twice and then give up. (Although that's kind of how it looked here.)

~ Then the wife dies too, at Rampart. This episode keeps the string alive—the paramedics rarely lose a victim at the scene. Now and then someone is already dead when they get there, but usually Roy and Johnny keep the patient alive and it's *Rampart* that loses them. You know, the fully-equipped hospital staffed by highly-trained experienced professionals.

(That reminds me of the real-life data about the outcome of patients who receive CPR. It's not encouraging, as the recovery rate of those patients is actually pretty small. Also, studies have shown that many times CPR is stopped too soon... if continued for at least 20 minutes—better: 30 minutes—there might be a dramatically improved success rate. I know I'm not explaining this well, but I promise, I've read reputable articles about this in the past few months.)

~ The last rescue, between the buildings. I'm surprised Cap didn't request a second engine company, if only for manpower. Three lives is a lot to chance on the efforts of four or even five guys (including Vince).

~ So this is the end of another season—and the series. Sadly, this episode wasn't on Netflix, so I only have a couple of screen shots of dubious quality and content. Does The Book mention a filming date for this one? I know the airing order of the last three or four episodes were all screwed up so I'm not sure which ones were filmed when. I think all data points to All Night Long *airing* last, but that doesn't mean it was filmed last. And I wonder if they knew when they filmed it that it *was* the last episode.

* * *

I meant to also mention that *if* Kevin was "paying tribute" in this episode (the name Fishburn, jazz musician, etc.) I think it's funny that in this episode he (and the show) acknowledged that Johnny often goes off on some obsession, or "kick." It was flat-out stated at least twice—he often gets on these "kicks" and goes overboard. Thank you, Show, for acknowledging that you do this to Johnny often enough that it became a 'thing.'

Also, I guess the episode title reflects Johnny's staying up all night creating his TV show. I wonder if Kevin gave it the title, or someone else??

Speaking of episode titles.... I wonder why this show (and Adam-12, for another example) even have episode titles to begin with. It's not like the title ever appears on screen at all, at any time. And this was before DVDs, so the viewers, who only saw one ep per week, had no need to know episode titles. It's not like they stood around the water cooler and said "Did you watch Emergency the other night? It was the 'Loose Ends' episode." They didn't know *any* of the titles. (Hmm, but they might have appeared in TV Guide, I guess.) Other than that, I can see titles maybe coming in handy for the producers/directors as they plan out the filming schedule and work with scripts, but I also think it would be just as convenient (if not more so) to simply refer to them as 6.15 or 6.21.

Oh well, just another strange thing for me to wonder about....

* * *

May Fair

> The book Gage was reading was, "Female Domination of Beasts, Vol 1".Interesting!!

Wow, how can you tell? Good eyes!! The cover was only visible for a fraction of a second as he opened the book... the title wasn't clearly seen, I didn't think. (But I wouldn't put it past the prop people to have a book of that title in its bookcase.)

~ ~ ~

Well, what can we say about this last, final episode of this fun series we love so well?? First of all, I have to admit that every time I think of it, I can't stop the Lionel Richie song from popping into my head—which kind of isn't fair, as this episode came first, years before the song. But as I watched it today I found myself wondering about Kevin writing this ep. Did he know it was going to be the finale of the season? (I'm pretty sure that when he wrote it, months earlier, he probably had no way of knowing the show wouldn't be renewed again. But who knows.)

In any case, watching this one, I admit I tried to get into Kevin's head to see if I could discern any patterns. Last time I think I mentioned how this (final) episode sort of mirrored the first episode, in which it was mentioned that Johnny went on some sort of "kick," so in that respect the series has come full circle. And of course the title is All Night Long, and the entire episode takes place All Night Long.

It begins at the station and it's after 9pm. Roy and Mike are in the apparatus bay playing Ping Pong as Cap stops by for a moment. Marco is in the dorm, and apparently Johnny and Chet are in the dayroom. Johnny is, believe it or not, reading (wha—??) and Chet is watching some sort of game show, which Johnny, believe it or not, says is the "dumbest thing I've ever seen," or words to that effect. Chet says there are worse game shows out there, and Johnny says he has half a mind to write one himself. It doesn't take a genius to figure out Chet's reaction to *that*. One thing that's interesting here is that Chet says he's known Johnny for "a long and arduous six years," which of course is more or less true in the 'real world' as we're finishing the sixth season. In any case, the die is cast and Johnny is determined to prove to his doubting co-worker that he *can* write a TV show. (By the way, Chet's hair isn't as curly in this ep as it used to be. I wonder why?)

First call is for a "man down," and this is where we meet Mr. Jefferson, a jazz musician, and his friend Julius, who's played by James McEachin (i.e., Detective Crockett). When they get the man to Rampart, Dixie does a mini-PSA explaining heart catheterization as she tells Julius that Jefferson needs the procedure done ASAP. I think I wondered last time if Kevin wrote about this "jazzy" guy as a sort of tribute to Bobby Troup and Julie. (Yeah, I'm probably reading *way* too much into that.) In any case the story sort of weaves throughout the whole episode as events take place throughout the night at Rampart, and after a successful bypass operation, Julius (hmm, Julius ~ Julie?) sits down with both Dr. Early and Dixie and they talk jazz.

Meanwhile, at the station, Johnny's hard at work with Cap's typewriter (although why he's in the dayroom and not in Cap's office—where he can close the door, since it's the middle of the night—is beyond me). Anyway, first Roy and then Chet come to visit and dig Johnny out from beneath the pile of crumbled up paper (really, do people actually do that?). There's a lot of trash talk in these scenes, but Johnny—since he *is* Johnny—is undeterred. Roy even points out Johnny's penchant (through six long seasons, no less) for mini-obsessions, how he obsesses non-stop for a while and then suddenly "bingo," he's over the fad, just like that. (Nice work pointing out the show's recurring trope, Kevin.) Johnny doesn't deny it, he just says "you just wait and see." His conversation with Chet gives Johnny yet another direction for his show—crazy people dressed in crazy clothes. That's as much of an explanation as he gives. (Congratulations, Johnny, you just invented The Gong Show! Or maybe Let's Make a Deal.)

In the middle of the night the station gets called out for an MVA. A car gets T-boned by a pickup truck. Roy looks after the truck driver ("It's not my fault!") who's not really injured except for a bump on his head—which, as usual, Roy bandages to within an inch of its life. At the car, Johnny and Vince manage to get the driver's door open and pull the man out, but Johnny can't find a carotid pulse. Just like last time I watched this episode, this bothered me. He checks twice for a carotid pulse and tells Vince "Cover him up," and walks away. Yeah, that doesn't seem to be a very thorough assessment; the *least* he could have done is have Roy check the man out as a sort of "second opinion." Instead, Johnny goes to deal with the car's passenger (the driver's wife), and with Marco doing the translating he finds out what's wrong, where she hurts, etc. Tenderness and pain in her abdomen suggest there could be internal injuries so once they get her out of the mangled car Brackett orders the anti-shock suit for her. So she's definitely alive upon arrival at Rampart, but unfortunately, despite having two doctors, two paramedics, and two nurses in the room… the woman dies. By the way, at the accident scene, after the ambulance arrives we see two men come with a gurney for the (supposedly dead) husband. Guess they're from the coroner's office; a white van-type vehicle is briefly visible in the background. I don't recall seeing that little detail any other time in this show. Another, similar detail is the arrival of a tow-truck as the ambulance is getting ready to drive off. It's refreshing to see these realistic touches, especially since I don't recall seeing the coroner's truck before.

Back at 51s, Johnny goes right back to the typewriter, even doing a bit of meta speculation about adding a dog to his show, a "dog who does nothing, but just sits there. People like that." And I'm sure people did; I'm sure Henry had fans, too. But to me, the big mystery is, when Johnny finally says, "I'm finished!" and goes over to the couch... where did the pillow come from? In that same scene when we see Henry, he's on the couch, no pillow. But when Johnny walks over to him, the pillow is there. He even says "That better not be my pillow." So who put it there, and when?

Final call comes very early, before shift change: man trapped between buildings. The scene is an apartment building shaped like an L, and the victim strung a line between the two farthest points and tried to climb across. Supposedly he hit his head on... something, although I can't imagine what... and is passed out, which seems (to borrow a familiar word) incredible. I think his friend says "he hit his head on the pole," but there's no pole within 20 yards of him. Maybe he says "pulley"?? That doesn't make a lot of sense, either. Anyway, our guys rig up their lines—and it's a *complicated* rigging!—and go out there to bring him in.

If you listen to the chatter the man's friend directs toward Cap, you can almost believe he's talking not about Mr. Crazy-Pants out there on the line, but about another character who's near and dear to our hearts. "He spent all night setting this up. ... He's done all sorts of crazy projects. ... I don't think anyone could have worked so hard to accomplish so little." Guess who he could be describing??

Anyway, we all know how it ends up. The man who's "dressed in crazy clothes" is going to try out for a "crazy" TV show. Now where have we heard *that* before?? Poor Johnny. And I do mean *poor* since he won't be getting rich from his great TV show idea. Roy suggests that Johnny can always come up with a new idea (or 'kick'?), but Johnny says "No more ideas!" (Actually, he says "*something* is gone, no more ideas," but I can't make out what that *something* is. And, again, since this episode isn't on Netflix, I don't have closed captioning.) I like when Roy says "You ever think about writing a show about firemen?" If *I'd* written this episode, Johnny would reply, "Firemen? Who'd want to watch a show about *that?*"

Oh Johnny, if you only knew…..

Final notes:

~ We've remarked that in some recent season 6 episodes Johnny has been looking a little tired, but I think he looked quite fresh and his usual adorable self in this one.

~ According to imdb trivia for this episode, there was originally a scene written that featured—of all people—Jamie Lee Curtis. But the scene, in which she supposedly played a "lethargic babysitter," was cut. I wonder why?? (Fun fact: before making a name for herself in Halloween, Curtis starred in a short-lived show we all might have heard of—Operation Petticoat.)

~ How does Johnny think he can write a TV show? I wouldn't have a clue how to go about writing a TV show, especially something like a game show. (Actually, now that I think about it, coming up with the idea and writing it out would be the easy part... selling it to the 'powers that be' and getting it made would be the *real* trick.)

~ At the car accident scene, Johnny's 'usual' response to the wife, that her husband is "fine, gonna be fine," is an outright lie. But since she probably doesn't understand him, maybe it doesn't count?

~ Who remembers those typewriter eraser pencils, with the eraser at one end and the brush at the other?

~ Love Chet's line to Johnny, something like, "You have your own special brand of crazy." Too true! But then, would we really want to change him?

Author's Note

So that's the end of the series. (Pass the tissues, please!) This groundbreaking show ran for six great seasons; I know many of us wish it could have continued for six more, but in the long run (heh: long run) I think it probably ended just when it should—with the viewers wanting more. It was a groundbreaking show at the time it aired, and it's amazing to think of the millions of lives that have been affected by it. I'm not talking about fans who watched every week, but rather of average citizens all across the country, whose lives were saved, touched, or somehow made better by the presence of paramedics, firefighters, EMTs, or other emergency personnel. Many of those who have provided emergency medical care over the past 30-40 years were inspired by this "little show that could." And even for those who never watched it, the fact is that the growth of the paramedic/EMT professions across the country might not have happened so quickly if not for this series.

In any case, if you enjoyed this rambling mess of commentaries, let the world know: leave a review on Amazon or Goodreads. Spread the word on Facebook and Twitter. If you did *not* like this book, you're welcome to announce that as well, in which case may I suggest Morse code and carrier pigeon? (Ha, just kidding! Well, not really.)

To contact me personally, e-mail can be sent in care of my publisher, who will weed out the death threats… I hope. That address is **jyharrisbooks@gmail.com**.

Thank you.

May Fair
KMG-365

Watching EMERGENCY! Seasons 4-6

If you're reading this, chances are you've already read the book about the first three seasons. If for some reason you haven't, what are you waiting for? Check out all the rescues and hijinks of Station 51 (and Rampart) and see how this show went from the somewhat-awkward pilot movie to the smooth, wonderful show we all know and love. **Now there's even an episode guide for the *cough*Emergency! movies*cough.***

P.S.: Special shout-out to J.Y. Harris Books for the assist with getting these episode guides out there into the world—not as easy as some might think! I'd like to return the favor by mentioning other books published by them. J.Y. Harris has written time-travel adventures geared toward tweens (ages 11 and up). The first is titled *__Timekeepers: A Revolutionary Tale__*. Check it out! Also under the J.Y Harris Books umbrella are a number of books by Jean Louise. *__It Takes a Thief__* (three novellas) is a series about a pickpocket and a security consultant who team up to right wrongs and help people—sort of like Robin hood, but with cellphones instead of swords. Jean Louise has also written some novelettes about two police officers. Classic TV fans might find it coincidental—or not—that the two partners in the **Boys in Blue** series are named Pete and Jim. (*wink***Adam-12***wink*) Anyway, check out these books.... (Oh, and the first book of Boys in Blue, titled *__Arrest Me__*, is FREE. Score! Although I personally recommend the later book, *__Suspect Behavior__*.)

www.ingramcontent.com/pod-product-compliance
Lightning Source LLC
Chambersburg PA
CBHW020624220526
45464CB00001B/13